A **HISTORY** OF **MEDICINE** IN
50
DISCOVERIES

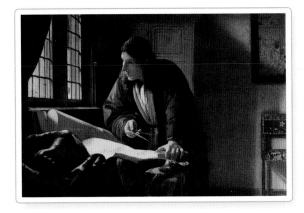

MARGUERITE VIGLIANI, MD AND GALE EATON

Series Editor PHILLIP HOOSE

Tilbury House Publishers
12 Starr Street, Thomaston, Maine 04861
800-582-1899
www.tilburyhouse.com

First hardcover edition: June 2017
ISBN 978-0-88448-400-4

Library of Congress Control Number: 2017933710

15 16 17 18 19 20 4CM 5 4 3 2 1

Interior designed by Jonathan Friedman, Frame25 Productions
Cover designed by John Barnett, 4 Eyes Design

Printed in Korea through Four Colour Print Group, Louisville, Kentucky

Table of Contents

Presenting the HISTORY IN 50 Series, by Phillip Hoose   ix

Introduction: What's a Discovery?   xiii

1. The Iceman: Forensic Analysis of a Neolithic Killing   1

2. A Parade of Ants: Magic and Folk Healing   5

3. Massage: Rubbing Out Demons and Kinks   9

4. Secrets of the Dead: Ancient Egyptian Mummifiers and Surgeons   13
   Applied Anatomy: Surgery in Ancient India   16

5. 170 BC: Sleep Therapy at the Temples of Asklepios   17
   The Myth of Asklepios   20
   The Placebo Effect and Double Blind Trials   21

6. AD 200: Galen Discovers Nerves and Humors   22
   How Many Elements and Humors?   26

7. 900: Al-Razi and Evidence-Based Medicine in the Middle Ages   27
   Jundi-Shapur and the Survival of Learning   30

8. 1508: Da Vinci's Heart   31
   Renaissance Anatomy   34

9. 1600: The Chamberlen Family Secret   35
   Caesarean Sections   38
   Midwifery and the Birthing Stool   39

10. 1670: Looking through Van Leeuwenhoek's Tiny Microscopes   40
    The Royal Society for Improving Natural Knowledge   43
    A Proto-Germ Theory in the Renaissance?   44

11. 1721: Fighting Smallpox and Public Opinion in Colonial Boston   45
    Vanquishing Smallpox for Good   48
    Royal Smallpox Treatments   49
    Infected Blankets and Germ Warfare   50

12. 1747: Limeys and the Conquest of Scurvy   51
    Nutritional Deficiencies   55
    White Rice Poisoning   56

13. 1776: A Folk Remedy for Congestive Heart Failure   57
   Ancient Pharmaceuticals   61

14. 1799: Heroic Bloodletting, Leech Mania, and
   Discovering What Doesn't Work   62
   Bloodletting in the Twenty-First Century   66

15. 1816: René Laennec Invents the Stethoscope   67
   Taking the Pulse   71

16. 1828: Cutting for Stone   72
   The Lancet: Outing an Incompetent Surgeon   75
   Extracorporeal Shock-Wave Lithotripsy: A Minimally Invasive Solution?   76

17. 1846: Laughing Gas   77
   Magic Mushrooms   81

18. 1847: Wash Your Hands   82
   Florence Nightingale Battles the Army   85

19. 1848: Monster Soup   87
   The Miasma Theory and Correlation vs. Causation   91
   Public Health in the Bronze Age   92

20. 1854: Cholera and Epidemiology   93
   Cholera Discoveries Lost and Found   96
   Cholera and the Third World   97

21. 1867: Gregor Mendel and Inherited Traits   98
   Sickle-cell Trait: Mendelian Inheritance Meets Darwinian Selection   102
   The Language of Genetics   103

22. 1870: Discovering Ancient Skull Surgeries   104
   The Legend of Hua Tuo and the Emperor's Headaches   107

23. 1881: Spontaneous Generation and the Germ Theory of Disease   108
   Joseph Lister Applies Germ Theory to Surgery   112
   Koch's Postulates   113

24. 1882: Tuberculosis Emerges from the Miasma   114
   Desperate Cures: The Royal Touch and Burning the Vampire's Heart   117

25. 1894: A Barrel of Snakes and an Antitoxin   118
   Resisting Poisons in Antiquity   121
   Science as a Competition   122

26. 1896: The Discovery of X-Rays   123

27. 1898: A Small-Game Hunter Fights Bubonic Plague   127
     Did Yersinia Pestis *Really Cause the Black Death?*   132

28. 1898: Viruses Borrow Life Support from Tobacco Leaves and Humans   133

29. 1900: Marie Curie's Lab Glows in the Dark   137
     Radiation Therapy: A Dangerous Panacea   141

30. 1901: Making Blood Transfusions Safe   142
     Blood Transfusions in War and Peace   146

31. 1905: Hormones and Endocrinology   147
     La Mujer Barbuda   150
     The Pineal Gland   151
     Serotonin: Not a Hormone   152

32. 1907: Typhoid Mary Becomes the World's Most Notorious Cook   153

33. 1909: Ehrlich's Magic Bullet and the Beginnings of Chemotherapy   157
     Medicine and Artificial Dyes   160
     Syphilis: Somebody Else's Disease   161

34. 1922: Controlling Diabetes   162

35. 1929: Fleming's Dirty Dishes Give Us Penicillin   166
     Molds and Folk Medicine   169

36. 1930: Psychosurgery   170

37. 1939 – 1955: Rat Poison for a U.S. President   174
     Vitamin K   177

38. 1944: Discovering DNA   178
     Watson and Crick Discover the Structure of DNA   182
     The Human Genome Project   183
     Genetic Counseling   184

39. 1945: A Miracle Drug in the Sewage   185

40. 1945: Saving Lives with Sausage Casings,
     Washing Machines, and Juice Cans   189
     The Iron Lung   192

41. 1951: Frankenstein and the Heart Machines   193
Alas, Poor Yorick!   196
Before Pacemakers: "I Sing the Body Electric!"   197

42. 1967: Baruch Blumberg Discovers a Cancer-Causing Virus   198

43. 1967: The First Heart Transplant   202
Ethical Issues in Transplantation   205
Microchimerism in Transplant Surgery   206

44. 1972: A Magic Bullet from Chinese Medicine   207
Chairman Mao, Biomedicine, and Traditional Chinese Medicine   212

45. 1978: The First Test Tube Baby   213
Whose Baby Is It?   217
Contraception   218

46. 1983: Preventing Cancers   219
The Ethics of Discovery: Informed Consent   222

47. 1998: MMR Vaccine, Autism, Discovery, and Fraud   224
Herd Immunity   228
Scientific Discovery and Fraud   229

48. 2011: Bionic Parts   230
Drug-Eluting Implants   234

49. 2013: Poop Therapy for the Human Microbiome   235

50. 2016: Researching the Zika Virus   238

Conclusion   243

Glossary   247

Sources   251

Endnotes   279

Index   298

Presenting the History in 50 Series

by Phillip Hoose

The *History in 50* series explores history by telling thematically linked stories. Each book in this series includes 50 illustrated narrative accounts of people and events—some well-known, others often overlooked—that, together, build a rich connect-the-dots mosaic and challenge conventional assumptions about how history unfolds. In *A History of Civilization in 50 Disasters,* for example, Gale Eaton weaves tales of the disasters that happen when civilization and nature collide. Volcanoes, fires, floods, and pandemics have devastated humanity for thousands of years, and human improvements such as molasses holding tanks, insecticides, and deep-water oil rigs have created new, unforeseen hazards—yet civilization has advanced not just in spite of these disasters, but in part because of them.

History in 50 is a canny, fun, and logical way to present history. The stories are brief, lively, and richly detailed. They work as narrative and also as bait to lure readers to well-selected source material. History in these books is not a stuffy parade of generals, tycoons, and industrialists, but rather a collection of brief, heart-pounding non-fiction narratives in which genuine calamities overtake us, genuine athletes leap skyward on feet of clay, and genuine discoverers labor bleary-eyed through the night to take us to the depths of the ocean, explore the vast reaches of space, unlock the genetic code, or develop a vaccine that saves millions of lives. It's history that bellows and shivers and roars.

And who doesn't love lists? Making a list of fifty great episodes of any kind invites—*demands*—debate. Even if the events aren't ranked (they're in chronological sequence), something always gets left out. I just finished reading *A History of Civilization in 50 Disasters*. I paged wide-eyed through plagues, eruptions, famines, microbes, and vaccines that worked or didn't. From my reading chair I took on dust storms, melt-downs, and epidemics at all scales that claimed my unwavering atten-tion. When I closed the book and looked up, blinking, my first thought was, "Unbelievable. How have we ever made it through all this?"

But these feelings quickly gave way to a surge of indignation: *Where was the Tri-State Tornado of March 1925?* It's my favorite disaster—one that hit home. Actually a series of twisters, the Tri-State storm ripped through Missouri and Illinois before closing in on my great-grand-parents in southwestern Indiana. Seven hundred people were killed in what is commonly ranked as the worst tornado ever. Contemporary meteorologists agreed that it was surely a category five twister, and yet it didn't make the top fifty disasters? I needed to lodge a protest.

But then I realized that my pique was a good thing. The book had made me care. The stories had swept over me and shaken my certainty like the 1906 San Francisco earthquake. And I realized that many read-ers will have the very same reaction: *Hey, where's my favorite episode?* It will spur debate. I imagine smart teachers asking students to describe their own favorite historical episodes, backing up findings with research. I imagine readers of all ages heading back to their bookshelves to support their arguments.

History is rewarding, but in my experience most people have to be led to it. So-called Reluctant Readers are mainly reluctant to be bored. They require, and deserve, historical material that meets them partway. History with menacing characters, even if some of them are invisible (germs); history replete with tough decisions; crisp episodes that leave you wondering what you would have done in that situation;

history moved by people just like us, often from the humblest of origins, struggling in their daily lives while reaching for greatness—that's the history that works for most readers. And that is the history we have in this brilliant new series. The writing is clear and exciting, punchy stories that are, on average, two pages long. I have high hopes for the *History in Fifty* series, and it gives me pleasure to enthusiastically endorse it. Why? Because it works.

PHILLIP HOOSE is the National Book Award–winning author of *Claudette Colvin: Twice Toward Justice* and *The Boys Who Challenged Hitler: Knud Pedersen and the Churchill Club.*

Introduction

What's a Discovery?

Medicine is an ancient art, and the first discoveries are long forgotten. Humans took care of the sick and treated illness thousands of years before anyone wrote things down. Sumerian and Egyptian doctors left their prescriptions, along with rituals for driving off demons and securing their patients' health, but said little about the process of figuring out what worked. Ancient medicine was a given. It was taught by the gods and handed on by revered authorities, and doctors who wanted patients to believe in a treatment would say it was very old. They would not have called it a new discovery.

And what is a discovery? Is it a creative leap, a novel idea that springs forth fully formed? Or is it a new way of seeing things that were always there? If there's a sudden insight, it usually flashes into a well-prepared mind. The Greek mathematician Archimedes struggled to figure out how to measure the volume of a gold crown without melting it into a regular shape. Setting the problem aside he sank into his bathtub, and water sloshed over the rim. "Eureka!" he cried, which means "I have found it!" And we picture him running down the street stark naked in his excitement at discovering the Archimedes principle: you can measure an object's volume by the amount of water it displaces.

The story of that original "eureka moment" survives because we like to believe discoveries can happen that fast, in a brilliant mix of accident and creative genius. Wilhelm Röntgen just happened to notice a flicker of light out of the corner of his eye and discovered X-rays. René Laennec watched children at play and invented the stethoscope. August Kekulé dreamed of a snake with its tail in its mouth and discovered the six-carbon ring structure of the benzene molecule. But the eurekas come after deliberate observations of something that cannot be understood, followed by multiple attempts to explain it, and finally by a process of thinking in a new way that explains all of the observed events.

Whether they were sudden inspirations or the result of long trial and error, ancient discoveries have often been forgotten and rediscovered. A good example is the development of sanitation by the Harrapans of the Indus Valley (in present-day Pakistan) around 2500 BC. Their engineers managed wastewater better than the later Romans; their houses had indoor plumbing. Did they know they were protecting communities against disease? Their civilization was wiped out by drought, famine, and climate change about 1800 BC, and after AD 1800, reformers like Edwin Chadwick had to fight for sanitation in England. Chadwick didn't know about germs but was sure filth was unhealthy. So who discovered sanitation? The Harrapans, or Chadwick?

Discoveries can be lost even when there is some continuity between civilizations. Roman army surgeons throughout what is now Europe knew about antisepsis for wounds, sterilization of instruments, and suturing of blood vessels. They knew the benefits of proper wastewater management, ventilation, and mosquito control to prevent disease. But medical knowledge was lost with the fall of Rome, and over the next thousand years Europe evolved a civilization with a whole new set of ideas, in medicine as in everything else.

The influence of a discovery depends largely on when and where it is made. William Harvey (1578–1657) discovered that blood circulates in the human body; Ibn Nafis of Damascus discovered the same thing in 1242, some 300 years earlier. Harvey didn't know about Ibn Nafis, so who made the discovery?[1] Harvey's work had more influence on modern medicine because he made it in seventeenth-century Europe, as the scientific method was gaining traction. His contemporaries were excited about observing natural phenomena and designing experiments. They soon built on Harvey's discovery and carried it forward, so it has not been forgotten.

By contrast, many discoveries are ignored or rejected because they do not fit the theories of their times. The Cuban doctor Carlos Finlay showed in 1881 that yellow fever was transmitted by mosquitoes, but nobody believed him until twenty years later. Walter Reed saw Finlay's paper, replicated his research, and is still remembered as the discoverer of mosquito-borne disease, although he cited Finlay. Fleming's discovery of

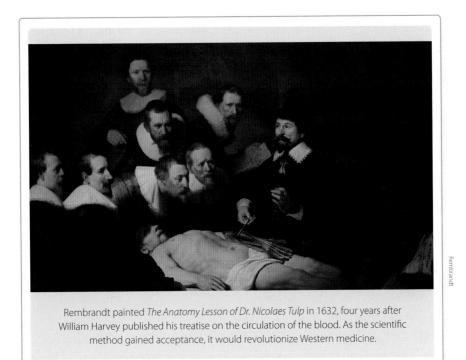

Rembrandt

Rembrandt painted *The Anatomy Lesson of Dr. Nicolaes Tulp* in 1632, four years after William Harvey published his treatise on the circulation of the blood. As the scientific method gained acceptance, it would revolutionize Western medicine.

penicillin and Mendel's discovery of the laws of inheritance were ignored for years; later readers saw their importance. Hungarian physician Ignaz Semmelweis became a virtual outcast for insisting that childbed fever was spread by doctors with dirty hands; today physicians wear gloves.

Resistance to discovery is only natural. Medicine is life-and-death work, and discarding time-honored treatments and theories in favor of new insights looks risky. It is, for example, very difficult to test the effectiveness of promising new cancer treatments against established treatments because the latter cannot in good conscience be withheld.

George Washington died in a world where all doctors were sure that disease was caused by an imbalance of the four humors: blood, phlegm, and black and yellow bile. The way to cure disease was to deplete excess humors by making the patient bleed, vomit, and defecate. As Washington struggled to breathe, his youngest doctor wanted to try a tracheotomy, opening his windpipe, but more traditional views prevailed. Washington was drained of nearly half his blood on that last day. Sometimes discovering what doesn't work is valuable, and we have included more than one failed discovery in this book.

On the other hand, working with colleagues who share a delight in learning and ideas is more fun. Centers of learning like Jundi-Shapur in Persia and Salerno in Italy supported discovery by acting as intellectual incubators. Medieval Arab scholars preserved and translated the knowledge of ancient Greece, then built on it. In the nineteenth century, teams of scientists competed to discover things first; Louis Pasteur's laboratory in France and Robert Koch's in Germany were powerful rivals.

It has been said that only the lens of time can reveal whether or not a discovery is false or true. Thus in the last century we have compiled a Diagnostic and Statistical Manual of Mental Disorders (DSM) to standardize the language of psychiatry so that research can be conducted. The DSM is a consensus document with 947 pages. The tome is as ponderous as any Islamic pharmacopoeia, but unfortunately none of the diagnoses in the DSM-5 correlate with any biomarker, mutation, or imaging finding by X-ray, MRI (magnetic resonance imaging), or PET (positron emission tomography) scan.[2] So, after almost a century of trying to medicalize madness, the DSM might end up in the dustbin of history, like Paracelsus's salt, sulfur, and mercury theory. On the other hand, Paracelsus was the first to introduce the idea that illness was caused by outside forces, a theory that later became the germ theory of disease.

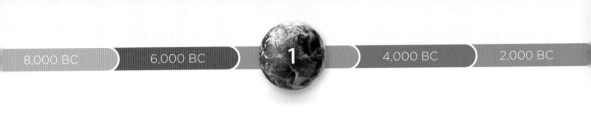

The Iceman

Forensic Analysis of a Neolithic Killing

More than 5,000 years ago, a man climbed high into the Alps. Enemies pursued him. His hand was cut to the bone, his skull fractured. Before he could reach safety, an arrow pierced a major blood vessel in his shoulder.[3] Did he fall from the path and freeze? Did he die in combat? We can't be sure.

When German hikers found his mummified body in 1991, they took a picture and reported to local authorities. Hikers do get lost in the Alps, but this one's clothes were made of animal hides, and his tools were copper—predating the Bronze Age.[4] He was dubbed Ötzi the Iceman, and the medical examiner handed him over to scientists for X-rays, DNA analysis, and other tests.

By 3200 BC, farmers and herders had lived in the Alps for centuries. Ötzi's mother may have been one of them. Researchers sequenced his mitochondrial DNA—the part that's transmitted only from mothers to their children—and couldn't find any living matches.[5] This could mean that Ötzi's mother came from a small population with no descendants in the direct female line, maybe an isolated mountain settlement. But Ötzi's father may have come from farther away; he has relatives today in Sardinia and elsewhere.[6]

Ötzi was about 46 years old and 5 feet 2 inches tall, with brown eyes, Type O blood, and lactose intolerance.[7] He ate well—his guts contained meat (including ibex and deer), grains (wheat and barley), and other plants—but he probably had bad digestion; he had ulcer-causing bacteria and a whipworm infection. He also had hardening of the arteries, three gallstones, Lyme disease, and a predisposition to heart problems.

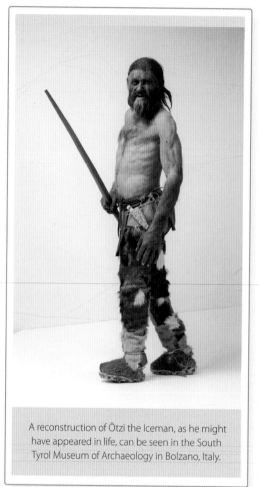

A reconstruction of Ötzi the Iceman, as he might have appeared in life, can be seen in the South Tyrol Museum of Archaeology in Bolzano, Italy.

Was he a farmer? Whipworm is common in soil fertilized with human waste; but it can easily be transmitted on unwashed food. He may have been a herder; he had the kind of arthritic knees you'd expect if he carried heavy loads on mountain trails.[8] He could even have been a coppersmith; his hair carried traces of copper and arsenic.[9] From his one remaining fingernail, scientists could tell he'd been ill three times in the months before he died.[10]

How did he treat his ailments? Maybe with tattoos. He had 61 of them, some invisible to the naked eye,[11] and most seem to match traditional acupuncture points. Were they meant to ease the pain of arthritis, gallstones, and whipworms? Some researchers suggest that the Iceman's people practiced a therapy "very similar to what we know as Chinese acupuncture."[12]

But he also used medicinal plants. Hanging from his belt were two walnut-sized pieces of fungus: *Piptoporus betulinus*, or birch bracket, which grows on tree trunks. It tastes awful and causes diarrhea. Ötzi could have been carrying it to start his fire, but he had better tinder in his pouch: *Chaga*, or tinder fungus, which ignites very easily and smolders for a long time.[13] Some researchers think he used *P. betulinus* to fight his whipworms.[14]

Did Neolithic humans discover medicinal fungi? Folk medicines around the world still grind mushrooms into powders for teas and poultices, and Ötzi's tinder fungus would cauterize wounds and stanch

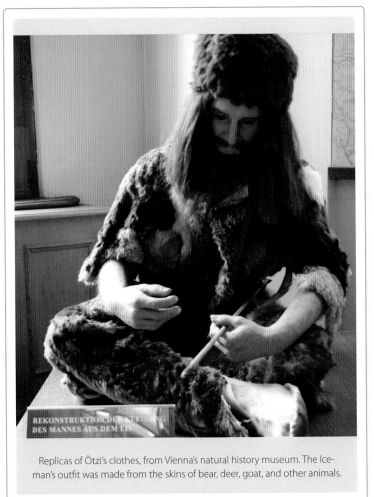

Replicas of Ötzi's clothes, from Vienna's natural history museum. The Iceman's outfit was made from the skins of bear, deer, goat, and other animals.

Sandstein/Wikimedia Commons

bleeding.[15] Today, more than 270 species are thought to benefit the immune system.[16] But perhaps Neolithic humans were born knowing this. Anecdotal evidence has long hinted that other animals instinctively eat medicinal plants when sick, and researchers now have begun to test the hypothesis that great apes and many other animals do self-medicate.[17] As for humans, remnants of chamomile and yarrow—bitter herbs with little nutritional value—have been found in tartar from 50,000-year-old teeth. They may well have been taken as medicine.[18] Were the first practices of medicine discovered, or did they evolve?

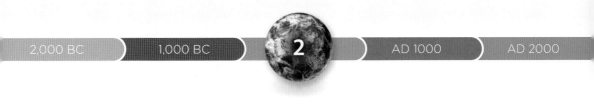
A Parade of Ants

Magic and Folk Healing

Far up the Amazon and away from Western medical resources, a boat's engineer had an abscessed tooth. There was no antibiotic aboard, and explorer Lyall Watson (1939–2008) couldn't pull the tooth with pliers. But the expedition didn't turn back to civilization. The captain (like the engineer, indigenous to the Amazon basin) knew a shaman, a little guy who agreed to cure the engineer for two packs of Marlboro cigarettes. He didn't look like a shaman—his T-shirt said "Property of the Louisiana Jail." But Watson and the captain watched as he slid the engineer's molar out easily, though it was not loose. Then he said, "That's not the problem. The problem has to leave." He swayed back and forth, and out of the engineer's mouth came first a trickle of blood and then a parade of large ants, hundreds of them. The captain and the engineer laughed at the shaman's joke; in their language, the word for that kind of ant meant "trouble."[1]

Was it magic? Sleight-of-hand? Theater? The engineer was cured by a healer whose role was to communicate with the spirit world—a shaman. We cannot know if prehistoric tribes had shamans, but today's world has some 5,000 indigenous groups,[2] and in many of them shamanistic traditions survive. They are not alike; Australian Aboriginals and Sámi reindeer herders in Scandinavia use different methods and

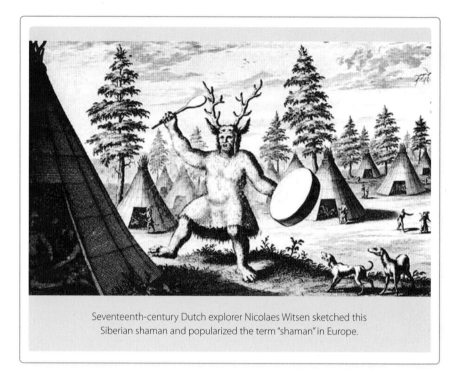

Seventeenth-century Dutch explorer Nicolaes Witsen sketched this
Siberian shaman and popularized the term "shaman" in Europe.

resources to deal with different conditions.[3] But in cities as well as remote areas, folk remedies are used in homes, and people still consult shamans and other folk healers when they need a cure.[4] Shared knowledge and participation keep folk medicine vital and adaptable,[5] and even children learn the basics.

Today's folk healings can't give us a perfect idea of prehistoric medicine. Shamans pass on their lore by example and word of mouth, changing it to fit a changing world. So, when Australian healers adopted the English "billy can" to boil herbs instead of steeping them in water overnight, the heat killed some active herbal ingredients and strengthened others.[6] Their cures changed.

But two basic aspects of folk medicine go straight back to Ötzi's time and before: first, folk healing is usually a community affair, and second, it often relies on magic and the supernatural.

Traditional healings may take place in forest clearings or sweat lodges instead of hospitals; healers may wear feathers instead of scrubs.

The whole community may join in ceremonial drumming and chanting.[7] In Korea, a shaman "unites the gathered people . . . through dance that leads to the bright spirit," so people and shaman share an ecstatic sense of insight and focused intuition.[8] The whole community is involved, and the whole community is in touch with something apart from ordinary experience, something that feels like magic.

The shaman, serving as a bridge to the spirit world, doesn't diagnose illness by reading X-rays or analyzing blood samples. Modern American and European physicians expect to find clues to a body's illness in the body; traditional healers, believing that illness is sent by angry gods, demons, or witches,[9] look for answers in the spirit realm instead. To get in touch with ancestors or other helpful spirits, shamans might put themselves into a trance or use divination bones.[10]

This is the biggest difference between Western medicine and the various folk medicines. In Western medicine, a new discovery has to be objectively tested using the scientific method. Researchers look inside

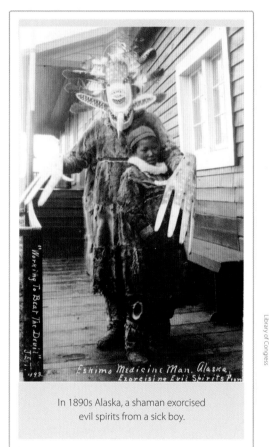

In 1890s Alaska, a shaman exorcised evil spirits from a sick boy.

bodies for the cause of illness, and they try to develop treatments that are of general use, helping more than one patient.

Shamans look for supernatural causes of illness and do not use statistics. "In fact," says one Western doctor who was initiated as a shaman

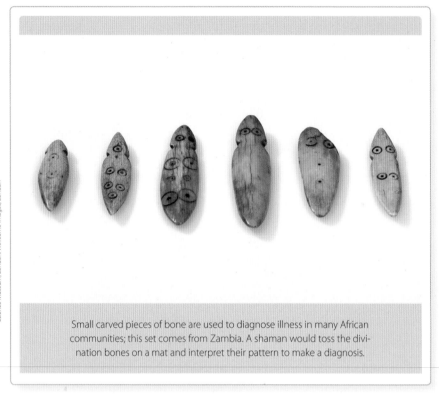

Small carved pieces of bone are used to diagnose illness in many African communities; this set comes from Zambia. A shaman would toss the divination bones on a mat and interpret their pattern to make a diagnosis.

Science Museum, London/Wellcome Images, London

in South Africa, "systematic inquiry gets in the way of the process. One has to put cognitive, left-brained intellect aside."[11] Traditional healing relies not on generalizable scientific discovery, but on the magical discovery of individual cures.

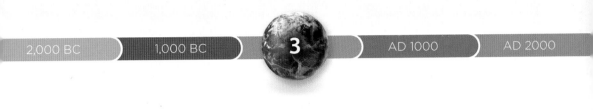

Massage

Rubbing out Demons and Kinks

In the seventh century BC, a Babylonian doctor makes a house call. The patient lies sick in bed, paralyzed by headache and pain. The *asipu*—the priestly magician and exorcist—has already diagnosed the illness: a demon is causing it. Now the *asu*—an attending physician—will drive out the demon with a 43-step ritual. First he anoints himself with oil, reciting the "pure oil, holy oil" incantation. Then, reciting the "to loosen evil muscle" incantation, he prepares salve to rub on the patient. Starting with the head and working out to the toes, he massages the demon out of the body and blocks its return with strings of amulet stones on the arms, legs, and torso. Finally he secures the patient's surroundings against the demon's return by sprinkling water, burning incense, tying knots, drawing protective circles, and reciting more spells.[1]

We know massage is an ancient art, because a Babylonian scribe wrote directions for this demon-eviction ritual on a clay tablet that ended up in the library of King Ashurbanipal (668 BC–ca. 627 BC). Centuries later a Roman author, Aulus Cornelius Celsus (ca. 25 BC–AD 50), wondered who discovered the "art of rubbing": Hippocrates (ca. 460–370 BC), who wrote about it first, or Asclepiades (ca. 124–40 BC), who explained it better?[2]

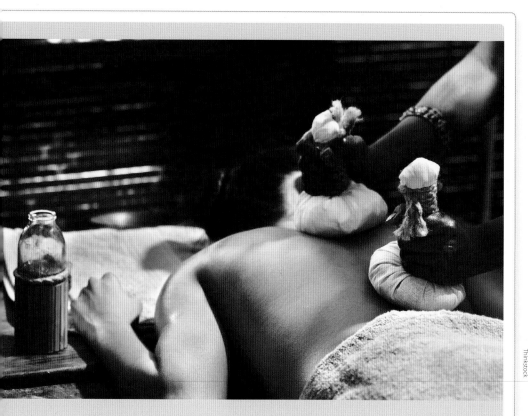

The ancient practice of massage is still associated with fragrant smells and soothing music. Candles and a rubbing ball filled with herbs add to the effect of a traditional Thai massage.

Thinkstock

So who really discovered massage? We've probably been stroking each other since before humans were human. Anybody who has patted a crying child on the back or rubbed a sore knee knows that massage comes naturally, and anybody who has watched a cat with kittens knows that humans aren't the only ones who soothe each other by touch.

Today, trained medical professionals still treat patients with massage therapy. They manipulate soft tissues,[3] often using scented oil or lotion. Sometimes their hands glide over a patient's skin; sometimes they knead tight muscles to release knots or break up scar tissue.[4] Massage may relieve pain and stress in patients with cancer, heart disease, or stomach problems.[5] It may help strained muscles recover.[6] It may even help premature babies grow.[7]

Yet medical researchers are still trying to discover exactly how and why massage works. Celsus didn't mention demons, but he did believe that rubbing worked by pushing something out of the body—something that was causing tightness or weakness.[8] Today's researchers want to observe and measure that unknown something. They find clues by comparing what happens to patients who are massaged with what happens to those who receive some other treatment or none at all. For example:

Babies: Premature babies need to grow, and several studies show that infants gain more weight in a week when they receive 15-minute massages twice a day. Also, their vagus nerves (which regulate heart rate) and their stomachs are more active. Does massage help babies absorb food better by stimulating their digestive systems?[9]

Patients suffering from pain and stress: Massage appears to increase the body's supply of serotonin—an anti-pain neurotransmitter—and decrease the amount of "substance P" (associated with pain) and cortisol (associated with stress) in the system.[10] Patients have reported for centuries that massage makes them *feel* better. Now researchers, using biological evidence, are backing them up.

Athletes: Researchers at a Canadian university biopsied the thighs of 11 young men who had exercised to exhaustion. Then they massaged one thigh each, waited 2.5 hours, and repeated the muscle biopsies. The massaged legs showed reduced levels of inflammatory proteins and more substances involved in muscle fiber maintenance.[11]

Celsus believed that massage could speed healing, and he was probably right. But there is not yet enough evidence to qualify it as a proven treatment; the National Institutes of Health advise using it to

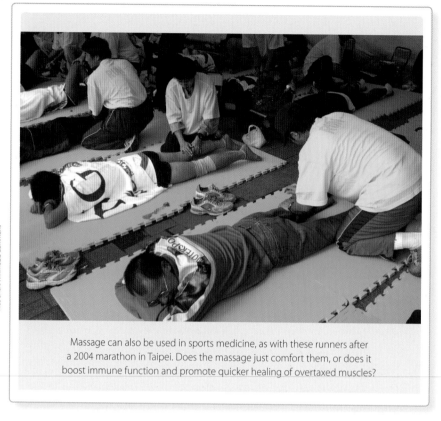

Rico Shen/Wikimedia Commons

Massage can also be used in sports medicine, as with these runners after a 2004 marathon in Taipei. Does the massage just comfort them, or does it boost immune function and promote quicker healing of overtaxed muscles?

complement rather than replace conventional care.[12] One obstacle to discovering the exact value of massage is that nobody yet has designed a double blind study (see Chapter 5) to test it.

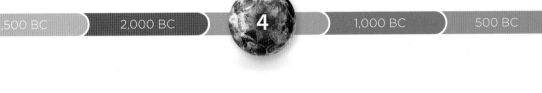
Secrets of the Dead

Ancient Egyptian Mummifiers and Surgeons

The ancient Egyptians should have been anatomy whizzes. For three thousand years their embalmers took bodies apart while getting them ready for the afterlife. Between 1570 and 1075 BC their expertise reached notable heights, and the bodies of pharaohs buried then are so well preserved that modern researchers can study their genetics and medical histories. But did the embalmers share anatomical information with doctors?

The bodies of nobles, commoners, and even animals were also preserved—although preservation quality might depend on ability to pay. Herodotus (484–425 BC) reported that a top-of-the-line mummification began with the removal of organs. He said embalmers even pulled the brain out through the nose with an iron hook—but they left the heart, the "seat of the mind,"[1] so the dead person would still be able to think in the afterworld. Then they washed out the empty abdomen with wine, filled it with spices, and dried the body for 70 days in natron—a salt that helped pull out moisture—before giving it a final wash, bandaging it in linen, and encasing it in a form-fitting coffin. But they took shortcuts with the remains of the poor, even substituting onions and garlic for high-end preservative spices.

Based on this description, early twentieth-century researchers tried removing the brains of dead animals. It was a time-consuming job,[2] and ancient embalmers likely skipped it when conditions warranted.[3] When they did remove the brains, they sometimes used the larger opening at the back of the head where the spine meets the skull.[4] One team of researchers found a wooden stick in a mummy's skull, and teased it out with CT (computer tomograph) images and an endoscope. It was probably left there by a careless embalmer, tired of brain removal duty.[5] So Herodotus oversimplified. Many elite mummies kept their brains, many common mummies didn't, and not all brain removal was done through the nose. But we continue to learn from mummies how much the Egyptians knew—and how much they didn't know—about medicine.

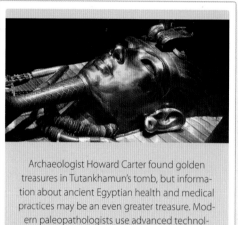

Egypt Archive

Archaeologist Howard Carter found golden treasures in Tutankhamun's tomb, but information about ancient Egyptian health and medical practices may be an even greater treasure. Modern paleopathologists use advanced technology to analyze Egyptian mummies.

While embalmers took care of Egypt's dead, priests and physicians took care of the living. Some of their prescriptions and case reports have survived on papyrus scrolls. The famous *Edwin Smith Papyrus* was probably copied around 1500 BC from an original text[6] written a thousand years earlier, near when the first pyramid was built. One of the earliest medical books ever written, it gives diagnoses and treatments for 48 injuries that could have been incurred by pyramid construction workers.[7] They ranged from simple fractures to head traumas and spinal cord damage.

Worksite doctors had to examine each injury, taking a pulse and looking for visual clues and odors to help with diagnosis. Based on the patient's chances of survival, doctors would decide whether and how to treat the injury. They used sutures, bandages, splints, and poultices. They applied honey to infections and stopped bleeding with raw meat.

The writer described outcomes for these cases, including neurological deficits.[8] So the *Edwin Smith Papyrus* is an early example of both occupational medicine and case reporting—a subject and a method that remain important today.

And yet Egyptians probably knew more about treating the outsides than the insides of living bodies. Embalmers were not medical doctors,[9] and they had no reason to study the structure of muscles, arteries, veins, or nerves. They clearly did not understand what the brain was for, and while physicians were highly regarded in ancient times, they may not have done everything writers have claimed. There is no solid evidence, for instance, that they did cataract surgery,[10] and even their bone surgeries were probably limited.[11] There is a limit to how much surgeons can learn if they are not allowed to dissect the human body.

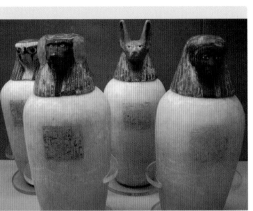

A set of canopic jars held organs and entrails from a noble lady in the tenth century BC. The jars represent the four sons of the god Horus, who had the heads of a falcon, a baboon, a jackal, and a human.

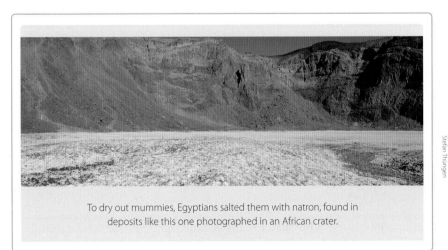

To dry out mummies, Egyptians salted them with natron, found in deposits like this one photographed in an African crater.

Applied Anatomy: Surgery in Ancient India

Nowadays if you see a man slashing watermelons or cucumbers with dazzling fast knives, he's probably a top chef. But in India around 600 BC, he might be a student of the legendary surgeon Sushruta.

Throughout the ancient world, study of human anatomy was hampered by ethical, religious, and aesthetic objections to the practice of dissection. Laws and taboos generally prevented cutting into the body.[13] In India, where a person could be made unclean for days even by carrying a body to be cremated, touching a corpse with a knife was unthinkable.[14]

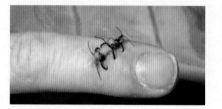

The *Sushruta Samhita* taught Indian doctors to staple wounds shut with army ants, as indigenous peoples still do in India, East Africa, and Brazil. Once the ants bite both sides of the wound, their bodies can be removed.[12]

Yet surgeons need to know anatomy, and Sushruta taught his students how to study it without becoming polluted. Take a corpse in good condition, wrap it in grass, put it in a cage to keep out scavenging animals, and immerse it in a rushing stream. When it begins to decompose, scrape off skin and flesh with grass brushes; you can observe how the body is made without actually touching the corpse or using a knife.[15]

Sushruta reportedly developed a number of advanced surgical techniques. He made an effective inhalation anesthetic from cannabis, wine, and henbane.[16] To suture wounds, he used the huge mandibles of soldier ants for staples.[17] For plastic surgery, he invented an absorbable suture made of sheep gut, similar to the catgut still used for fiddle strings.[18] Before Hippocrates, Sushruta and other ancient Vedic physicians achieved levels of sophistication the West would not reach for two thousand years, like restoration of a normal appearance to the face after a nose had been cut off as punishment for adultery.

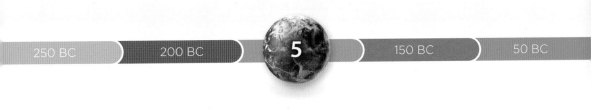
170 BC

Sleep Therapy at the Temples of Asklepios

Imagine you are ill, and doctors cannot help you. The cause of your illness is unclear. Family and friends think you must have offended some god, and only divine intervention will restore your health. So you make a pilgrimage to the Asklepieion at Epidauros, the most famous temple of the Greek god of healing, Asklepios.

This is around 170 BC, and all around the Mediterranean sick men, women, and children are being treated at hundreds of Asklepieia.[1] Many of these temples stand on the sites of older shrines, scenic places with natural springs. Athens built an Asklepieion in 420 BC and Rome in 293 BC, both after disease outbreaks devastated their populations. But the most famous temples are at Trikka, Kos, and above all Epidauros.

You wait in line with other seekers to enter the Asklepieion. Even if you cannot read, big marble slabs with images of previous miracle cures show you what to expect.[2] Seekers who are dying will be turned away, but complaints from deafness to tapeworm will be treated. The god even performs surgery as patients sleep. One man carried the point of a spear in his jaw for six years; another had an abscess in his belly. The god cured them both,[3] and he will cure you.

You are admitted to the outer part of the complex to pray, make sacrifices, and bathe—rituals that prepare you to be healed.[4] In your leisure, you enjoy spa-like amenities: a gymnasium, special diet, and

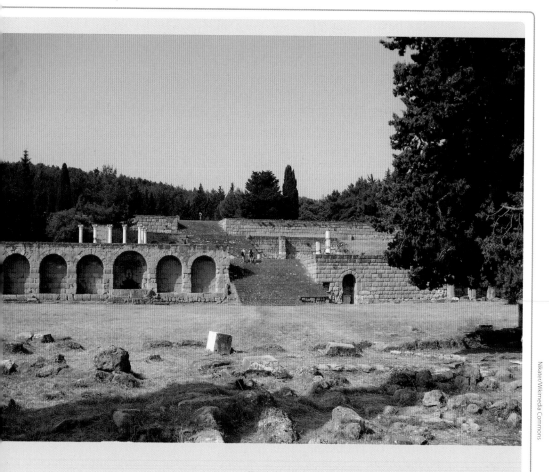

The Asklepieion at Kos.

pure water, as well as fresh air, sunshine, music, and medicines. You are encouraged to be cheerful.[5]

The priests know from your dreams when you are cleansed in body, mind, and soul. Now you enter the *abaton*, the sacred hall. You sacrifice a ram, spread its skin on your *cline* or couch, and lie down to sleep. Lights dim. You experience what the Romans call *incubatio* and the Greeks *enkoimesis*, a trance-like sleep in a holy place. The god is present. His holy animals, the dog and the snake, may lick you with their healing tongues;[6] the god himself may touch you. And your dreams, carefully interpreted by the priests, bring healing insight.[7] You will be cured.

Evidence suggests that Asklepios and his priests cured almost every patient admitted to these temples, which some scholars consider the first hospitals.[8] How was this possible? Selection, patient expectation, and effective treatment must all have contributed to their miraculous cure rate. Selection was clearly a factor, since hopeless cases were not accepted for treatment.

Expectations also mattered. The mind affects the body, and seekers who believed in the healing powers of the sanctuaries were open to healing. Like medieval pilgrims to the shrine of Thomas à Becket and modern pilgrims to Lourdes, they had religious faith to strengthen their expectations. Some research-ers also suggest that up to a third of the patients had psychosomatic ailments and would have been especially suggestible.[9]

And the treatments were effective. There were herbal remedies, and for pain relief there was hypnosis as well as opium. Priests kept their secrets, so we don't know details, but surgeries must

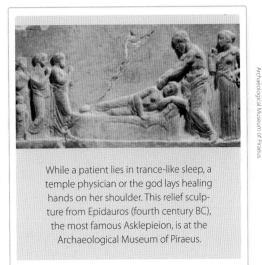

While a patient lies in trance-like sleep, a temple physician or the god lays healing hands on her shoulder. This relief sculpture from Epidauros (fourth century BC), the most famous Asklepieion, is at the Archaeological Museum of Piraeus.

Archaeological Museum of Piraeus

have been performed on anesthetized patients.[10] Overall, the clinical environment was surely healing. Bathing, massage, sunshine, exercise, and a healthy diet are still recommended for good health, and sleep is essential. Modern research shows that sleep boosts the immune system,[11] and lack of it increases your risk of illness.[12]

So did Greek temple physicians discover anesthesia, or surgery, or psychoanalysis? Did they discover the placebo effect or the importance of inspiring confidence in patients? It is easier to find out what they knew than how they discovered it. Today, complementary medicine includes yoga and Tai Chi, diets, massage, meditation, and other practices that seem to balance mind and body. The effectiveness of such therapies hasn't been conclusively proven by modern research, but the priests of Asklepios knew they would work.

The Myth of Asklepios

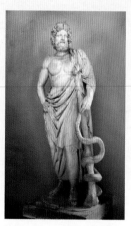

Michael F. Mehnert/Wikimedia Commons

This statue of Asklepios, exhibited at the Museum of Epidauros, shows the serpent coiled around his staff. Associated with healing since at least the sixteenth century BC, the ancient site of Epidauros was dedicated to Apollo around 800 BC; the Asklepieion there was of central importance.

Asklepios was rescued from his dying mother's womb by his father, the sun god Apollo. From the great centaur Chiron he learned to heal "many painful diseases." Patients would come to him "afflicted with congenital sores, or with their limbs wounded by gray bronze or by a far-hurled stone, or with their bodies wasting away from summer's fire or winter's cold." He tended "some of them with gentle incantations, others with soothing potions, or by wrapping remedies all around their limbs, and others he set right with surgery."[13] He became revered as a god, and his human descendants became famous healers. His sons ministered to the wounds of their fellow Greeks in the Trojan War,[14] and even the legendary Hippocrates (c. 460–c. 370 BC) claimed descent from him.

The Placebo Effect and Double Blind Trials

A placebo is a harmless substitute for a genuine medical intervention. The classic example is a sugar pill—an inert pill with no active ingredients. Sham operations and other procedures can also be placebos.

Placebos have an important role in testing the safety and effectiveness of therapies. When a new drug is tested in a double blind trial, it is given to half the volunteer patients in the study. The rest receive a placebo. Neither patients nor their doctors are told who is receiving which treatment, because their expectations might influence outcomes. (Thus the term "double blind": the patients are blind, and so are the doctors.) Researchers want to know if the new drug will help significantly more patients than the placebo will.

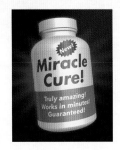

With no medically active ingredients, a placebo should have no medical effect. Yet many patients improve when treated with placebos. Is the "placebo effect" an example of mind over matter?

But these trials are complicated by the "placebo effect." Placebos work approximately 35 percent of the time to relieve conditions ranging from the common cold to chest pain.[15] The effects of placebos vary. Patients respond better to injections than pills[16] and better to expensive interventions than to cheap ones,[17] and they can even be influenced by pill color.[18]

There is also a "nocebo effect": people have negative side effects from placebos.[19]

All this makes it harder to interpret the results of double blind trials. Sometimes sham treatments or placebo pills even turn out to be more powerful than effective, proven treatments.[20] For purposes of therapy evaluation, the placebo effect is a nuisance.

But in actual therapy, placebos can help. Some researchers now use the term "context effect" instead, because a health care environment can have therapeutic effects in and of itself.[21] Others use the term "care effect" for therapeutic benefits that follow medical consultation and can't be fully explained by the actual medical treatment given.[22] The Asklepieia, with their spa-like environments and attentive priests, were ideally designed to maximize the placebo effect.

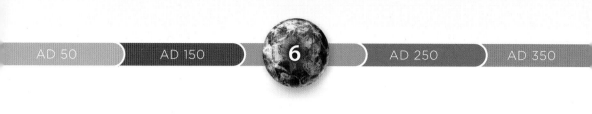

AD 200

Galen Discovers Nerves and Humors

The ancient Romans loved a good show. They crammed into the Colosseum to watch gladiators fight lions, crocodiles, and ostriches. They packed chariot races at the Circus Maximus like NASCAR fans. They staged concerts and talent shows. Intellectual Romans would even watch a famous Greek doctor do surgery on a live pig.

They would not be a respectful audience. Conservative Romans scorned doctors and were suspicious of Greeks. One famous writer saw Greek medicine "on the same level as see-through dresses . . . on the index of moral depravity."[1] But inscriptions show that when Galen (AD 129–c. 216) arrived in Rome, 75 percent of the doctors had Greek names. Galen was a celebrity, physician to gladiators and emperors, and author of many books. But as a Greek doctor he faced Roman prejudice, and he might have had a chip on his shoulder.

His pig operation was a demonstration of experimental anatomy. Galen knew that some nerves control sensation and others control movement. By doing systematic experiments, he could show how injuries at different points on a nerve's path from the brain can affect sensation and motion beyond those points.[2] As he prepared this operation, he told the audience what to expect: the pig would squeal until he cut the nerves to its larynx. Then it would go silent, because the brain's signal could no longer reach its vocal cords.

A rude Roman philosopher, Alexander Damascenus, interrupted Galen's talk. Aristotle knew best, said Damascenus: the heart, not the brain, is what controls human thought and speech. Pigs are not human. Showing that the brain controls a pig's voice doesn't prove it controls a human's.

Galen stomped out. He wasn't about to perform for boorish skeptics. Other members of the audience scolded Damascenus and prevailed on Galen to return and teach them more. The show went on.

But Damascenus had a point: pigs are not human. Galen honed his surgical skills and investigated the body by performing a dissection almost every day, but dissecting humans—living or dead—was strictly forbidden. He made do with monkeys, pigs, sheep, goats, and the

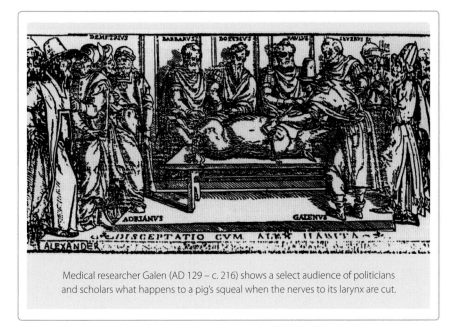

Medical researcher Galen (AD 129 – c. 216) shows a select audience of politicians and scholars what happens to a pig's squeal when the nerves to its larynx are cut.

emperor's pet elephant. So his anatomy was flawed: a dog's womb and a cow's brain are not exactly like their human equivalents.[3] Many of his conclusions were wrong, but he filled the gaps in observation with logic. It all made sense, and doctors followed Galen for centuries.

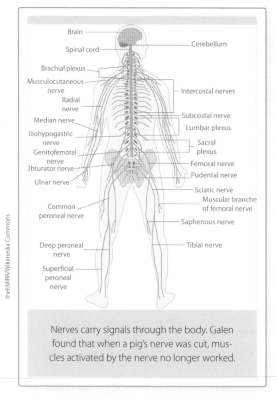

Brain
Cerebellum
Spinal cord
Brachial plexus
Musculocutaneous nerve
Intercostal nerves
Radial nerve
Subcostal nerve
Median nerve
Lumbar plexus
Iliohypogastric nerve
Sacral plexus
Genitofemoral nerve
Femoral nerve
Obturator nerve
Pudental nerve
Ulnar nerve
Sciatic nerve
Muscular branche of femoral nerve
Common peroneal nerve
Saphenous nerve
Deep peroneal nerve
Tibial nerve
Superficial peroneal nerve

Nerves carry signals through the body. Galen found that when a pig's nerve was cut, muscles activated by the nerve no longer worked.

Galen himself tried to follow Plato, Aristotle, and Hippocrates.[4] To make sense of all he learned, he relied on the theory of the four humors, which he attributed to Hippocrates. Humors were bodily fluids, and ancient Greek doctors had competing ideas about how many there were and how they had to be balanced to maintain health. By Galen's time, the Hippocratic camp held just four fluids—blood, bile, black bile, and phlegm—to be the essential humors. Galen's version of the theory finally prevailed in Europe, shaping medical thinking throughout the Middle Ages and beyond.[5] So for hundreds of years, scientists and doctors believed that:

* The universe was made up of four elements: earth, air, fire, and water.

* In these elements four qualities were combined: hot, cold, wet, and dry.

* The body had four essential humors: blood, phlegm, black bile, and yellow bile.[6]

* The essential humors also combined the four qualities, and corresponded to the four elements.

This theory was not correct, but it was appealingly tidy.

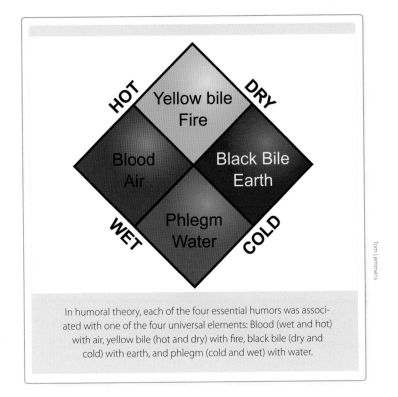

In humoral theory, each of the four essential humors was associated with one of the four universal elements: Blood (wet and hot) with air, yellow bile (hot and dry) with fire, black bile (dry and cold) with earth, and phlegm (cold and wet) with water.

Tom Lemmens

In the process of becoming the chief medical authority of the Middle Ages, Galen was simplified. His medieval followers usually didn't read the fat volumes he had written in Greek, settling instead for summaries in Latin or Arabic. Centuries later, when thinkers like Vesalius (AD 1514–1564) and Harvey (AD 1578–1657) went back to the original Greek, it spelled the end of Galenic medicine. They revived Galen's experimental methods, made new discoveries, and left his theories behind.[7]

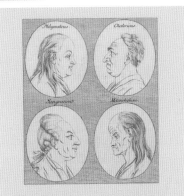

This eighteenth-century woodcut illustrates four dispositions associated with the four humors. Clockwise from upper left, phlegm dominates in the phlegmatic (unemotional) man, yellow bile in the choleric (angry) one, black bile in the melancholic (depressed) one, and blood in the sanguine (cheerful, optimistic) one.

Physiognomische Fragmente zur Beförderung der Menschenkenntnis und Menschenliebe, by Johann Kaspar Lavater

How Many Elements and Humors?

Prehistoric medicine relied on the supernatural: disease was caused by angry gods, ghosts, or witches. But as civilization advanced, the Greeks were not the only ones who began explaining disease by imbalances in the body instead.

In India, Ayurvedic doctors were medical professionals, not priests, and they thought health was influenced by individual circumstances and environmental stresses.[8] They based their diagnoses and treatments on physical examinations and patient histories. The major Ayurvedic texts (600–400 BC) described a humoral system, explaining health and disease as the result of imbalance among five essential elements (earth, air, fire, water, and space) that flow through the human body and the world. If that balance gets out of whack, people get sick.

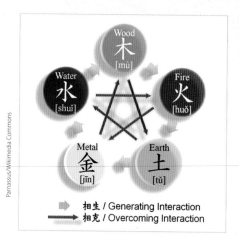

Chinese humoral theory involves five elements: wood, earth, water, fire, and metal.

Similarly, around the sixth century BC, a variety of humoral theories developed in China.[9] The third-century *Yellow Emperor's Classic of Internal Medicine* explained disease rationally in terms of diet, lifestyle, emotions, environment, and age—all of which affected the balance of five humors.[10] Chinese humoral theories persist to this day in traditional Chinese medicine.[11]

Did all these civilizations develop similar concepts independently, or did ideas travel along their far-flung trade routes?

We now know they were right about some things. Bodily fluids really do need to be kept in balance—not just four or five essential humors, but more than 50 hormones that act as chemical messengers. The body really is made up of elements found throughout the universe in different combinations. The ancient humoral theories were based on intuition and speculation, not data, but they contained seeds of truth.

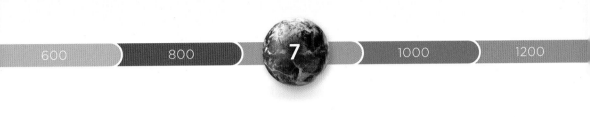

900

Al-Razi and Evidence-Based Medicine in the Middle Ages

There's an old story that gets repeated: when the great caliph Harun Al-Rashid decided to establish a hospital in Baghdad, he asked the physician Abū Bakr Muhammad ibn Zakariyyā al-Rāzī (854–925) to choose the site. Al-Razi proceeded with his usual logic: he placed cuts of meat around the city to see how fast they would spoil. The spot where meat remained unspoiled the longest was the place with the freshest air, and obviously the best site for a hospital.[1]

This can't be fact, since Harun died nearly a century before al-Razi was called from Persia to head a Baghdad hospital. But it's a lovely story, exemplifying Harun's support for public welfare and al-Razi's evidence-based approach to medicine. It helps us imagine the thriving civilization of Islam at a time when Europe lagged behind.

Between 622 and 750, Islam conquered territories from the Atlantic Ocean to the Indus River—lands that had belonged to the Byzantine and Persian empires. Intellectual life continued, and Muslim scholars absorbed the traditions of Greek, Jewish, and Iranian learning in the lands they had conquered.[2] Then they carried science and medicine forward to new heights.

Harun really did establish a hospital at Baghdad, recruiting physicians from the vibrant interfaith medical center of Jundi-Shapur in Persia.[3] Islamic hospitals were well funded, with endowments from the rich and powerful and supplemental allocations from state budgets. Some doctors charged fees, but hospitals could usually admit patients free of charge. There were hospitals for the blind, disabled, and mentally ill; there were hospitals in leper sanctuaries and prisons.[4] And throughout Islam, great teaching hospitals nourished medical research. Doctors had traditionally learned through apprenticeships, with ambitious students traveling to learn the skills of masters.[5] In teaching hospitals, student interns had well-stocked libraries,[6] pharmacies, lecture halls, and

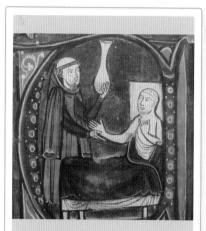

A thirteenth-century European image of al-Razi shows the surgeon at a sickbed, holding a vessel for collecting urine.

Recueil des traités de médecine, Gerardus Cremonensis

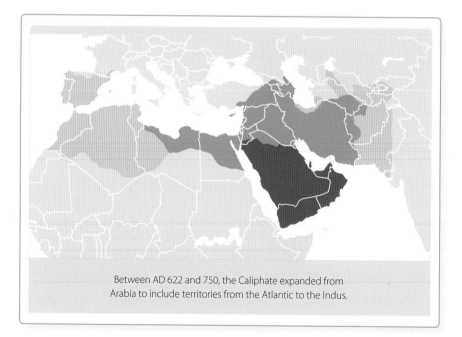

Between AD 622 and 750, the Caliphate expanded from Arabia to include territories from the Atlantic to the Indus.

master physicians qualified to teach a range of specialties.[7] They could consult archived case reports and hear new findings presented at medical conferences.[8]

Al-Razi, known in Europe as Rhazes, was one of the most influential physicians of the Middle Ages. He was born near Tehran, worked as a musician and moneylender until his thirties,[9] and went on to become an astute medical clinician and prolific writer. He is famous for his careful observation of the differences between smallpox and measles.[10] In his 25-volume *Comprehensive Book of Medicine*, he transmitted the works of many Greek physicians, but not uncritically—he interspersed material from other Greek and Iranian thinkers and from his own practice.[11] Handing on a prescription for gout,

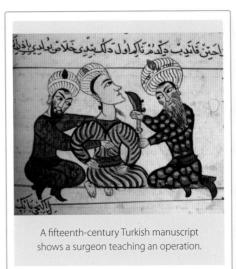

A fifteenth-century Turkish manuscript shows a surgeon teaching an operation.

he commented, "The drug is said to be effective within the hour, but I need to verify this."[12] He followed Galen's humoral theory of medicine, but he wrote a book called *Doubts about Galen*.[13]

In Europe, al-Razi's influence increased in the Renaissance. The *Comprehensive Book of Medicine* was translated into Latin in the thirteenth century, and the fifteenth-century invention of printing carried it to a wide audience.[14] Would he have been pleased?

Maybe not. He emphasized the importance of keeping up with current research, and one of his true legacies may have been teaching his readers the value of logical inquiry. To evaluate the toxicity of mercury, al-Razi experimented on an ape. He recommended treating epilepsy with a sneeze-producing substance because he'd tried it on one group of patients but not another; he could testify that sneezing helped.[15] In another clinical trial, he compared two groups of patients

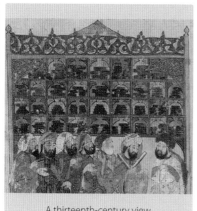

A thirteenth-century view of students in a library.

with symptoms of the onset of meningitis, and concluded that they could be saved by bloodletting.[16] For centuries, European medicine relied more on reverence for old sources than on new research. But "Rhazes" was one of the revered sources, and eventually scientific learning revived in Europe. Did the inquiring mind of al-Razi, with his pioneering use of clinical trials, help kindle new discoveries?

Jundi-Shapur and the Survival of Learning

When Muslims conquered Persia in AD 636, they found a treasure trove of medical texts in the city of Jundi-Shapur.[17] Founded in the third century by Shapur the Great, Jundi-Shapur was the intellectual center of the Sassanid Empire.[18] Greek physicians and Nestorian monks, driven out of Byzantium as heretics in the reign of Justinian, established a medical school there. The Nestorians were scholars, teachers, and translators, so Jundi-Shapur was rich in Syriac translations of Hippocrates, Galen, and their schools.[19] The medical school and its associated hospital were a cultural crossroads for Persians, Greeks, Indians, Zoroastrians, Jews, and Nestorians.[20]

Much of ancient Greek science would have been lost forever if it had not been translated into Syriac and Arabic by Muslim scholars. What the Muslim world learned in places like Jundi-Shapur, Europe began to learn again centuries later. Late in the Middle Ages, ancient European works and newer Muslim ones reached Spain (under Islamic rule) and the great medical school at Salerno (influenced by Islam). They were translated into Latin, sowing the seeds for a revival of learning.

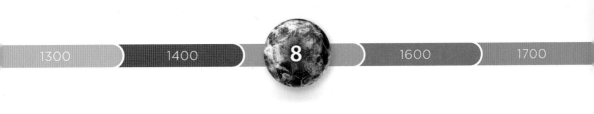

1508

Da Vinci's Heart

More than a century before William Harvey discovered the circulatory system, a famous artist stopped to chat with a patient in a Florence hospital. The patient claimed to be a hundred years old, and said he didn't feel "any bodily ailment other than weakness."[1] And then, quietly, he died.

The artist at his bedside was Leonardo da Vinci (1452–1519), at the hospital to continue his lifelong study of anatomy. Leonardo dissected the old man's body and found that he had died because his arteries, narrowed with age, blocked the flow of blood to his tissues.[2] Comparing his thickened blood vessels with those of a recently deceased toddler, Leonardo discovered age-related hardening of the arteries.[3]

Before Leonardo, human dissection was taboo in most times and places. There were exceptions—Herophilus dissected human bodies in the third century BC—but for ages, physicians and artists alike had to learn about anatomy from books.[4] Leonardo wanted to paint humans in natural motion, not standing stiff as medieval cartoons or bulging with muscles like "a sack of walnuts."[5] He studied the outward motion of bones and muscles, and then—in love with motion—he studied the inward motion of blood through veins and arteries.

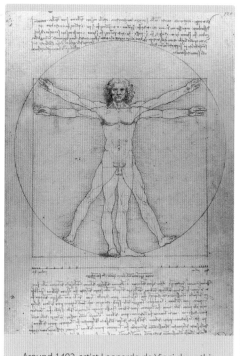

Around 1492, artist Leonardo da Vinci drew this illustration to illustrate the geometric balance of human proportions. The picture is often called "Vitruvian Man," because it refers to ideas on proportion held by the Roman architect Vitruvius.

Leonardo was the original "Renaissance man," curious about almost everything and competent in many areas. He trained as an artist in Renaissance Florence,[6] but when he went job-hunting, he showcased his skills as a map-maker, an engineer, and a military architect. Italian princes were always making war; if they didn't need an artist, they might need a guy who could invent new weapons. On the side, Leonardo dabbled in science. His notebooks, written backward, teem with ideas and inventions. (His helicopters couldn't be built for centuries after his time, but think what an advantage flight would have given a warring Renaissance prince.)

Over fifty pages of Leonardo's diaries are devoted to study of the heart, a project on which he collaborated with a professor of medicine, Marcantonio della Torre.[7] Leonardo's knowledge of hydrodynamics (the flow of water) helped him understand the flow of blood. He came up with an experiment, letting water flow through glass tubes shaped like the valves of a heart. Would blood eddy and curl through the heart like water through river channels? Da Vinci drew his hypotheses with swirling lines to represent blood flow and marginal notes to explain what was happening.[8]

He observed that water rotated in circular vortices behind the valves, helping to close them. A 1969 experiment with a transparent model of the aorta showed that Leonardo was right,[9] and twenty-first century MRI scanning confirms it: blood flows through the heart in the patterns Leonardo predicted.[10]

Yet Leonardo never realized that blood circulated through the body in a circle.[11] Following the teaching of Galen, he believed that blood formed in the liver, went to the lungs for oxygen, and then was pumped to the rest of the body. He had never heard of Ibn Al-Nafis (1213–1288),[12] a great Arab physician who understood that blood flows in a circuit, from the heart to the tissues and then back from the tissues to the heart.

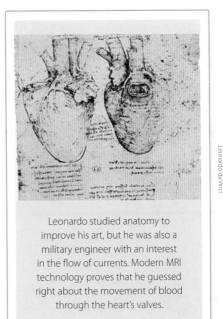

Leonardo da Vinci

Leonardo studied anatomy to improve his art, but he was also a military engineer with an interest in the flow of currents. Modern MRI technology proves that he guessed right about the movement of blood through the heart's valves.

Why do some discoveries change history, while others go unnoticed? Timing matters. Europe was not ready to learn from Ibn Al-Nafis. Centuries later, in England, William Harvey (1578 – 1657) rediscovered the circulatory system—and even then, Harvey's work was rejected by the medical community because it contradicted the work of Galen. Only after other scientists and researchers confirmed his views was Harvey recognized as a medical pioneer.[13]

But publication matters, too, and Leonardo's scientific work

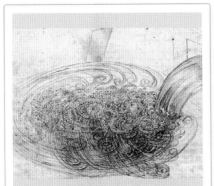

Leonardo da Vinci

Leonardo sketched the way moving fluids encounter barriers, eddying and swirling in dynamic vortices.

went unpublished until the late nineteenth century.[14] He left thousands of pages of barely decipherable notes; his literary executor was overwhelmed.[15] Thus Leonardo's discoveries had no impact on the history of medicine.

Renaissance Anatomy

The Renaissance began as a cultural movement in fourteenth-century Italy. Renaissance artists and thinkers questioned authority, and medical authorities were certainly open to question. After all, about a third of Europe's population had died in the Black Death (1347–1351), and doctors hadn't been able to stop it. Eager for knowledge they couldn't find in ancient texts, medical schools began to encourage direct observation.

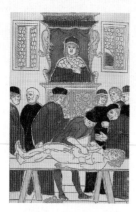

In this 1495 illustration of an anatomical dissection, the lector is reading from an anatomy book (probably by Galen), while the sector makes an incision. The ostensor points to direct students' attention.

Most doctors had learned their anatomy from unillustrated copies of Galen. Even after Frederick II (1194–1250) ordered all medical students to attend at least one dissection,[16] hands-on learning opportunities were scarce. Students craned their necks to see the surgeon's knife, while one professor read aloud to them from an anatomical text and another pointed to the part of the body being cut.[17]

Andreas Vesalius (1514 – 1564) helped change this. As an anatomy teacher at the University of Padua, he introduced a new approach: he performed dissections himself and recorded his observations with illustrations. Soon he discovered Galen's anatomical errors.[18] In 1543 he published *The Fabric of the Human Body*, and the printing press—still a fairly new invention—made his accurate illustrations available for medical education. Vesalius opened the door to a new era in medicine, where doctors trusted direct observation and critical thinking instead of blind obedience to tradition.

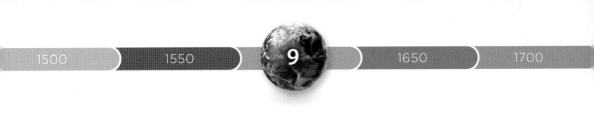
1600

The Chamberlen Family Secret

Imagine a carriage arriving at an upscale address in London, in the reign of King James I. Inside the house, a wealthy woman is in labor. The surgeon arriving at her door is one of two brothers, Peter Chamberlen the Elder (1560 – 1631) or Peter Chamberlen the Younger (1572 – 1626). He brings a gilded box, carried by two men; it must hold a great machine, but nobody is allowed to look. The woman's relatives are banned from her room, and she is blindfolded.[1] She only knows that the Chamberlens' secret will help her and her child survive.

Childbirth has always been risky. Between 1400 and 1800, an estimated 1 to 3 percent of deliveries resulted in the mother's death. Women averaged five pregnancies each, so approximately 10 percent died in childbirth or soon afterward.[2] Babies were even more likely to die.

Sometimes a woman's pelvis was too narrow for a baby's head, or the baby arrived in an awkward position and got stuck. An obstructed labor could go on for days, until either the baby or the mother died.[3] If the baby died first, midwives would call a doctor to save the mother by removing her child. Doctors used various surgical instruments—crochets, perforators, and cranioclasts—to hook the skull of the dead baby, pierce it, crush it, and haul it out.[4] If the mother died first, the living baby had to be removed immediately by Caesarean section.

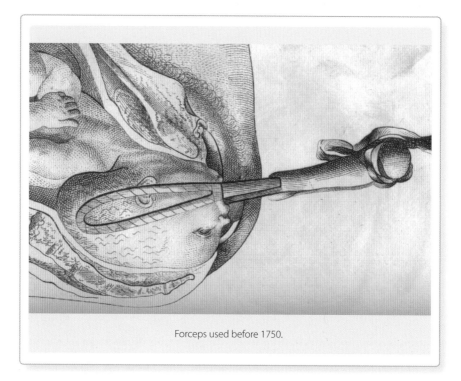

Forceps used before 1750.

But hidden in the Chamberlens' box was a new tool, designed to pull the baby out of the birth canal without damaging either mother or child. One of the brothers had designed an obstetrical instrument we call a forceps. It was rather like two spoons, one to fit over each side of a small head, so the surgeon could ease the baby out of the birth canal.

The two Peter Chamberlens guarded their secret invention closely, and it served them well. They were barber surgeons, licensed to do surgical procedures but not to prescribe medicines.[5] Physicians still had higher status than surgeons, and if there was any medical specialty less prestigious than surgery, it was midwifery. Yet the Chamberlens became wealthy and enjoyed royal patronage. Peter the Elder attended both Queen Anne and Queen Henrietta Maria in their pregnancies.[6] The Chamberlen family kept the forceps secret for a century, handing it down to new generations of doctors and man-midwives: Peter the Younger's son Dr. Peter, his grandson Hugh the Elder, and his great-grandson Hugh the Younger.[7] Hugh the Elder (1630 – ca. 1720) once tried to sell the secret in France, but the deal fell through, and instead of money he went home with a French textbook on midwifery. He translated that and published it as *The Accomplish't Midwife*, with a sly hint in the foreword about the secret he wasn't telling.

Hugh the Younger (1664 – 1728) probably leaked the secret, and in the early eighteenth century other forceps came into use. The Van Roonhuysen family developed a flexible model with a lever, and kept it secret for many years.[8] William Smellie (1697 – 1763) discovered that the baby's head normally rotates through the birth canal; he used forceps to help with this natural rotation.[9]

Childbirth, no longer supervised by midwives and matriarchs, was becoming the responsibility of male physicians. Women lay in bed, modestly covered in blankets, rather than sitting on birthing stools and letting gravity help the process. Physicians used forceps and other instruments more than midwives, often without sanitizing them. Rich women, attended by doctors, were for the first time likelier to die in childbirth than poor women, who could afford only midwives.[10] New discoveries in obstetrics brought unintended results.

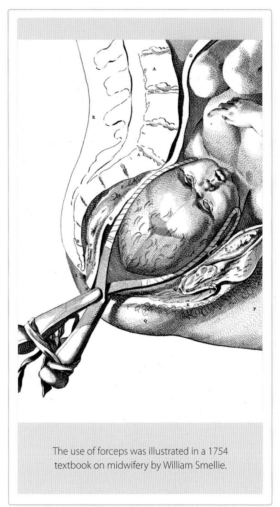

The use of forceps was illustrated in a 1754 textbook on midwifery by William Smellie.

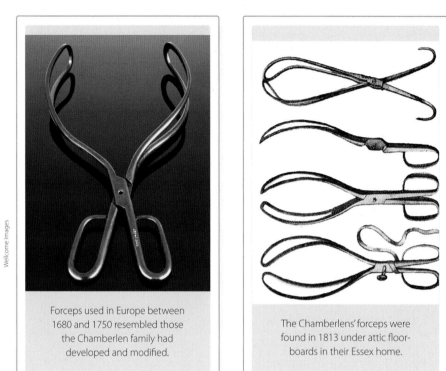

Forceps used in Europe between 1680 and 1750 resembled those the Chamberlen family had developed and modified.

The Chamberlens' forceps were found in 1813 under attic floor-boards in their Essex home.

Caesarean Sections

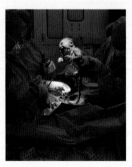

Obstetricians delivering a baby by Caesarean section.

The Caesarean section—cutting through the skin and the uterine wall to deliver a baby from the abdomen—probably wasn't named in honor of Julius Caesar. Under Roman law, he would have been cut from his mother's womb if she had died in childbirth. But Caesar's mother, Aurelia, was still alive when he was 45.[14] More likely the term comes from the Latin "caedere," meaning "to cut."

Midwifery and the Birthing Stool

Midwives are health care professionals who care for women during and after pregnancy. They help mothers deliver, care for, and breastfeed their babies.

There have always been midwives. References in *Exodus* and the *Ebers Papyrus* date back to the Bronze Age, and the occupation itself is surely rooted in prehistory. Typically, midwives were mothers themselves; they used their own experience, with what they'd learned from elders, to help new generations of mothers.[11] Yet Agnodice, a Greek maiden remembered as the first midwife, was said to have learned her skill from male doctors.[12] According to Hyginus (64 BC–AD 17), Agnodice disguised herself as a man to study medicine from Herophilus (335–280 BC), and once her masquerade was discovered, she helped overturn an Athenian law forbidding women to become doctors. But she probably wasn't real.

A more reliable source of information on classical midwifery is Soranus of Ephesus, who practiced gynecology in Greece, Egypt, and Rome around AD 98–138. In his four-volume treatise on womens's health,[13] Soranus advised the pregnant woman to prepare for labor by bathing in wine, then letting the midwife rub her belly with oils to lessen stretch marks. The midwife should have all the necessary equipment to ensure a safe delivery: goose fat to soften the birth canal, herbs to anoint its opening, clean olive oil, sea sponges, pieces of wool bandages to cradle the infant, a pillow, strong smelling herbs in case of fainting, and, most important, a midwife's birth stool.

The birth stool made it easier for a woman to sit up while giving birth, so gravity could help the delivery. The seat had a crescent-shaped hole through which the baby would be delivered. There were armrests for the mother to grasp during the delivery. Most birth stools had backs, which the laboring mother could press against; otherwise, Soranus advised, an assistant should support the mother from behind.

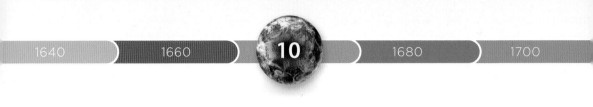
1670

Looking Through Van Leeuwenhoek's Tiny Microscopes

Antonie van Leeuwenhoek (1632–1723) was not educated to be a scientist. Science was a new field, just developing from natural philosophy. Indeed, when his English contemporaries chartered something like an Academy of Science, they called it the "Royal Society for Improving Natural Knowledge."

And before scientists, there were certainly no microbiologists. Microbiology needs microscopes, and microscopes were still just "executive toys" at the time.[1] Yet Van Leeuwenhoek peered through his home-made lenses at microbes and bacteria. He called them "animalcules"—tiny animals—and stubbornly maintained their existence when more established scientists ridiculed his reports. He also observed spermatozoa in semen (he was surprised how big flea sperm turned out to be). He is called the "Father of Microbiology."

Van Leeuwenhoek grew up in the Netherlands, in a middle-class family. He didn't learn Latin;[2] his scientific communications would have to be translated from his colloquial Dutch. Instead of studying at a university, he apprenticed as a bookkeeper in Amsterdam. Back in Delft, he set up a fabric shop. He also served as a minor city official,

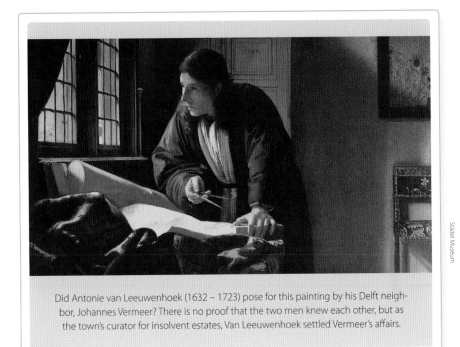

Did Antonie van Leeuwenhoek (1632 – 1723) pose for this painting by his Delft neighbor, Johannes Vermeer? There is no proof that the two men knew each other, but as the town's curator for insolvent estates, Van Leeuwenhoek settled Vermeer's affairs.

Städel Museum

exercising his mathematical ability—his duties included calculating volumes of wine and settling the estates of citizens who died insolvent.[3]

He encountered Robert Hooke's *Micrographia*, published in 1664. Hooke, the Royal Society's "Curator of Experiments," used microscopes to enlarge common things: fleas, leaves, needles, and even cloth. Van Leeuwenhoek could see that a microscope would help him inspect fabric. He began making his own lenses, which enabled him to look at nature on a new scale.[4] In 1673, encouraged by a young physician, he wrote the first of his more than 190 letters to the Royal Society in London.[5] In 1680, he was elected to membership in the society. He never attended a meeting or learned English; Hooke learned Dutch so he could read Van Leeuwenhoek's letters.[6]

In his spare time, the sketchily educated Van Leeuwenhoek was becoming a scientist. His approach was bottom-up.[7] Some investigators begin with guiding questions, and design experiments to answer those questions. Van Leeuwenhoek began with tools, just looking through

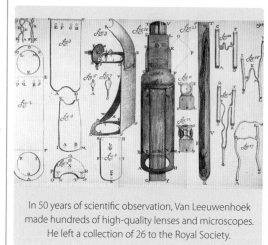

In 50 years of scientific observation, Van Leeuwenhoek made hundreds of high-quality lenses and microscopes. He left a collection of 26 to the Royal Society.

lenses to see what he could see. But correspondence with other scientists helped him focus. The Royal Society's secretary, Henry Oldenburg, published Van Leeuwenhoek's letters and also suggested things for him to study, including fertilized eggs, muscle fibers, and saliva.[8] Van Leeuwenhoek examined his own saliva and scrapings from his teeth, and in 1676, he reported the first unmistakable observations of bacteria.[9]

The discovery of bacteria would have huge significance for medicine, but nobody understood that at the time. People were still arguing about questions like spontaneous generation. Do maggots have maggot parents, for instance, or do they emerge from dead flesh? The question had philosophical and even religious implications.[10] Van Leeuwenhoek, if he thought about it before picking up his microscopes, probably held with folk wisdom: fleas emerged from dust. All fleas were the same size; which were the parents? But then he enclosed a few fleas until they laid eggs, and carried the eggs around in his pocket until they hatched larvae. He observed larvae spinning cocoons,

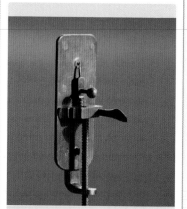

Replica of a Leeuwenhoek microscope. The tiny lens is near the top; the sample on its sharp-tipped holder could be brought into focus with the key-like knob. Van Leeuwenhoek also had to arrange a steady light source at the right angle for his observations.

and recognizable fleas developing in pupae. It must have been an itchy pocket, but Van Leeuwenhoek discovered the life cycle of insects.[11]

Van Leeuwenhoek is remembered for making hundreds of microscopes, but he didn't invent the microscope or teach others to improve it. He left twenty-six of his instruments to the Royal Society,[12] but almost all the lenses he made have since been lost.

His true legacy was to look through lenses with an open mind and try to understand what he saw. "He held and practiced the values of empiricism, objectivity, and openness," points out one scholar. "He changed his ideas based on new evidence. He was . . . an important participant in what we now call the Scientific Revolution and the Enlightenment."[13] Van Leeuwenhoek's gift to medicine was not just his discovery of microbes or sperm, but his commitment to the process of discovery.

The Royal Society for Improving Natural Knowledge

The Royal Society was chartered in London in 1662.[14] It had its roots in groups of physicians, natural philosophers, and experimenters who had been meeting more or less informally. Some had met at Gresham College as early as 1645,[15] and the "learned society" formed there after a November 1660 lecture by Christopher Wren.

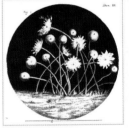

Robert Hooke

England had just been through decades of civil war; Parliament men had overcome Royalists for a time, and King Charles I had been executed in 1649. The legal and religious underpinnings of society had been contested. The monarchy was restored in 1660, but the men of the new Royal Society—both Royalists and Parliamentarians—would question intellectual authority. The Society's motto is "Nullius in verba," or "Take nobody's word for it."[16]

Robert Hooke's *Micrographia* (1664) has been called the first book of popular science. It revealed worlds invisible to the naked eye, like this colony of mold growing on leather.

The Royal Society was an important institution in the development of modern science. Both in its meetings and in its publications, it brought inquiring minds together and fostered the exchange of ideas.

(Continued on next page)

(Continued from previous page)

It published books—including Hooke's *Micrographia* and Isaac Newton's *Principia Mathematica*—but starting in 1665 it also published *Philosophical Transactions*, "now the oldest continuously-published science journal in the world."[17]

Van Leeuwenhoek's letters reached the world through *Philosophical Transactions*—at least when the journal was edited by scientists open to Van Leeuwenhoek's ideas. Volumes 16, 17, 29, and 30 were edited by comet-discover and mathematician Edmond Halley, who limited communications to "Discourses or Relations concerning Physical, Mathematical, and Mechanical Theories or Observations."[18] This included astronomy, not biology; the peer review process under Halley ruled out Van Leeuwenhoek, who ended up self-publishing many of his letters.

The Royal Society and its journal were not perfect, but they were in the vanguard of the Scientific Revolution. Other scientific societies followed. Like the medical schools at Jundi-Shapur and Salerno, the new societies inspired generations of thinkers.

A Proto-Germ Theory in the Renaissance?

As early as 1546, a Renaissance Italian physician proposed the idea that epidemic diseases could be caused by tiny particles or spores—although it is not clear whether he believed the "spores" were living things. Girolamo Fracastoro (ca. 1476 – 1553) thought that infections could be transmitted by direct or indirect contact, or even without contact over long distances; also, things like clothes or linen could transmit "the seeds of contagion" from one person to another.[19] Fracastoro's ideas were influential; maybe that's why in 1631, as another wave of plague hit Italy, Tuscany set up a special pest-house for fumigating silk.[20] But without powerful microscopes or a well-developed experimental method, Fracastoro could not prove or refine his hypothesis. Until the nineteenth century, the miasma theory (see Chapter 19) remained the standard explanation for much disease transmission.

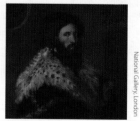

National Gallery, London

Renaissance physician and scholar Girolamo Fracastoro may have been too far ahead of his time when he proposed that disease could be caused by tiny particles.

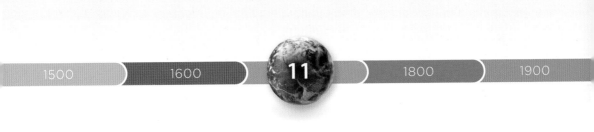
1721

Fighting Smallpox and Public Opinion in Colonial Boston

I t was 1721, and passions were running high in Boston. Before dawn one November morning, somebody lobbed a firebomb into the home of Puritan minister Cotton Mather. It failed to detonate, so the attached note could still be read: "Damn You, I will Inoculate You with this, and a Pox on You."[2] People distrusted Mather. As a young expert on witchcraft he had influenced the 1692 Salem witch trials. Twenty people were executed as witches, largely on the basis of "spectral evidence"—their accusers "saw" them performing evil magic while they were invisible to others. Mather supported the use of spectral evidence, but eventually it was ruled inadmissible in court. The trials and executions ended; jurors and a judge apologized for the injustice. Mather did not. Now, thirty years later, some thought his newest cause was another dangerously irrational delusion.

Smallpox was loose in town. Older residents had survived earlier epidemics, and many bore the scars: those who didn't die of smallpox were often disfigured, blind, or disabled for life. To save lives in this new epidemic, Mather urged Boston's doctors to inoculate children and other vulnerable people. Inoculation was a form of deliberate infection, giving patients a milder—more survivable—form of the disease. Mather had learned about it first from his slave, Onesimus, who had been inoculated as a child in Africa,[3] and later from a journal article.

In much of Asia and Africa, inoculation had long been common. It was risky. Inoculation made people sick, and about 2 percent of them died.[4] But the death toll from naturally acquired smallpox was about 30 percent,[5] and people knew that even a mild case of smallpox left its survivor immune for life. When a rising epidemic struck, inoculation might be safer than hoping to avoid infection. So in Sudan, the mother of a healthy child would "buy the smallpox" from the mother of an infected child, haggling over the price of each pustule and carrying the germs on a cloth to tie over her child's arm.[6]

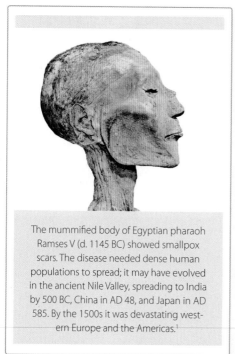

The mummified body of Egyptian pharaoh Ramses V (d. 1145 BC) showed smallpox scars. The disease needed dense human populations to spread; it may have evolved in the ancient Nile Valley, spreading to India by 500 BC, China in AD 48, and Japan in AD 585. By the 1500s it was devastating western Europe and the Americas.[1]

In Boston, only one doctor was willing to try the procedure: Zabdiel Boylston. He was unusually daring; in 1718 he performed the first recorded mastectomy in America. He was skilled; patients survived his surgeries. He was open to non-European ideas, with genuine respect for Native American medicine.[7] And he was motivated to fight smallpox. He had nearly died of it himself, and it had killed most of his wife's family. Like Mather, he worried about the fate of his children in this new epidemic.

Boylston's inoculations were fiercely opposed by his colleagues—especially Dr.

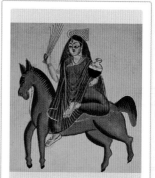

From Pakistan to Bengal, people prayed to Shitala—goddess of sores, pustules, and ghouls—for protection from smallpox.

William Douglass, who wanted to study the natural progression of smallpox through the Boston population. The government ordered Boylston to stop inoculating patients, and public opinion targeted him as well as Mather. In one satiric editorial, Douglass claimed that inoculation was so dangerous it could be used as a way of "reducing the Eastern Indians"[8]—a cruel joke, since Native Americans had already lost as much as 90 to 95 percent of their population to smallpox

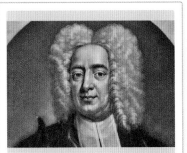

The Reverend Cotton Mather, a Puritan minister who goaded and abetted the Salem witch trials in 1692, met with distrust when he recommended inoculation against the 1721 smallpox epidemic. Was this another of his dangerously irrational ideas?

Columbia University

introduced accidentally, and sometimes deliberately, by white settlers.[9]

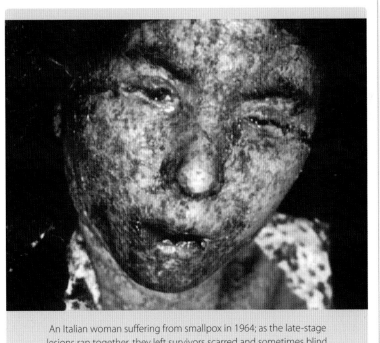

An Italian woman suffering from smallpox in 1964; as the late-stage lesions ran together, they left survivors scarred and sometimes blind. The last naturally transmitted case of smallpox occurred in 1977.

Centers for Disease Control and Prevention

Because of the controversy, Boylston went in fear of his life. But he inoculated 248 patients, cared for them while they were quarantined, and lost only six,[10] just over 2 percent. Meanwhile smallpox infected 5,889 people—over half the population of Boston—and killed 844. The epidemic raged through London, too, and while Mather and Boylston advocated inoculation in the colonies, Lady Mary Wortley Montagu advocated it in Britain. An ambassador's wife, she had seen it done in Turkey, publicized

Vanquishing Smallpox for Good

L'ORIGINE DE LA VACCINE.

The origins of the vaccine: a milk-maid with a mild case of cowpox is visited by eager physicians.

Wellcome Images

Edward Jenner, FRS (1749 – 1823), is credited with discovering smallpox vaccine, but his breakthrough was just one victory in the long fight against a dreaded disease. Like most successful scientists before and since, he built on the work of others.[15] He knew about inoculation, which remained controversial because of the 2 percent fatality rate and the risk of contagion from patients undergoing the process. But Jenner noticed that cowpox, a much less dangerous disease, also gave its survivors immunity from smallpox. So in 1798 he tried a less dangerous inoculation, using pus from cowpox, and experimented to prove that his inoculated patients were indeed immune to smallpox. This procedure was called "vaccination," from the Latin word *vacca*, for cow. Jenner published his findings, leading eventually to the acceptance of his comparatively safe vaccine.[16]

Over the next two centuries, mass vaccination programs and other strategies interrupted the ancient chain of smallpox infections.[17] As recently as the 1950s, smallpox still infected 50 million victims a year.[18] Then the World Health Organization launched an all-out global immunization campaign, and the disease was eradicated by 1980.[19] The virus survives only in laboratories in the U.S. and Russia.[20] Should the last specimens be destroyed?

her four-year-old daughter's inoculation,[11] and persuaded her friend Princess Caroline to have two of the royal princesses inoculated.[12] News of Lady Mary's activities eased the governmental pressure on Boylston. When the danger passed, he was seen as a medical hero, invited to speak to the Royal Society, and urged to publish a report of his activities.[13] If Boston authorities had mandated inoculation instead of forbidding it, Boylston calculated 726 lives would have been saved. His comparative statistical analysis made Boylston a pioneer yet again; if not the first, he was one of the first to evaluate a medical intervention this way.[14]

Royal Smallpox Treatments

Smallpox was an equal-opportunity scourge—it attacked rich and poor alike, and attempts at curing it were just as misguided for royalty as anybody else. Take the red cure. After Charles V of France (1364 – 1380) caught smallpox, he was dressed in red; when Elizabeth I of England (1358 – 1603) caught it, she was wrapped in a red blanket.[21] How could this help?

Since there was no cure, prevention was the best bet. Kings, like anybody else who could manage it, would leave smallpox-stricken towns as fast as they could. They would impose quarantines to keep the disease from spreading. But these barriers didn't always work. What if somebody in the king's household was already infected, and the symptoms just weren't yet visible? What if somebody sent a gift contaminated with smallpox virus?

In China, the first Manchu emperor died of smallpox in 1661 despite quarantine measures. His son Kangxi (1654 – 1722), scarred but alive, was chosen emperor partly because of his painfully acquired immunity, and a new policy mandated inoculation for family members and the nobility. Contemporary Chinese sources describe three methods: putting a piece of cotton imbued with pox pus into the nostril of a healthy child, having the child inhale dried pulverized pox scabs, or having the child wear a piece of clothing from an infected child.[22]

Infected Blankets and Germ Warfare

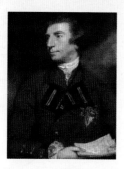

Lord Jeffrey Amherst fought ruthlessly for British dominance in North America, even using germ warfare. "Could it not be contrived to send the small pox among the disaffected tribes of Indians?" he asked a subordinate in 1763. The results: a gift of infected blankets and an epidemic among the Delaware and Shawnee.

Columbus stumbled onto America in 1492, and by the 1500s European explorers and settlers were infecting its people with deadly diseases to which they had no natural immunity: typhus, influenza, diphtheria, measles, and—worst of all, over and over—smallpox.[23] Epidemics swept across Central and South America almost immediately, killing a larger percentage of the population than the fourteenth-century Black Death had killed in Europe. Civilizations never recovered. In the beginning this was probably accidental; later there were at least some instances of deliberate germ warfare, and those have been remembered ever since.[24]

Lord Jeffrey Amherst authorized the distribution of infected blankets in 1763, but there is evidence that others before him did the same. Throughout the Americas, one tribe after another tells a story of deliberate infection, often by blankets. The Incas told of a mysterious box given to them by the Spaniards in 1493.[25]

The idea of toxic gifts is ancient. Poisoned cloaks and shirts, tiny boxes, and infected dresses appear in Greek myth, Arthurian legend, Hindu stories, and fairy tales.[26] And smallpox was a known contaminant. In India, one method of inoculation was to wrap healthy children in victims' blankets, in hopes that they would catch a mild version of the disease and survive.[27] Jenner stored pus in a feather quill for later use.[28] Humans had the imagination to carry out a genocidal plot, and smallpox was a perfect weapon.

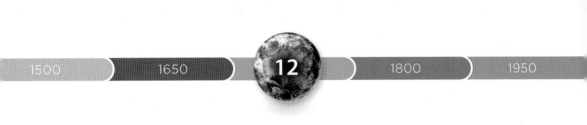

1747

Limeys and the Conquest of Scurvy

In 1535, a crew of French explorers were dying of scurvy in the Quebec ice. First their gums bled and their teeth fell out. They bruised all over. "Some lost their very substance and their legs became swollen and puffed up while the sinews contracted and turned coal-black," said their captain, Jacques Cartier.[1] Columbus had discovered America in 1492, and now European explorers were poster children for malnutrition. Sailing for months without refrigeration, they had no fruits or vegetables to eat. Luckily for Cartier, a Native American cured his men with cedar beer.

Nobody realized scurvy was caused by malnutrition, but cures around the world were rich in vitamin C. Evergreens worked in the frozen north and citrus fruit in the south. In 1497, Portuguese explorer Vasco da Gama spent a record three months out of sight of land, and about 100 of his 170-man crew died of scurvy. The survivors met Moorish traders, bargained for oranges, and recovered their health.[2]

Centuries passed. Scurvy deaths mounted, and the idea of curing it with fruit was repeatedly forgotten. In the early 1600s East India Company officials used lemon juice; but lemons were rare in Britain, and nobody knew *why* they worked. Was it because they were acidic? A

1740 British expedition tried substituting vitriol (sulfuric acid),[3] which didn't go bad on long voyages. The expedition lost 1,767 of 1,955 men.[4]

In 1747, naval surgeon James Lind investigated the effects of six acids on scurvy.[5] His test subjects were twelve sailors with scurvy, with two in each treatment group. All the sailors received the same diet, but each group got its own daily treatment:

1. a quart of cider;

2. twenty-five drops of elixir of vitriol;

3. six spoons of vinegar;

4. half a pint of seawater;

5. two oranges and one lemon;

6. a spicy paste plus a drink of barley water.

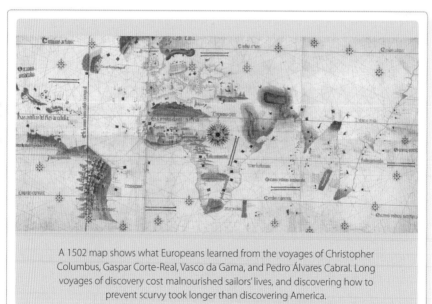

A 1502 map shows what Europeans learned from the voyages of Christopher Columbus, Gaspar Corte-Real, Vasco da Gama, and Pedro Álvares Cabral. Long voyages of discovery cost malnourished sailors' lives, and discovering how to prevent scurvy took longer than discovering America.

Group Five ran out of fruit in six days, but already one sailor was fit for duty and the other mostly recovered. The other groups did poorly.[6]

Lind's experiment showed the value of citrus fruits, but not understanding nutritional deficiencies, he didn't know why the cure worked.[7] Eighteenth-century explanations for scurvy echoed traditional medical theories. The humoral theory seemed plausible: salt thickened the spleen, causing black bile to stagnate.[8] The "bad air" or "miasma" theory could also be true; crews were packed into poorly ventilated quarters, and ship's officers, who had more spacious cabins, were less affected by scurvy. Of course, the officers also got the best food.

Lind left the navy, became a medical doctor in Edinburgh, and kept thinking about how to keep sailors healthy. He reviewed all the literature on scurvy and concluded that diet, foul air, and lack of exercise all helped cause it. He noted that citrus fruits had proved

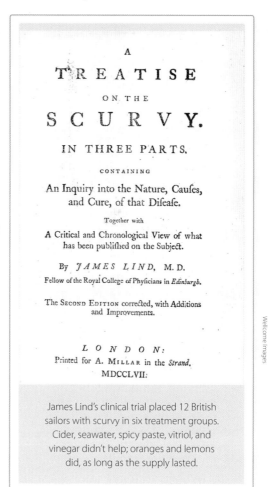

A

TREATISE

ON THE

SCURVY.

IN THREE PARTS,

CONTAINING

An Inquiry into the Nature, Causes, and Cure, of that Disease.

Together with

A Critical and Chronological View of what has been published on the Subject.

By JAMES LIND, M.D.

Fellow of the Royal College of Physicians in *Edinburgh*.

The SECOND EDITION corrected, with Additions and Improvements.

L O N D O N:

Printed for A. MILLAR in the *Strand*. MDCCLVII.

James Lind's clinical trial placed 12 British sailors with scurvy in six treatment groups. Cider, seawater, spicy paste, vitriol, and vinegar didn't help; oranges and lemons did, as long as the supply lasted.

Wellcome Images

effective against scurvy for "nearly 200 years," and he later used them successfully to cure hundreds of men in a large hospital.[9] But his findings were based on a tiny study and were out of step with prevailing medical theories.[10]

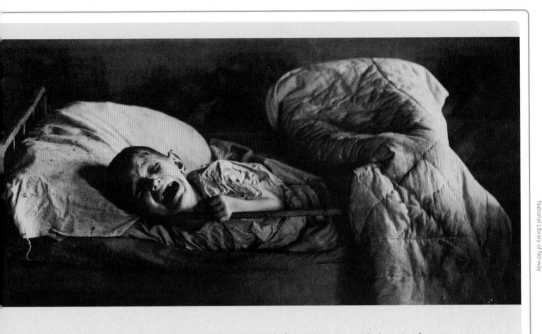

National Library of Norway

A malnourished child sometime before 1921, crying with the pain of scurvy.

Economics finally swayed the Royal British Navy. Thomas Trotter, surgeon on a slave ship, found a better way to preserve lemon juice and make it cheap enough for regular use. Meanwhile, Sir Gilbert Blane pointed out that disease—mostly scurvy—was killing 26 men for every one the enemy killed. Buying 50 oranges or lemons was as good as having an extra fighting man, Blane argued; it was money well spent.[11] In 1795, lemon juice finally became standard issue.[12] Later, to save money, the navy substituted lime juice, and Americans started calling British sailors "limeys."

Lind is remembered for saving men from scurvy by giving them citrus fruit, a good source of vitamin C, but vitamin C was not discovered for more than a century after his experiment. Probably Lind's greatest accomplishment was his experimental approach to a medical problem. By comparing six remedies in a fair trial, and attempting to hold other variables steady, he was moving toward evidence-based medicine.

Nutritional Deficiencies

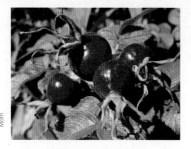

Rose hips have even more vitamin C than oranges and lemons.

Between 1928 and 1932, Albert Szent-Györgyi and Charles Glen King discovered why Lind's advice worked.[13] Scurvy is caused by a severe deficiency of vitamin C, a water-soluble nutrient needed for normal growth and development. Without it skin, tendons, ligaments, and blood vessels cannot remain healthy; wounds cannot heal; bones, cartilage, and teeth weaken.[14] The human body cannot make its own vitamin C and must rely on dietary sources, including fresh fruits, vegetables, and certain meats and fish. Scurvy is rare these days, and doctors may forget to look for it, but approximately 6 percent of Americans tested between 1999 and 2006 had vitamin C deficiencies.[15] Alcoholics, fussy eaters, and people who live on fast foods are at risk.

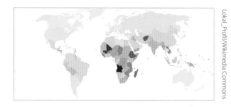

Deeper reds show where protein-energy deficiency causes more ill health, disabilities, and early deaths.

Scurvy is but one of many diseases that are caused by nutritional deficiencies. Iron deficiency causes anemia, protein deficiency causes kwashiorkor, iodine deficiency causes goiter, and vitamin D deficiency causes rickets. Beriberi is caused by thiamine (B1) deficiency, and pellagra is caused by niacin (B3) deficiency. Each of these diseases can be prevented by a well-balanced and nutritious diet. In parts of the world where there is insufficient food, more people suffer from nutritional deficiency diseases, and sometimes multiple dietary deficiencies.

White Rice Poisoning

In 1897 Dutch physician Christiaan Eijkman, head of a medical lab in what is now Jakarta, discovered the cause of beriberi. Neurologists had linked it to a rice-based diet and were entertaining two possibilities: either rice was somehow poisoning people, or a rice-based diet was too low in protein and fat.[16]

No bacteria or parasites were found to explain the problem, and the investigation was stymied. In July the lab's chickens came down with what looked like the same kind of nerve disease, a mysterious epidemic that suddenly cleared up in November. Why?

Starting in mid-June, the lab keeper had been saving money by feeding the chickens leftover cooked rice from the kitchen of the attached military hospital. But a new cook arrived in November and laid down the law: no military rice for civilian chickens. When the chickens' supply of polished rice was cut off

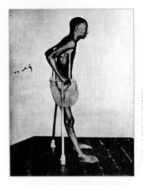

This man's strength has been sapped by beriberi, which causes muscular atrophy and paralysis.

National Institutes of Health

and they had to make do with brown, they recovered within a few days. Eijkman's research soon showed that a substance in the husk of the rice counteracted the illness. This substance—now known as thiamine, or vitamin B1—is present in brown rice but not in the more refined white rice. A white rice diet was poisonous, not because of a toxin it included, but because of a vital nutrient it excluded. Eijkman was awarded a Nobel Prize for his discovery.

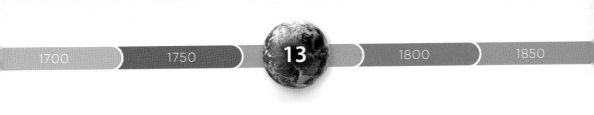
1776

A Folk Remedy for Congestive Heart Failure

It was July 1776. Across the ocean in Philadelphia, colonists were declaring independence from Britain; the American Revolution was beginning. Near Birmingham, England, William Withering was fighting to save a life. A woman in her forties had been attacked some weeks earlier by "a severe cold shivering fit" and then a fever. She had great pain in her left side, shortness of breath, and a desperate cough.[3] Withering's colleague Erasmus Darwin had tried everything; could Withering help?

The woman was turning blue. Her pulse was weak and jagged, her legs and stomach were hugely swollen, she couldn't pee, and every breath was a struggle. The treatments they'd learned in medical school weren't working—even ipecac no longer made her vomit, because her stomach was too empty. Clearly there was nothing to lose. So Withering suggested a folk remedy, and Darwin agreed. They cured her with an infusion made from a common flower: foxglove, or *Digitalis purpurea*. She lived for years.

Withering (1741 – 1799) was a respectable doctor. He had earned his M.D. at the University of Edinburgh, entered practice in 1767,[4] and moved his practice to Birmingham in 1775. He kept up with research in medicine and other sciences. Darwin had drawn him into the Lunar

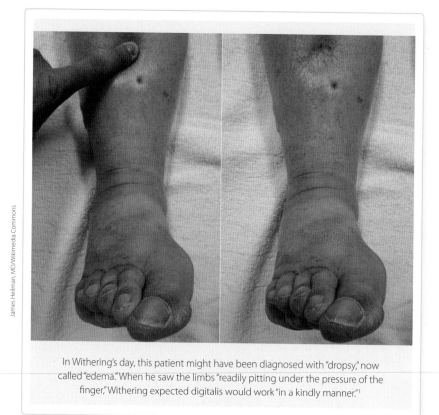

James Hellman, MD/Wikimedia Commons

In Withering's day, this patient might have been diagnosed with "dropsy," now called "edema." When he saw the limbs "readily pitting under the pressure of the finger," Withering expected digitalis would work "in a kindly manner."[1]

Society—an informal learned society that included chemist Joseph Priestley, inventor James Watt, and other innovators.[5]

It wasn't his scientific colleagues who first brought the foxglove to Withering's attention in 1775. Somebody asked his opinion of a family cure for dropsy, an old woman's secret recipe. Dropsy was a common name for fluid retention: it made ankles and fingers swell, abdomens balloon, eyes puff. The old woman's cure induced vomiting and purging (known treatments for dropsy) and urination (the real key to a cure, Withering believed).

The recipe involved twenty herbs. Withering knew herbs; his father was an apothecary, an early pharmacist.[6] He quickly realized "the active herb could be no other than the Foxglove,"[7] and he began investigating. He gathered reports on foxglove from published literature and the hearsay accounts of other physicians, and when other remedies failed, he tried it on his own patients.[8]

Over the next ten years, he learned to make a controlled dose by harvesting the leaves when they were most potent, drying them, and infusing them in liquid. Boiling destroyed their potency.[9] He learned to use the minimum effective dose, stopping when the patient vomited or urinated or the pulse slowed.[10] He learned to recognize which patients would respond.

Some 57 of his 158 carefully documented cases did not respond, either because they were too sick or because their illnesses were not related to the heart.[11] Swelling and edema can be caused by various underlying problems, from malnutrition to liver failure, but what foxglove really helps with is congestive heart failure. The active ingredient is digitalis, which works by strengthening and regulating heart rhythm.

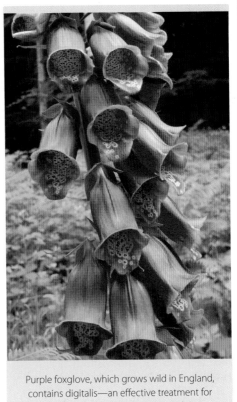

Purple foxglove, which grows wild in England, contains digitalis—an effective treatment for edema caused by congestive heart failure. The plant was used in traditional remedies, and its name may come from "folk's glove," evoking the fairies or "fair folk."

Not knowing this, Withering thought digitalis could be "used with advantage in every species of dropsy," with few exceptions.[12] But he noticed that "it has a power over the motion of the heart, to a degree yet unobserved in any other medicine," and he hoped that would prove beneficial in the future.[13] Withering's empirical study laid the groundwork for figuring out how

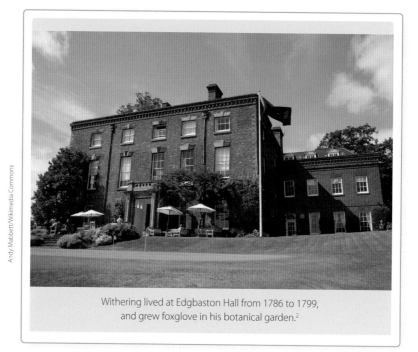

Withering lived at Edgbaston Hall from 1786 to 1799, and grew foxglove in his botanical garden.[2]

digitalis works. He published *An Account of the Foxglove and Some of Its Medicinal Uses* in 1785, the year he was elected to the Royal Society. For the sake of "Truth and Science," he reported "every case in which I have prescribed the Foxglove, proper or improper, successful or otherwise."[14] He believed it was important to document even mistakes. The facts would stand, while opinions would be corrected "with the detection of error, or the improvement of knowledge."[15] His

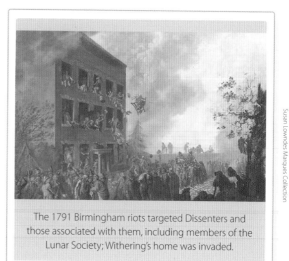

The 1791 Birmingham riots targeted Dissenters and those associated with them, including members of the Lunar Society; Withering's home was invaded.

contribution to medicine saved many lives, and digitalis-based heart medications are still in use today.

Ancient Pharmaceuticals

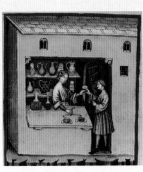

from *Tacuinum Sanitatis*

A fourteenth-century Italian pharmacist would have remedies on hand, and some of them would work. The process of discovering what worked and why was not yet very scientific.

What if you had an eye infection, and your doctor's prescription contained pig's eyeball, black eyeshadow, incense, dried crocuses, insect intestines, and powdered gazelle dung? Gross! But ancient Mesopotamian and Egyptian pharmacists used weird ingredients to drive the demons out.

Early Sumerian clay tablets describe more than 250 medicinal plants, 120 mineral substances, and 180 other drugs. The leaves, roots, bark, sap, and seeds of plants were all used and crushed into powders.[16] The powders were then soaked in wine or beer to make a mixture that could be added to massage oil, used in wound dressings, or diluted with milk or honey for a syrup. Ingredients often had symbolic significance for the disorder being treated; if you coughed up blood, your treatment might include red flowers. We cannot identify all the Sumerian plants named in the older tablets, but we can translate animal and mineral ingredients such as snakeskin, turtle shell, salt, and saltpeter,[17] and we recognize their uses.[18]

In Renaissance Europe, drugs were still connected with magic and ritual. Paracelsus (1493 – 1541) believed that medically useful plants looked like the body parts they could cure. Hepatica, or liverwort, has a lobed leaf that resembles a liver and was prescribed for liver ailments. Lungwort has spotted leaves that reminded people of diseased lungs, so naturally it was used to treat pulmonary infections.[19]

Ancient ingredients such as castor oil, gentian, opium, and colchicum are still used today because they work. Others have been found unsafe or ineffective and have been replaced by new prescriptions. But maybe the biggest change in pharmaceuticals is the discovery process. When William Withering saw the old woman's secret cure for dropsy, he did not look for the ingredients that would drive off demons or the ones that looked like swollen body parts. He looked for what would actually work, and he kept records to figure out what conditions would make it work best.

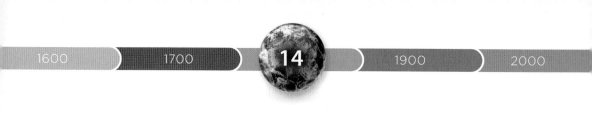
1799

Heroic Bloodletting, Leech Mania, and What Doesn't Work

George Washington (1732–1799) was a hero. In 1755, dashing back and forth across a French and Indian War battlefield, he had two horses shot from under him; four bullets pierced his coat.[1] Years later, he led America to victory in the Revolutionary War and served as the nation's first president. And in his last illness he asked for the leading heroic measure of his era: bloodletting.

On December 12, 1799, Washington worked outside in snow, hail, and freezing rain. Next day he did it again, in spite of a scratchy throat. By December 14, he could barely speak or breathe. He choked on a home remedy of molasses, vinegar, and butter. So between 7:30 a.m. and 4:00 p.m. he was bled four times, yielding a total of at least 80 ounces. He also received calomel and tartaric emetic[2] to make him defecate and vomit. Weak and dehydrated, he died at 10:20 p.m.

Was this a case of gross malpractice? No. His physicians were following the best practices of their time. The famous Dr. Benjamin Rush advocated "copious depletion," draining fluids from the body by bloodletting, purgatives, emetics, and cold. Galen's humoral theory still influenced physicians, who counted on these aggressive treatments to remove toxins from the body and restore a natural balance.[3]

Metropolitan Museum of Art

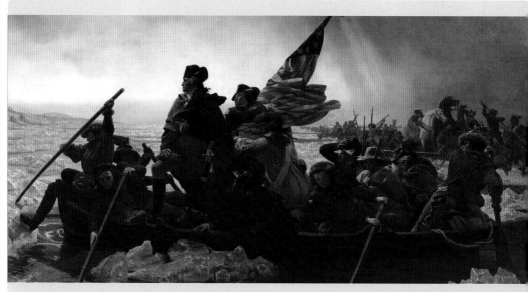

As commander-in-chief of the Continental Army, George Washington led American forces through harsh winter campaigns to gain independence from Britain. The nation's hero did not expect to be defeated by sleety weather and heroic medicine on his own property.

Yet Dr. Rush had been accused of "killing patients" by bleeding them. Rush had sued his accuser, and was awaiting a verdict on that very December 14.[4] Although he won his case, public opinion was shifting. Some of Washington's contemporaries thought bloodletting killed him.

It may have hastened his end. The average adult has about 160 ounces of blood; a modern doctor would hesitate to take 80 ounces in a day. Washington's attendants had limited options. His throat was swollen almost shut, and they may have hoped dehydration would reduce the swelling. Nobody had heard of antibiotics. The youngest doctor wanted to try a new procedure, tracheotomy (an incision in the windpipe), but he was overruled.[5]

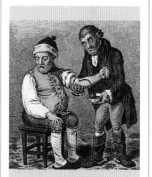

Wellcome Images

An unhappy patient is bled; his physician, still wearing spurs, must have been called in haste.

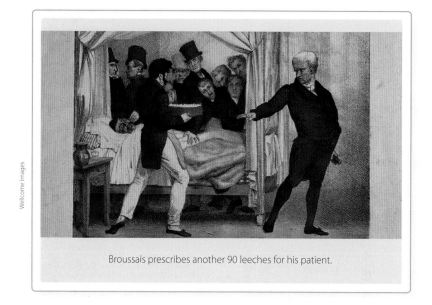

Wellcome Images

Broussais prescribes another 90 leeches for his patient.

Bloodletting remained standard practice for decades. Andrew Jackson (1767–1845), America's seventh president, even practiced it on himself when no doctor was handy; he used the cupping method,[6] mobilizing blood flow by creating suction on the skin.

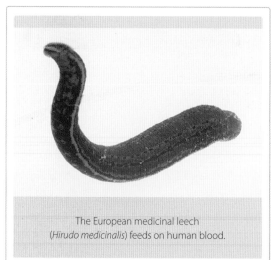

Karl Ragnar Gjertsen/Wikimedia Commons

The European medicinal leech (*Hirudo medicinalis*) feeds on human blood.

A third method of bloodletting achieved great popularity when French physician François-Joseph-Victor Broussais (1772–1838) started a "leech craze" in Europe.[7] Medicinal use of leeches, which suck blood from the body, wasn't new—they show up on wall paintings in Egyptian tombs[8]—but Broussais used them so enthusiastically that he was called the "vampire of medicine."[9] In 1833, France alone imported 42 million leeches.[10]

But another French doctor, Pierre-Charles-Alexandre Louis, put Broussais's theories to the test, and his results—published in the U.S. in 1836—shocked the medical world. Of 77 pneumonia patients at a Paris hospital, 41 had been bled in the first four days of their hospital stays; the other 36 had not been bled until the fifth day or after. Those who were bled sooner tended to recover sooner—if they recovered at all. But 44% of them died, compared to 25% of those who were bled later.[11] Louis looked for other factors that could have affected outcomes. Was one group older, on the average? Was one group sicker to start with? But he concluded that the time of bloodletting was the critical difference.

James Jackson, co-founder of the Massachusetts General Hospital, could hardly believe this, so he reviewed his own records. He found no evidence that bloodletting helped pneumonia patients.[12]

Louis and Jackson were not the first doctors who ever tried to base their practice on evidence. Case notes had been carefully recorded and

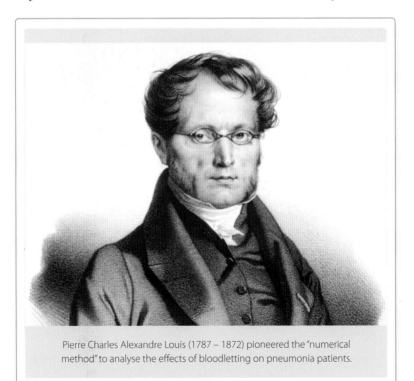

Pierre Charles Alexandre Louis (1787 – 1872) pioneered the "numerical method" to analyse the effects of bloodletting on pneumonia patients.

handed down for millennia. But single cases yield anecdotal evidence, and it's easy for doctors and patients to remember the cases that support a theory and forget the others. This is called "confirmation bias." By tabulating cases and analysing them numerically, Louis and Jackson were taking steps toward more powerful statistical studies that would yield better evidence.

Bloodletting in the Twenty-first Century

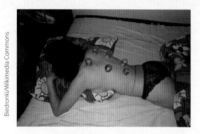
Biedronki/Wikimedia Commons

Cupping in progress.

Cupping, derived from folk traditions of sucking out poisons with the lips or through a horn, is probably the oldest bloodletting technique; it is referenced in ancient Greek, Chinese, and Hindu medical texts,[13] and is still used in China, Southeast Asia, and America. "Hijama," or wet cupping, is used in Morocco, Algeria, and Oman,[14] while many Ethiopians pierce the skin to let out "black blood."[15] Eskimos of Northwest Alaska use "poking" to let out bad blood, pus, and other substances.[16] And champion athletes at the 2016 Olympics used cupping to encourage blood flow to muscles that had been subjected to lactic acid build-up, although we have no scientific proof that this works.

We know today that leeches are helpful for certain delicate plastic surgeries, like reattachment of an amputated finger. We also know that bloodletting is a good treatment for iron overload and other disorders where the bone marrow makes too many red blood cells. In some parts of the world today, doctors in hospitals are still using leeches to bleed patients for treatment of heart problems, arthritis, gout, chronic headaches, and sinusitis.[17] New theories of health and disease do not support bloodletting, and controlled scientific trials have shown that it is ineffective for most purposes. If it helps Olympic athletes, could that be because of the placebo effect?

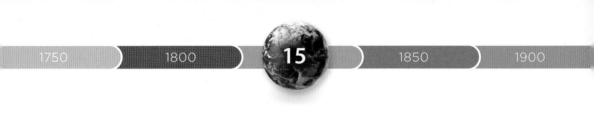

1816

René Laennec Invents the Stethoscope

One important medical advance was inspired by children at play. Dr. René Laennec (1781–1826) was running late, and his short-cut took him through a courtyard where teams of street children played happily in a pile of litter. As some knocked and scratched at one end of a wooden beam, others pressed their ears to the far end and listened. Laennec must have smiled; he remembered how much fun it was to hear sounds changed and amplified through wood. But he hurried on to meet his patient,[1] a young woman with heart trouble.

It was 1816, and European ideas about medicine were changing. The old humoral medicine was patient-specific. Patients differed in their dominant humors—sanguine or melancholy, bilious or phlegmatic—and so, even if their symptoms were identical, humoral theory might lead their doctors to treat them differently. Now, more detailed knowledge of the body suggested more disease-specific approaches. The Italian anatomist Giovanni Morgagni (1681 – 1771) asked, "Where is the disease?" And after doing hundreds of autopsies, the French doctor Xavier Bichat (1771–1801) could point to the exact spot; various illnesses left their own distinctive lesions or marks in victims' hearts, lungs, and other organs.[2]

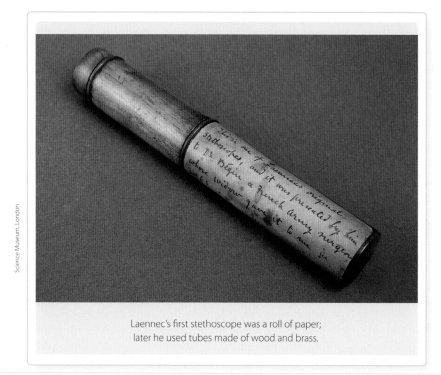

Laennec's first stethoscope was a roll of paper;
later he used tubes made of wood and brass.

The patients had to be dead before Bichat could autopsy them, though. Pinpointing the disease in a living patient was harder. Unable to see inside the body, doctors relied on other senses, especially touch and hearing: they felt the pulse, and they listened to the patient's lungs in action. Listening was called "auscultation," and physicians went beyond ordinary listening to decipher the lung sounds. Laennec was good at it. Planting his ear between a patient's shoulder blade and spine, he might hear something like a voice from the roots of the lung: "bronchophony," he called it, and it usually meant serious pneumonia. Or he might hear a "sonorous rhonchus," like a loud snore; this could mean that passageways to the lungs were enlarged.[3] Laennec might also tap a patient's chest and listen for fullness; he knew the art of percussion,[4] which Leopold Auenbrugger, an earlier physician, had developed to diagnose diseases of the heart and lungs.[5]

But it was hard even for an experienced doctor to figure out what the lungs were saying, and when the patient was fat it was even harder. Listening to a woman's heart could also be embarrassing; a modest nineteenth-century woman didn't like having a doctor's ear jammed between her breasts.

Laennec's patient that day was a fat young woman, and he didn't want to lean on her bosom. The children's game and his knowledge of acoustics gave him an idea. He rolled paper into a tube, placed one end on the woman's chest, and listened at the other end. To his pleasure, he could hear the heart's action better than he ever had with his ear directly on a patient's body.[6] The stethoscope was born. Soon Laennec was making his cylinders of wood instead of scrap paper, and in 1823 he published a book on his methods.

Laennec carefully linked what he heard in patients' bodies to the hidden lesions that would become visible only in autopsies. This experience

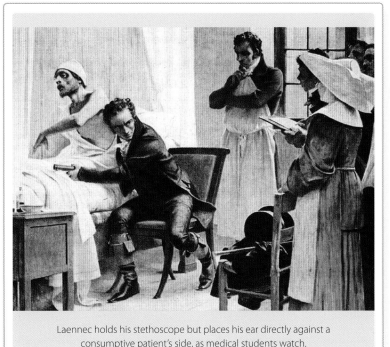

Théobald Chartran painting

Laennec holds his stethoscope but places his ear directly against a consumptive patient's side, as medical students watch.

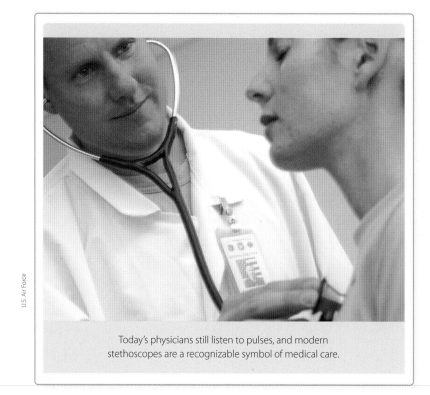

Today's physicians still listen to pulses, and modern stethoscopes are a recognizable symbol of medical care.

helped him locate problems when patients complained of illness, but it also revealed problems the patients hadn't yet noticed. So Laennec became the first to diagnose latent illnesses—conditions that were already doing damage before they caused any symptoms.[7]

Since disease could be present without causing symptoms, it couldn't be defined by symptoms. Based on Laennec's work, other doctors came to think of diseases as the result of organic lesions.[8] So Laennec's improvised tube of

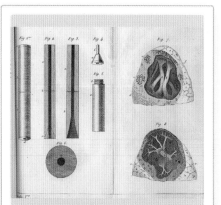

Drawings from Laennec's 1819 book show a simple stethoscope design (left) and cross-sections of the lungs (right). Physicians had begun to link specific diseases to specific evidence of damage seen in autopsies; the stethoscope made it easier to hear the damage happening.

paper, inspired by children at play, helped move Western medicine away from the old humoral theory of disease to a new focus on the specific causes of individual illnesses. The stethoscope was a game changer.

Taking a Pulse

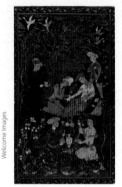

A physician takes a woman's pulse in this illuminated manuscript of Avicenna's *Canon.*

Ancient Egyptians[9] and Chinese alike would feel their patients' wrists and check whether the pulse was strong or weak, regular or erratic, deep or shallow, quick or slow,[10] "smooth as a flowing stream" or "light as flicking the skin with a plume."[11] The Roman Galen was famous for using the pulse in his diagnoses;[12] he could identify 27 characteristics in a single heartbeat.[13] The medieval Arabic physician Ibn Sīnā (Avicenna) focused on irregular rhythms.[14]

Nineteenth-century physicians knew far more about the circulatory system than their ancient and medieval forerunners, but observing its action in living patients was still a problem. Then in 1831 Jules Hérrison invented the sphygmometer, which helped doctors measure the force, regularity, and rhythm of a pulse more accurately. In 1860, Etienne Marey improved on it and added a sphygmograph with graphic recording capabilities.[15] They paved the way for the sphygmomanometer, or blood pressure cuff, which we still use today.

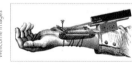

Marey's sphygmograph in use.

Hérrison's sphygmometer helped doctors measure the force, regularity, and rhythm of a pulse.

71

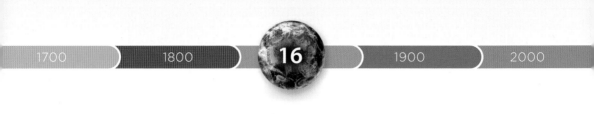

1828

Cutting for Stone

Stephen Pollard was still strong at 53, but he went to London so the nephew of a famous surgeon could take out his bladder stone.[1] Having a lithotomy, or stone removal, could kill a patient or leave him sterile. But Pollard already had six children,[2] and modern innovations had cut fatalities for the procedure from about 30 percent to less than 10 percent. Patients typically healed in less than 3 months.[3] Sadly, Pollard died; he became the subject of a libel suit when his surgeon was publicly accused of malpractice.[4]

Pollard certainly was not the first to suffer from a stone—one was found in the pelvis of an Egyptian mummy buried in 4800 BC.[5] Small mineral deposits can form in a kidney, break loose, and scrape against the insides of the urinary tract as they make their way out. Some pass without complication; others result in such pain that patients cannot sit still. Bloody urine is a bad sign.[6]

The ancients avoided operating. In Mesopotamia the doctors prescribed swallowing black saltpeter, ostrich egg shells, turpentine, and the sexual part of a she-ass to dissolve the stone.[7] In India, Sushruta massaged the perineum—the area around the anus and urethra—and treated the bladder with medicated milk, clarified butter, and alkalis. To prevent recurrence, he called for a vegetarian diet.[8] Sushruta's approach could work: alkalis would dissolve the stone, a buttery lubricant would help it slide out, and the diet would reduce stone formation. He recommended surgery only as a last resort.

In Greece, the Hippocratic Oath forbade lithotomy: "I will not cut for stone, even for patients in whom the disease is manifest; I will leave this operation to be performed by practitioners, specialists in this art."[9] What did this mean? Should physicians leave this operation to surgeons because surgeons are better qualified, or because only practitioners as disreputable as surgeons would stoop to lithotomy? Itinerant surgeons would reportedly wander into a town, taking fees for as many operations as they could do before the angry relatives of dead patients drove them out.

But maybe Hippocrates tried lithotomy himself. He wrote about the heartbreak of reaching into a bladder but not being "able to locate the stone."[10] And that's what happened to Pollard's surgeon, Bransby Cooper. Pollard lay strapped down before an audience of medical students as Cooper made an incision, fumbled with the forceps, and grabbed a

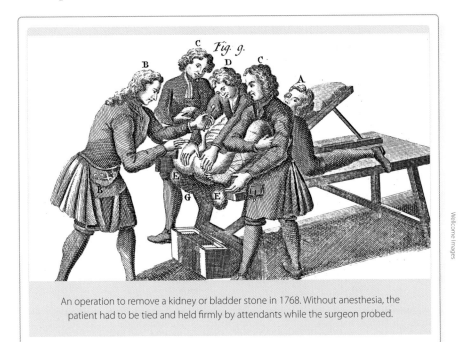

An operation to remove a kidney or bladder stone in 1768. Without anesthesia, the patient had to be tied and held firmly by attendants while the surgeon probed.

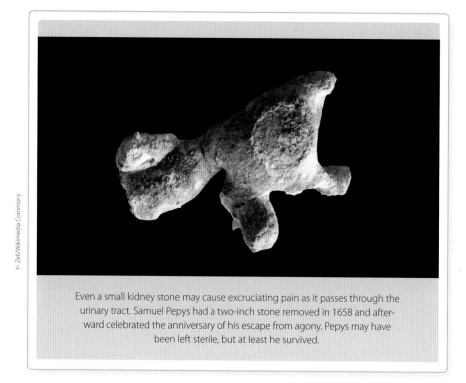

H. Zell/Wikimedia Commons

Even a small kidney stone may cause excruciating pain as it passes through the urinary tract. Samuel Pepys had a two-inch stone removed in 1658 and afterward celebrated the anniversary of his escape from agony. Pepys may have been left sterile, but at least he survived.

knife to enlarge the opening. He tried one tool after another. "It's a very deep perineum," he exclaimed. "I can't reach the bladder with my finger. . . . O dear! O dear!"[11] Pollard begged him to stop. A typical lithotomy took less than five minutes, but Cooper struggled for nearly an hour before triumphantly brandishing the stone over his head. Pollard "was put to bed much exhausted, but rallied a few hours afterwards, and leeches were applied"; he died the next day.[12]

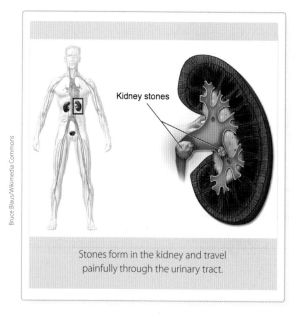

Bruce Blaus/Wikimedia Commons

Kidney stones

Stones form in the kidney and travel painfully through the urinary tract.

The operation for stone had been refined by anatomists and surgeons over thousands of years. Anatomist and surgeon William Cheselden (1688–1752) had introduced many refinements, including a hollow grooved staff to guide the grasping forceps. Cheselden could do a lithotomy in less than a minute, with good odds of survival, but his inventions were not foolproof.

The Lancet: Outing an Incompetent Surgeon

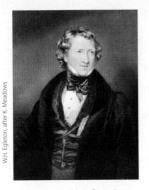

W.H. Egleton, after K. Meadows

Thomas Wakley, founding editor of *The Lancet*, ridiculed Bransby Cooper's panicky conduct of Pollard's lithotomy.

Poor Bransby Cooper. It was bad enough for a surgeon to flub an operation, but worse to do it while a reforming gadfly named Thomas Wakley (1795–1862) was watching. Wakley had trained as a surgeon himself, but found his real calling when he befriended a group of radical journalists and politicians. In 1823 he started *The Lancet*, a weekly newspaper dedicated to attacking all the weaknesses of the medical establishment and advocating for evidence-based medicine.[13] Long before the internet, Wakley reviewed doctor performance. Each issue of *The Lancet* carried recaps of notable operations, hospital by hospital. His coverage of the Pollard case was so sensational that Cooper sued for £2,000 in damages for libel. The facts were clear. The operation really did last a tortured 55 minutes, the patient really did die, his perineum really was not very deep, and whether or not Cooper owed his position to nepotism, he really was the nephew of King George's scalp surgeon. The jury found for Cooper, but awarded only £100 in damages. Wakley paid £400 in legal fees, donated what was left of his defense fund to Pollard's widow and children, and kept on overseeing the medical profession.

Extracorporeal Shock-Wave Lithotripsy: A Minimally Invasive Solution?

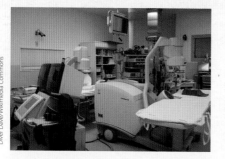

Diver Dave/Wikimedia Commons

The lithotriptor machine in this hospital operating room can be rolled into place when needed; there is a gurney for the patient to lie flat as extracorporeal electro-shock waves are aimed at a kidney stone.

By the late twentieth century, more people than ever had kidney stones, and operations, although we no longer have to live through them without anesthesia, are still worth avoiding. One alternative is extracorporeal shock-wave lithotripsy (ESWL), introduced in the 1980s. From an energy source outside the body, pulses are sent into a fluid chamber and then through the patient's soft tissues to crumble the stone.[14] This might seem like the answer to everything. The word lithotripsy means "stone pulverizing" in Greek, and if stones can be broken up so they pass easily through the urinary tract, no operation is needed.

Over time questions have arisen, however. For instance, ESWL may leave stone fragments in the urinary tract. Most flow through without any complications, but about one in five patients develops new stones at the site of residual fragments, so close follow-up is important.[15] And if ESWL fails, it may be more difficult to clear up the problems using percutaneous nephrolithotomy (PCNL, a procedure for removing kidney stones through a small skin puncture) than if PCNL had been the original therapy.[16] In some cases, at least, cutting for stone may be safer and more effective than the alternative.

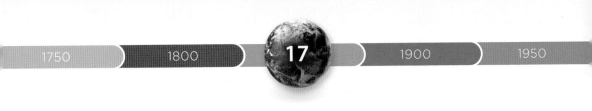

1846

Laughing Gas

Surgery hurts. Without effective pain control, patients avoided even minor operations. When they finally sought help, strong men pinned them down on the operating table. Who could help jumping and wincing at the sight of the surgeon's knives? Medical students heard tales of patients who struggled free, grabbed the knives, and attacked their surgeons before trailing blood out of the operating theater.[1]

Naturally, doctors have always tried to relieve pain. The ancient Egyptians used pressure on arteries to induce temporary numbness, especially in limbs.[2] The Greeks and Romans steeped mandrake, belladonna, and similar drugs in wine. In the Middle Ages a *spongia somnifera* (sleep-bearing sponge) soaked with opium and heart-slowing drugs was held to the patient's nostrils.[3] This worked some of the time, and killed the patient some of the time. Paracelsus (1493 – 1542) used tinctures of opium in alcohol, which became standard practice for the next 300 years.[4]

But surgeons still had to operate fast. British surgeon Robert Liston, known as the fastest knife in the West End, could amputate a leg in under three minutes, but speed cost accuracy. He once cut off an assistant's fingers along with the patient's leg, in an operation so bloody that a bystander died of fright; the patient and assistant died later, of gangrene.[5]

The nineteenth century brought new possibilities. Nitrous oxide, first synthesized by Joseph Priestley in 1772, was introduced to the British public in 1799 by Sir Humphry Davy. What a gas! Although Davy thought it might relieve the pain of surgery, nitrous oxide caught on first as a recreational drug. Itinerant chemists gave demonstrations, inviting volunteers on stage to inhale the gas and act silly in public. Nitrous oxide parties became popular, as did "ether frolics."[6]

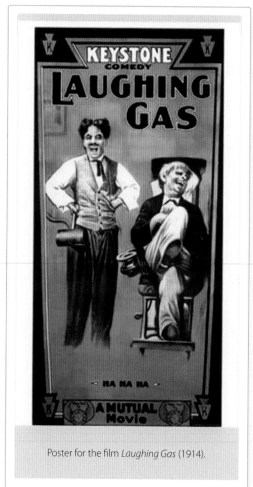

Poster for the film *Laughing Gas* (1914).

©1914 Keystone Studios

At a nitrous oxide demonstration in Connecticut, dentist Horace Wells saw one volunteer gash his shin on the furniture without noticing. The next day, Wells arranged to inhale "laughing gas" himself before having a tooth extracted. The experiment worked, and painless dentistry became a feature of his practice.[7] In 1845 he gave a demonstration at the Massachusetts General Hospital. The patient groaned during the procedure, and the audience hooted at Wells: "humbug!"[8]

But the discovery of anesthesia was now inevitable. In 1846, dentist William T. G. Morton and chemist Charles Jackson published their successful use of ether during surgery, and in 1847, James Young Simpson used chloroform as an anesthetic in childbirth.[9] There was controversy.

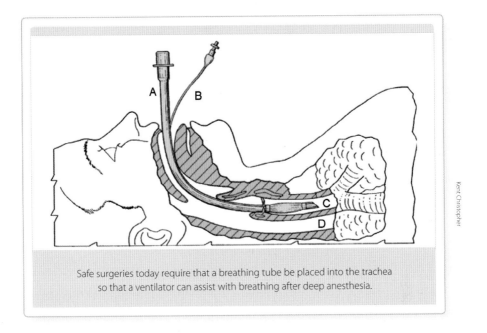

Safe surgeries today require that a breathing tube be placed into the trachea so that a ventilator can assist with breathing after deep anesthesia.

Kent Christopher

With her eighth child, Queen Victoria herself took chloroform, but by 1863 at least 123 deaths were associated with it.[10]

One reason for anesthesia-related fatalities was probably poor sanitation, but another could have been dosage. In Philadelphia, Dr.

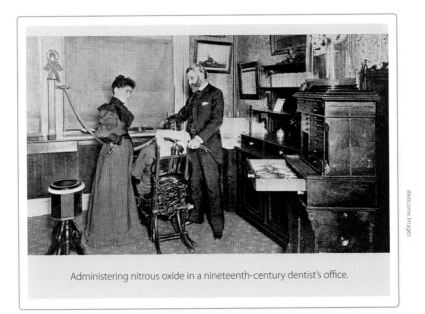

Administering nitrous oxide in a nineteenth-century dentist's office.

Wellcome Images

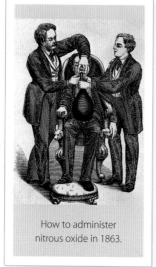

How to administer nitrous oxide in 1863.

Thomas Mütter struggled to control the concentration of ether; the dose could even be affected by temperature. In 1854 his student Edward Robinson Squibb perfected an apparatus to deliver "ether of uniform strength by using steam," and followed it up with an "ether mask" to save doctors from accidental inhalation.[11]

Anesthetics that could be inhaled or injected would change surgery. With less pressure to rush, surgeons could do more than amputate limbs and remove external growths. Today, anesthesiologists are important members of surgical teams, and complex operations may last for hours. Brain surgeries, organ transplants, and other lifesaving procedures became possible only after the development of reliable anesthetics.

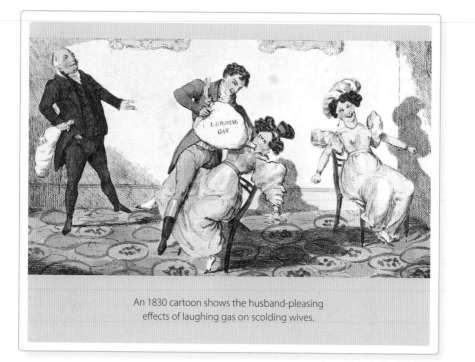

An 1830 cartoon shows the husband-pleasing effects of laughing gas on scolding wives.

Magic Mushrooms

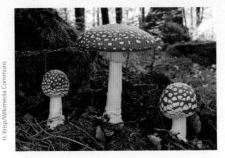

Beautiful fly agaric are poisonous, though rarely fatal, and were used by shamans in Siberian and other indigenous cultures.

Nitrous oxide was not the first substance people have enjoyed for its effects on the nervous system. People around the world have discovered substances—usually plants—that change their moods and perceptions of reality. Mushrooms, for instance, are famous not only for healing but for helping people reach altered states of consciousness, whether calm (traditional Chinese medicine values the reishi mushroom, or *Ganoderma lucidum*, for its calming effects[12]) or excited.

In many cultures sacred mushrooms have been used as entheogens—which means, in English, substances that "generate the divine within." As early as 4500 BC, Egyptians depicted mushrooms and other fungi on walls and in hieroglyphic texts, and shaped temple pillars like huge mushrooms.[13] In sixteenth-century Mexico, Spanish colonists tried to eradicate use of entheogenic mushrooms in the religious and healing rituals of the Nahuatl culture, but the ceremonial and shamanistic use of mushrooms continues in remote Mexican highlands.[14] In the 1950s Timothy Leary and Richard Alpert experimented with mushrooms containing psilocybin, which induced altered states of consciousness. The two lost their faculty positions at Harvard but became counterculture heroes as a result. Psilocybin was made illegal.

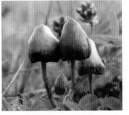

The psilocybin mushroom is used as an entheogen or recreational drug, bringing euphoria, altered perceptions, and spiritual experiences.

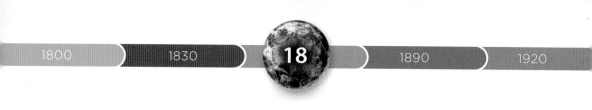
1847

Wash your Hands

Ignatz Semmelweis was appalled. The Vienna hospital where he worked was world famous for its obstetrics department,[1] but women would rather give birth outside on the street. It was safer.[2] Inside, more of them died of childbed fever, especially if they were put in First Clinic. The two maternity wards or clinics accepted patients on alternate days, but whenever their babies arrived, mothers begged to be put in Second Clinic. The death rate there was lower.[3]

Childbed (or puerperal) fever was a bacterial infection common in nineteenth-century hospitals and even after doctor-assisted home births. It tore through the reproductive systems and blood streams of women exhausted by childbirth. In America, Oliver Wendell Holmes Sr. announced in 1843 that the disease was carried on the unwashed hands and clothes of doctors, but he was largely ignored.[4]

In 1847, Semmelweis came to the same conclusion. As assistant to Professor Johann Klein, he was put in charge of First Clinic and found the patients were right about it. His ward's 1841–1846 death rate was 9.92 percent, compared to 3.88 percent in Second Clinic.[5] Was it because of miasma? No. The two clinics were under the same roof and shared an anteroom; all patients breathed the same air. Overcrowding?

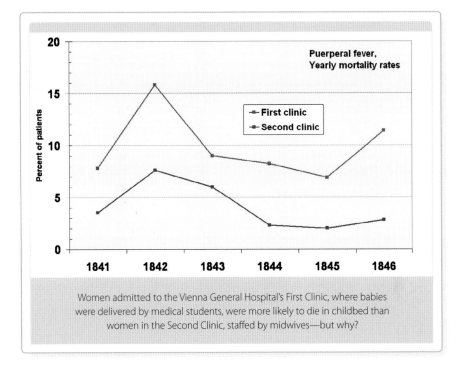

Women admitted to the Vienna General Hospital's First Clinic, where babies were delivered by medical students, were more likely to die in childbed than women in the Second Clinic, staffed by midwives—but why?

No. Second Clinic was more crowded. Semmelweis ruled out one hypothesis after another.[6]

Reluctantly, he concluded that sickness was being carried to First Clinic from the morgue. Up until 1840, the two clinics were alike in both staffing and death rates. After 1840, medical students trained in First Clinic and midwives in Second. Medical students did autopsies; midwives did not.

Then one of Semmelweis's friends died after cutting himself with a scalpel during an autopsy. He had all the symptoms of puerperal fever. Semmelweis reasoned that some particle from the cadaver had transmitted the disease to his friend—and particles from cadavers, on the hands of professors, assistants, and students, could be transmitting it to patients.[7] In May he began requiring everyone to wash their hands, not just with soap and water but with chlorinated lime. The mortality rate in the First Clinic dropped from 7.82% for the first half of 1847 to 3.04% for the second half.

Two incidents persuaded him that the fever could be spread by discharges from living tissue as well as corpses. In October, a woman with a discharging uterine cancer lay in the bed where rounds always began; of twelve women delivering on the ward just then, eleven died. Semmelweis made everyone wash with chlorine after examining patients with infected discharges. But in November, a woman with an oozing knee somehow infected the whole ward. Semmelweis did not believe her infection was spread on attendants' hands; he thought it must have been airborne, and childbirth made her neighbors tragically vulnerable to it. From then on, he isolated patients with discharging wounds.[8]

Although Semmelweis cut hospital mortality rates, he failed to influence medical opinion. He was a bad communicator, tactless, undiplomatic, and reluctant to publish or lecture.[9] He wrote angry letters to prominent obstetricians, denouncing them as murderers because they would not wash their hands. They were annoyed.

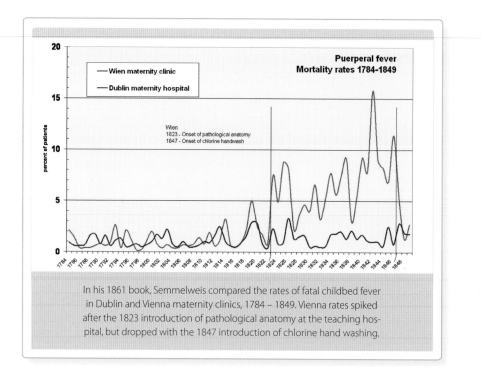

In his 1861 book, Semmelweis compared the rates of fatal childbed fever in Dublin and Vienna maternity clinics, 1784 – 1849. Vienna rates spiked after the 1823 introduction of pathological anatomy at the teaching hospital, but dropped with the 1847 introduction of chlorine hand washing.

Besides, they believed in established theories: infection was caused by contagion and miasma. Semmelweis argued that childbed fever was not contagious. Smallpox was contagious; exposure to it caused "only smallpox and no other disease." Childbed fever could "be caused in healthy patients through other diseases." And it was not miasmatic; it was transmitted by "decaying animal-organic matter," airborne or not.[10]

History supported Semmelweis. In 1867 James Y. Simpson reviewed more than 1,800,000 deliveries and found that mothers died in 3.4 percent of hospital births but only 0.47 percent of home births. His report was bitterly attacked, but Lister's antisepsis and Pasteur's germ theory soon gave doctors new ways to explain and control infections. Things improved.

Florence Nightingale Battles the Army

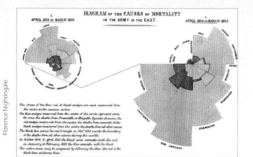

Florence Nightingale

Statistics became an increasingly important tool of scientific discovery in the nineteenth century—and also a tool of persuasion. Florence Nightingale devised this polar area graph to show that many more British soldiers died of preventable diseases (blue) than of wounds (red) or any other cause (black).

Florence Nightingale (1820–1910) was a statistics geek. At 22, she read an *Inquiry into the Sanitary Conditions of the Labouring Population of Great Britain*, by reformer Edwin Chadwick, who used statistics to show that unsanitary conditions lowered life expectancy.[11] So 11 years later, British fatalities in the Crimean War made Nightingale think of sanitation. Four of every five British deaths were caused by infectious disease. The military hospitals at Scutari were filthy and overcrowded; the *London Times* accused the army medical corps of negligence.[12]

(Continued on next page)

(Continued from previous page)

The public was outraged. Nightingale was outraged, and she did something about it. She stormed off to Scutari with 38 nurses in 1854 and set about reforming the hospitals, with considerable opposition from the doctors in charge. She directed nurses to wash and bathe wounded soldiers, clean their wounds, give them clean clothes, and feed them healthy diets. She established a system for removal of human waste and raw sewage from the wards, fixed the plumbing systems and the latrines, got windows that opened, and boiled hospital linens to destroy the lice.[13]

She recorded everything she did and saw. After the war, she remained an active political force, working behind the scenes for reforms in hospitals, nursing, and nursing education. She used statistics to rally support. Today's hospital sanitation practices were advocated by Florence Nightingale twenty years before the discovery of microbes. She never did believe in germs.

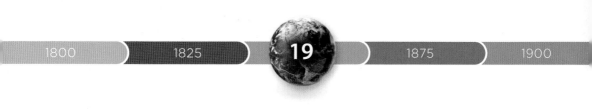
1848

Monster Soup

The stink of London worried Edwin Chadwick (1800–1890). "All smell is disease," he told Parliament in 1846; when you breathed the horrid miasma, you were breathing death. And if foul-smelling air was killing Londoners, the way to save them was obvious. Public health had to begin with getting rid of the stench.[1]

Public health was Chadwick's top priority in life. He was a lawyer, not a doctor, and he was more of a social reformer than a lawyer. He spent time researching the conditions of the poor, then drafting and campaigning for laws to improve those conditions. In 1832 he joined a royal commission charged with updating the ancient Poor Law. Chadwick studied workers' living conditions and soon became convinced that physical environment determined health. Cramming into filthy slums made people sick, and society had to support their hospital care, burials, widows, and orphans. The commission's doctors reported that sanitation to prevent disease would cost less. In 1848, largely because of Chadwick, Parliament authorized Britain's first Public Health Act.[2]

It was the Year of Revolutions, and the 1848 Public Health Act was revolutionary. Government agencies could now be responsible for anything from water and food supplies to garbage removal. Chadwick was appointed a commissioner of the General Board of Health (until

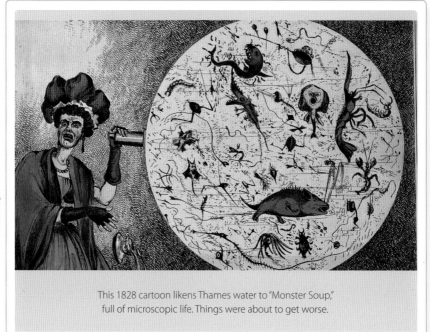

This 1828 cartoon likens Thames water to "Monster Soup," full of microscopic life. Things were about to get worse.

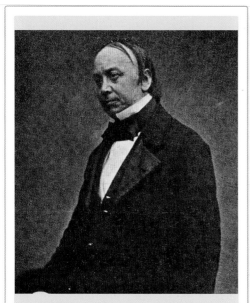

Sir Edwin Chadwick (1800–1890) persuaded British lawmakers to pass the groundbreaking Public Health Act of 1848.

1854) and the Metropolitan Commission of Sewers (until 1849),[3] and he was determined to use his new authority for the public good. Unfortunately, some of his efforts backfired.

He wasn't completely wrong to associate smell with disease. Nineteenth-century cities were filthy, and metropolitan London had become the world's largest city. With ever more people, horses, and other animals came ever more turds in the streets. London's waste management relied on an army of scavengers, from pure-finders (who collected dog poop) to mudlarks (who combed the river's edge for dropped coins and trinkets). The sewers historically handled storm run-off, while household waste ran into cesspools or piled up in cellars and back yards.[4] This could not be healthy.

So Chadwick and his allies abolished 30,000 cesspools, diverting house and street refuse into the Thames. Chadwick was a firm believer in the miasma theory. He believed disease was picked up from bad air— air that smelled of rotting waste and rubbish. If nothing else, noxious smells might affect the body by "depressing the system and rendering

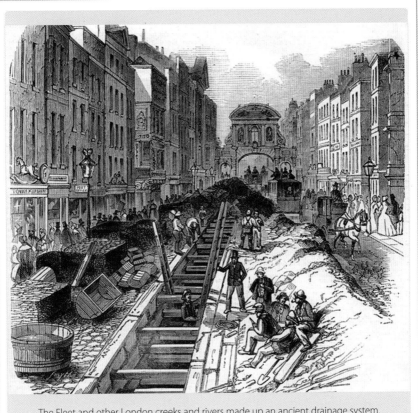

Illustrated London News, October 4, 1845

The Fleet and other London creeks and rivers made up an ancient drainage system. By the 1840s, the system was receiving raw sewage as well as storm run-off. When the sewers were deepened, some worried: would the corpses of 1665 plague victims be disturbed, releasing new contagion into the air?

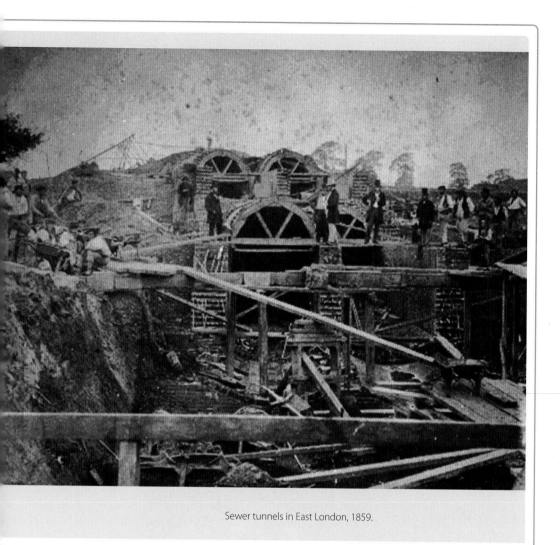

Sewer tunnels in East London, 1859.

it susceptible to the action of other causes."[5] In light of this theory, cleaning up the cesspools made sense. But as neighborhoods began to smell better, the river smelled worse. Untreated waste from households, slaughterhouses, chemical works, and other industries flowed into the city's drinking water.[6] Neighborhoods downstream from the sewer outlets suffered from worse than bad air; alcohol was a safer drink than Thames water.[7]

The miasma theory was wrong, but it was consistent with a strong public health infrastructure that tended to reduce mortality rates over time. Unfortunately, it led Chadwick to pay more attention to clean air than clean water, thus contributing to epidemics of cholera—a water-borne disease—in 1849 and 1854. Parliament did not renew the Public Health Act, and Chadwick was forced out of office in 1854. But largely as a result of his work, we now take it for granted that government has a role in providing paved streets, clean water, garbage removal, and sewage disposal.

The Miasma Theory and Correlation versus Causation?

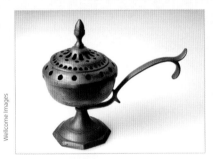

This nineteenth-century fumigator was made to counteract the foul smells of miasma with healthier-smelling herbs.

Wellcome Images

The ancient miasma theory was believed until the 1880s, when the germ theory provided a better explanation for disease. The idea of miasma made intuitive sense, because people who lived in dirty areas with poor sanitation really did seem to be at higher risk for disease. Bad smells were correlated with sickness.

But correlation is not causation. If X and Y are strongly correlated, it's possible that X causes Y, but there are other possibilities, too. Could Y cause X? Could X and Y both be caused by Z? Could the correlation be a coincidence?

When people believed that miasma (X) caused disease (Y), they avoided swamps at night. This was not a bad idea, since mosquitoes (Z) are likely to bite in swamps at night, infecting people with malaria (which means "bad air") and other dangerous germs.

Public Health in the Bronze Age

Indoor plumbing and flush toilets weren't standard operating equipment for working people in Chadwick's London. But between 2600 and 1900 BC, at the peak of the Harappan civilization, water management and urban planning flourished in the Indus river valley. Archaeologists have found cities and towns built on great artificial

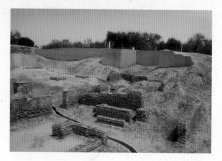

This 2014 view of an archaeological dig at Harappa, Pakistan, shows an ancient drain.

terraces there,[8] with essential goods and services—including water storage units and public bathing facilities—housed above flood level. In residential neighborhoods below, one- or two-story brick buildings lined the streets.

Water was supplied from large reservoirs[9] or vertical networks of private and public wells,[10] and houses had bathrooms and latrines. Wastewater from rooftops, kitchens, and bathrooms was channeled into covered street drains.[11] Public lavatories were also well drained, and gutters were carefully designed and maintained to prevent blockage.[12] Usually, wastewater and garbage were emptied between the inner and outer walls of the city. In some cities the mains directed wastewater outside the walls, where it could be used to fertilize surrounding agricultural fields.

The Harappans may have been the best prehistoric water managers, but they were not the only ones. Minoans, Assyrians, and Babylonians also had sophisticated sewerage and drainage systems, terra-cotta pipes, clean running water, fountains, bathtubs, and flushing toilets between 3000 and 2000 BC.[13] Yet Sir John Harington did not invent Britain's first flush toilet until 1596.

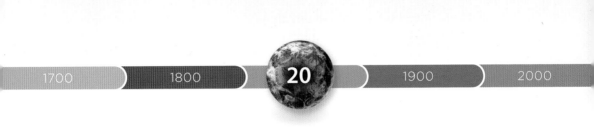

1854

Cholera and Epidemiology

It was 1854, and cholera—which had killed more than 14,000 Londoners in 1849[1]—was loose again.[2] This year's deaths were concentrated in Soho, and the National Board of Health sent a committee to investigate. They had a long list of things to check, starting with "nuisances"—a polite term for piles of excrement. Investigators were supposed to sniff grates, examine basements, and observe crowding and ventilation.[3] Meant to reveal risk factors for cholera, the list reveals Board of Health preconceptions: they expected confirmation of the miasma theory.

To understand epidemics, nineteenth-century physicians used new tools like statistics, maps, and other graphics. Yet they interpreted data in the light of old theories. Dr. Lewis Beck mapped the 1832 epidemic's progress along North American rivers and canals, and rejected the obvious conclusion that cholera was a waterborne contagion. It affected mainly the poor, he concluded, because the poor were most likely to be morally corrupt and therefore susceptible to miasma. (The gluttons in one poorhouse had binged on cucumbers and other vegetables.)[4]

In London, official mortality statistics were kept by William Farr, a colleague of Edwin Chadwick (Chapter 19) and an early member of London's Statistical Society. His data showed that some neighborhoods

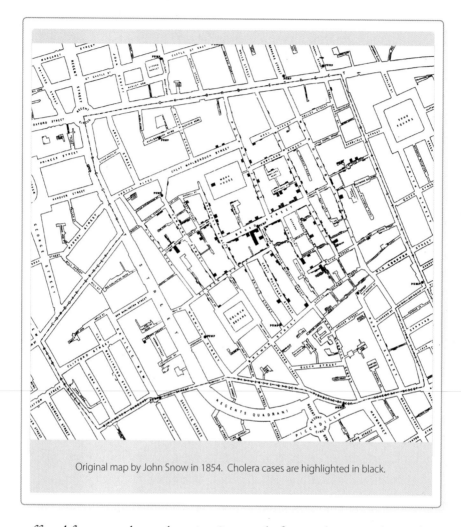

Original map by John Snow in 1854. Cholera cases are highlighted in black.

suffered far more than others in 1849, and after analyzing eight explanatory variables, he concluded that elevation was the important one. Living higher above the miasma was safer.[5] But Farr's analysis was contested by physician John Snow.

Snow was an anesthetist—he had been asked to administer chloroform to Queen Victoria during childbirth—and his understanding of gases made him doubt the miasma theory. He suspected cholera was waterborne. By August 1849, more people had died in London's southern districts (which had a death rate of 7.96 per 1,000 inhabitants) than in the other districts combined (with a death rate of 2.4 per

1,000). Snow's explanation: water for the southern districts came from the lower reaches of the Thames, downstream from the sewer outlets.[6] Farr disagreed, but kept providing Snow with data.

The 1854 outbreak struck near Snow's office. He mapped the streets, carefully marking the local pumps. Without indoor plumbing, people used those pumps for everything from drinking water to laundry, and they had their favorites. The Broad Street pump had a reputation for good water.[7]

Snow and Henry Whitehead, a local clergyman, interviewed residents at 83 addresses where people had died of cholera. Seventy-three of the dead lived closer to the Broad Street pump than any other, and of those, 61 were known to favor the Broad Street water.[8] An isolated death in Hampstead also had links to Broad Street; the victim liked the pump water so much that her family brought it to her after she moved away.[9] But there were surprisingly few deaths at a crowded workhouse

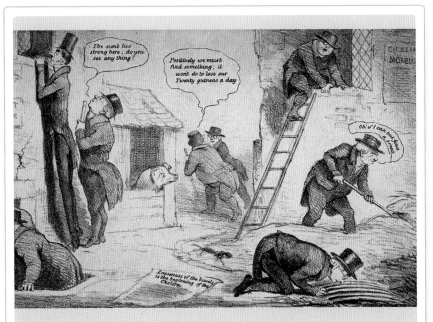

A committee from the Board of Health, sent to inspect the cholera-stricken Soho neighborhood, was instructed to look for ventilation issues, "nuisances," and smells.

and a brewery near the pump: the workhouse used its own well, and employees at the brewery preferred their daily rations of malt liquor.[10]

Afterward, people said Snow stopped the epidemic single-handed by stealing the handle of the Broad Street pump.[11] Not true. He did persuade local officials to disable the pump, but deaths were already declining then. The outbreak had begun when an infected baby's diapers leaked into the pump, and was almost over before anyone acted on Snow's findings.[12]

Snow's legacy is epidemiology—his systematic method of mapping and tracking cases. Today this method is used to track epidemics all around the world.[13] His waterborne theory of cholera, though unpopular in his own time, became more plausible in the 1880s in light of work by Louis Pasteur and Robert Koch.

Cholera Discoveries Lost and Found

John Snow was right: cholera is waterborne. He made his discovery using an epidemiologist's maps, not an experimenter's lab equipment, and he made it when other scientists were not ready to accept it.

It wasn't the only cholera discovery to be made and forgotten. In 1832, Scottish physician Thomas Latta used intravenous saline injections on fifteen dying cholera patients; five survived. He was criticized for not using approved therapies such as bloodletting, emetics, and cathartics—heroic remedies that lead to dehydration. The idea of fluid replacement finally took hold in the 1890s.[335]

Vibrio cholerae itself, the comma-shaped bacillus that causes cholera, was identified by Filippo Pacini in 1854, but his paper, "Microscopical observations and pathological deductions on cholera," was hardly noticed. Robert Koch had to discover the bacillus again in 1884.

Cholera in the Third World

Since 1817, seven cholera epidemics have swept the world,[14] spreading from seaports along inland waterways. Victims are seized with vomiting and diarrhea that soon becomes watery; clinicians in 1854 called it "rice water stool," after the rice-like flakes of small intestine in it. Dehydration comes quickly. The volume of blood circulating in the body plummets, lips turn blue, and organs fail.[15]

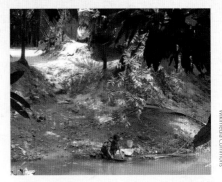

Washing clothes in a Bangladeshi village.

Cholera remains a serious problem today, with an estimated 3 to 5 million cases and 100,000 deaths each year.[16] Most cases occur in places lacking safe drinking water.

The *Vibrio cholerae* organism often lives unnoticed in tidal estuaries such as the Ganges River, the Bay of Bengal, and even the Chesapeake Bay.[17] Endemic cholera breaks out seasonally when water temperatures rise and rains wash nutrients downstream to the estuaries, where microscopic plankton bloom, nourishing tiny crustaceans called copepods, which in turn host *V. cholerae*. When the climate conditions are right, epidemics strike. Although boiling water would kill the bacteria, the people affected often cannot afford wood to boil water.[18]

Village women in Bangladesh have a cheap folk solution: they filter water by running it through an old sari folded four to eight times. Researchers discovered that folding the sari this way provides a 20-micron filter, small enough to remove plankton, copepods, and more than 99 percent of the *V. cholerae*. (A micron is one-thousandth of a millimeter, and there are 25 millimeters in an inch.) They compared the effectiveness of a sari filter, a nylon filter, and no filter, and found that filtering the water with either a sari or a nylon filter reduced the rate of cholera by half.[19]

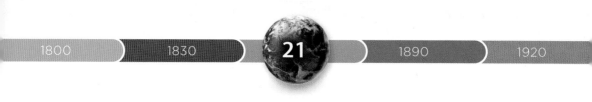
1867

Gregor Mendel and Inherited Traits

Gregor Johann Mendel (1822–1884), the father of genetics, did not use the word "genes." In 1865 he explained how traits are passed from one generation to the next, but his insight was so new there was no word for genes. He had to talk about "discrete, particulate factors" instead.[1] When he presented his "Experiments in Plant Hybridization,"[2] the audience drifted away without discussion.[3] Long after his death, Mendel's 1866 paper was recognized as "one of the three most important publications in the history of biology."[4]

Another of the top three, Charles Darwin's *On the Origin of Species*, came out in 1859. Darwin thought in terms of geologic time.[5] His theory was about inheritance at the species level: individual members of a species will survive longer and have more offspring if their traits are better adapted to their environment. But exactly how do individuals transmit traits to their offspring? Mendel, a farmer's son with experience in selective breeding, was equipped to investigate.[6]

A brilliant young man who suffered periods of depressive illness,[7] Mendel joined the scholarly Augustinian Abbey of St. Thomas in 1843. Shyness unfitted him for parish work, and he failed teaching examinations, but he pursued his scientific work with the abbot's support.[8] He was given a greenhouse, the monastery gardens, and help with his experiments.

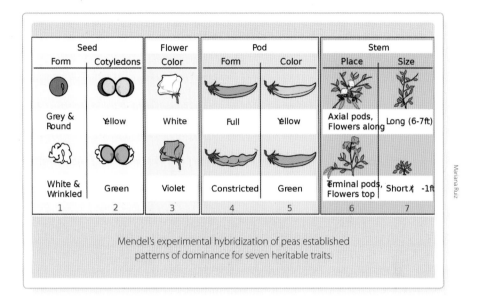

Seed		Flower	Pod		Stem	
Form	Cotyledons	Color	Form	Color	Place	Size
Grey & Round	Yellow	White	Full	Yellow	Axial pods, Flowers along	Long (6-7ft)
White & Wrinkled	Green	Violet	Constricted	Green	Terminal pods, Flowers top	Short -1ft
1	2	3	4	5	6	7

Mendel's experimental hybridization of peas established patterns of dominance for seven heritable traits.

Mariana Ruiz

He needed help—he counted more than 30,000 peas and pea plants.[9] In 1854 and 1855, he tested seeds from 34 varieties. From 1856 to 1863 he cross-pollinated them, testing the heritability of one trait at a time, then two, and finally three. He would open a partly developed blossom, remove its anthers, dust pollen over its stigma with a camel's hair brush, and tie a bag over it to keep insects from tracking in different pollen.[10] Mendel crossed round peas with wrinkled peas, tall-stemmed with short-stemmed peas, and so on, for a total of seven traits.

One value of each trait was expressed in the first child generation (f1). When green-seeded and yellow-seeded peas were crossed, for instance, all their offspring had yellow seeds. But in the next generation (f2), some offspring from yellow-seeded peas had green seeds. As he examined more peas, the ratio of yellow- to green-seeded peas in the f2 generation approached 3:1. Noticing this, Mendel called yellow the dominant value for seed color, and green recessive. Repeating the experiment with other traits, he got the same results. In the f1 generation, the recessive value of a trait would disappear, but in the f2 generation, it would show up in approximately one plant of every four—or 5,000 of every 20,000.

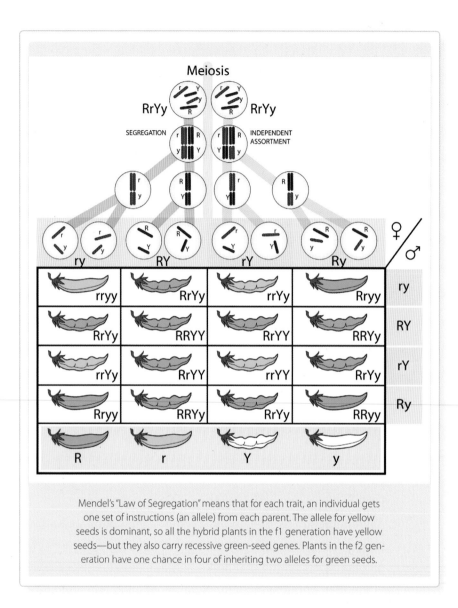

Mendel's "Law of Segregation" means that for each trait, an individual gets one set of instructions (an allele) from each parent. The allele for yellow seeds is dominant, so all the hybrid plants in the f1 generation have yellow seeds—but they also carry recessive green-seed genes. Plants in the f2 generation have one chance in four of inheriting two alleles for green seeds.

Mendel explained his observations by proposing that adult traits were inherited through discrete particulate factors that existed in pairs in all individuals. He understood plant fertilization, and he reasoned that for reproduction to occur, each individual would form its own germ-cells which contained only one discrete particle for each trait. He called these germ-cells "gametes." Thus, with one gamete from each parent, the offspring would have paired particles for each trait—one from the mother, one from the father.

His observations also led him to conclude that each pair of discrete particles segregated independently into either pollen or egg, a conclusion that later became known as the "Law of Independent Assortment."[11] Peas could be tall and purple or short and purple, tall and white or short and white. The more traits you look at, the more ways they can be recombined.

Mendel had studied probability—then a new science—and knew he needed large numbers for a reliable ratio. No doubt he was the first person to apply probability to the study of inheritance,[12] and in the 1930s a new generation of scientists (including Sir Ronald Fisher, J.B.S. Haldane, and Sewall Wright) built on his work to develop a new understanding of population genetics and a whole new vocabulary of terms to communicate about heredity and traits.

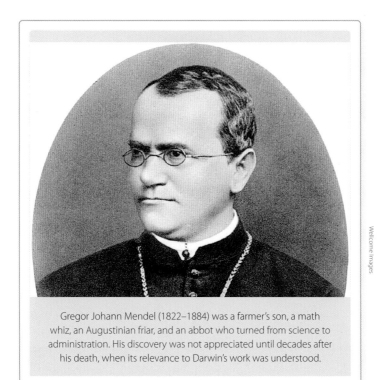

Gregor Johann Mendel (1822–1884) was a farmer's son, a math whiz, an Augustinian friar, and an abbot who turned from science to administration. His discovery was not appreciated until decades after his death, when its relevance to Darwin's work was understood.

Wellcome Images

Sickle-cell Trait: Mendelian Inheritance Meets Darwinian Selection

Sickle-cell disease is a painful inheritance. Literally. It is a genetic blood disease that affects the red blood cells—a hemoglobin disorder.[13] It afflicts millions of people worldwide with crippling bouts of pain and shortens their lifespans; even in wealthy countries, people with sickle-cell disease have a life expectancy of only 40 to 60 years. American children with sickle-cell disease are more likely than their classmates to have their spleens removed as preschoolers, and to be on first-name terms with emergency room personnel.

So if Darwinian evolution tends to weed out hereditary traits that lead to early death, why does 5 percent of the

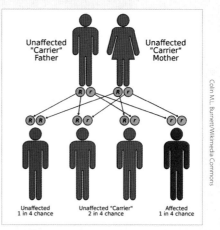

Unaffected "Carrier" Father

Unaffected "Carrier" Mother

Unaffected 1 in 4 chance

Unaffected "Carrier" 2 in 4 chance

Affected 1 in 4 chance

Colin M.L. Burnett/Wikimedia Commons

Sickle-cell disease is inherited in a recessive pattern. It protects against malaria, and so is more commonly found among populations exposed to malaria.

world's population carry trait genes for hemoglobin disorders? Because sickle-cell carriers are somewhat protected from an even more lethal threat: malaria, a mosquito-borne parasite that thrives in healthy red blood cells. In 2015, malaria killed an estimated 438,000 people—306,000 of whom were under five years old.[14]

In 1949, geneticist J.B.S. Haldane predicted that a hemoglobin disorder might help populations resist malaria. His reasoning: 1) a highly lethal type of malaria, *Plasmodium falciparum*, is believed to have infected humans for hundreds of generations—long enough for evolution to take place; 2) malaria fatalities are most common among children, before they reproduce—giving an evolutionary edge to a trait that prevents such early deaths; and 3) the *Plasmodia* parasites spend much of their lives in red blood cells, so an abnormality in the red blood cells might create an environment in which it would be harder for the parasite to survive.[15]

As it turns out, healthy carriers of the sickle-cell trait do get malaria, but fewer of their red blood cells are infected. They are less likely to get cerebral malaria or severe anemia, and less likely to die.[16] Siblings who inherit two copies of the sickle-cell allele face double jeopardy, since both sickle-cell disease and malaria cause anemia. But on average, twice as many carriers should be born as children affected with a recessive genetic disease; mathematically, sickle-cell trait is more of an advantage than a disadvantage to populations living with malaria.

The Language of Genetics

Since Mendel's time, a whole new language has evolved to talk about the science he helped invent—including the word "gene" in 1909. The word "allele" has been used since the 1930s for an alternative form of the same gene; Mendel hypothesized correctly that his peas had two copies of each gene, but he didn't have such convenient words for the concept. Now we can say that pea plants have two alleles at each gene locus, which makes them "diploid." A cell with only one allele for each gene (such as a gamete) is "haploid."

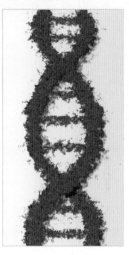

Shutterstock.com

If its alleles for a specific gene are the same, an individual organism is "homozygous" with respect to that gene; if the alleles are different, the individual is "heterozygous." Yellow-seeded pea plants that carry the recessive allele for green seeds are "heterozygotes," as are healthy carriers of the recessive sickle-cell trait. Like the medieval Arab translators who salvaged Greek science and built on it, modern scientists are constantly in need of precise, economical words.

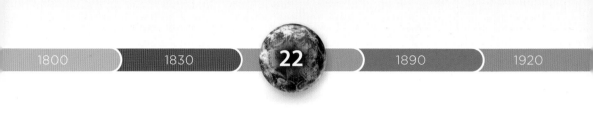
1870

Discovering Ancient Skull Surgeries

Why are there so many tidy round holes in prehistoric skulls? Possible answers might include sword punctures, falling rocks, acid drips in tombs, or beetles and rodents gnawing at the skull after death. Paul Broca (1824–1880) had a different explanation: surgery, done on living patients. Even in the Stone Age, humans performed an operation called *trepanation*, drilling a hole in the patient's skull.

Broca was a French doctor famous for work on the brain. He understood that different parts of the brain have different functions, and he developed a way of using landmarks on the skull to locate parts of the brain. When one of his patients had trouble talking after a closed head injury, Broca found the problem, trepanned the man's cranium, and drained an underlying abscess. He reported the case in 1876; it was the first "neurosurgery based on the new theory of cortical localization of function."[1]

Since he was also a famous anthropologist, it was only natural that anyone who wanted a second opinion on a prehistoric skull would turn to Broca. George Squier (1821–1888) did just that to resolve controversy over a skull he'd acquired in Peru. Squier thought the hole in this skull was made by an ancient American surgeon during the patient's life; members of the New York Academy of Medicine thought it was done after death. So in 1867, Squier asked Broca to examine the skull.[2]

Broca concluded the operation had been done a week or two before the patient's death; it had begun to heal. But why was it done? Squier thought it might have been a response to head trauma, but no visible cracks in the skull confirmed that idea. Had there been a closed head injury? Maybe the Incan surgeon had operated to relieve pressure, just as Broca himself would have done.[3]

The Peruvian skull excited French anthropologists, and soon they were unearthing ancient skulls in France. Broca's friend P. Barthélemy Prunières discovered many with large openings, and near them he found rondelles—round pieces of cranial bones, polished and shaped like amulets. Broca came to believe that Neolithic humans had practiced trepanation, largely on children, to cure some problem; he thought the rondelles were "tied to primitive religious beliefs."[4] Many researchers

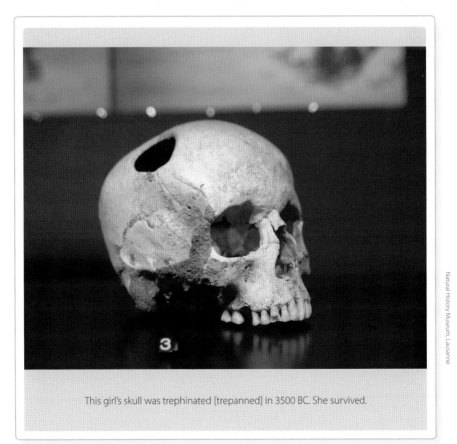

This girl's skull was trephinated [trepanned] in 3500 BC. She survived.

Natural History Museum, Lausanne

have accepted Broca's ideas. If Neolithic humans thought seizures were caused by demons that escaped through the holes, maybe they also thought children who survived were sacred, and amulets made from their skulls had power. It's a theory.

Since Broca's time, anthropologists around the world have found hundreds of trepanned skulls. Some European examples are more than 10,000 years old, and North African ones are even older.[5] Broca was right to think cranial surgery dates back to the Stone Age.

But was he right about why it was done? Answers may vary with culture. Some trepanations may have relieved pain or pressure in the head. In ancient Peru, Denmark, and China, it seems likely that war-riors were trepanated after right-handed enemies bashed them on the left side of the skull.[6] In today's Kenya, the Gusii people remove fractured bone after head trauma.[7]

Classical Greek and Roman writ-ings recommended trepanation for head injuries with or without fracture,[8] and we now regard putting holes in the head as the correct way to release a buildup of old blood or pus under the skull.[9] Trepana-tion may have been humanity's first sur-gical discovery.

And Paul Broca, investigating early examples of it, was pioneering a new area of medical research: paleopathology, or the study of ancient illnesses. Broca was a physician, an anatomist, and an anthro-pologist; today's paleopathologists are trained in even more disciplines. Using research tools that range from DNA sequencing to CT scans on the remains of ancient humans, they find new answers to old questions.

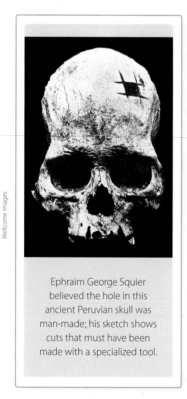

Ephraim George Squier believed the hole in this ancient Peruvian skull was man-made; his sketch shows cuts that must have been made with a specialized tool.

The Legend of Tuo Hua and the Emperor's Headaches

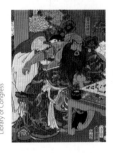

Statue of the legendary physician Hua Tuo at Longshan temple in Taiwan.

Old Chinese stories tell of the surgeon Hua Tuo (c. AD 140–c. 208), known as the Chinese "Father of Medicine."[10] Tuo was legendary for his ability to diagnose and cure all manner of ailments. His special anesthetic, Ma Fei San, was so powerful that patients could sleep through surgery and feel no pain; it was probably made of boiled cannabis dissolved in wine, though other traditional ingredients have been suggested.

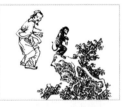

Hua Tuo was said to have based his system of exercises on ancient teachings and observation of animal movements. Here he imitates the posture of a monkey.

According to legend, the Emperor Cao Cao was struck by unbearable headaches and called on Tuo for help. Tuo said the headaches were caused by the pressure of air and fluid building up inside the skull. To relieve the pain, he would have to anesthetize the emperor and open his skull. But Cao Cao, fearing assassination, had Tuo executed.

Although Hua Tuo was said to have pioneered the use of anesthesia for surgery, a fourteenth-century romance described how the macho Guan Yu refused painkillers and just kept playing a board game while Hua scraped poison from his arm bone.

His medical secrets did not survive him. Tuo had a book—by some accounts, he received it from mysterious old men, clearly immortals, in a cave that collapsed right after he left it. Whether he relied on their magical secrets alone or added to the book from his own observations and experience, it was a valuable thing, and he left it to his kind jailer. But the jailer's wife burned it; being a great doctor was all too likely to get a man executed.

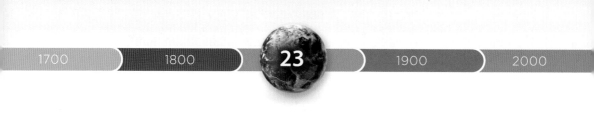
1881

Spontaneous Generation and the Germ Theory of Disease

G erm theory is common knowledge now; almost everyone believes that infectious diseases are caused by living organisms that are too small to see. But as recently as the late nineteenth century, scientists and physicians resisted this idea because it contradicted what they knew, not only about the transmission of disease but about the nature of life itself. Aristotle held that while some plants and animals grow from the seeds (or germs) of like plants and animals—wheat from wheat, pigs from pigs—others arise from spontaneous generation.[1] So maggots were believed to come from putrefying meat, and fleas from dust.

Then Italian physician Francesco Redi (1626 – 1697) showed by experiment that maggots come from flies. He put raw meat or dead fish in covered and uncovered jars; maggots developed in open jars but not covered ones. If he covered jars only with gauze, so flies could smell meat but not land on it, he got dead maggots on the gauze.[2] Redi published his findings in 1668, using Biblical references to support his conclusions.

Van Leeuwenhoek (Chapter 10) saw Redi's work by 1675. Though he could not read Latin, all the creatures he observed (including fleas and eels) had parents of their own kind.[3] But what about microbes? He called them "animalcules," and little was known about them.

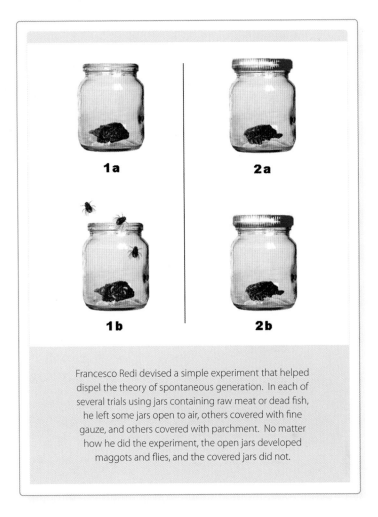

Francesco Redi devised a simple experiment that helped dispel the theory of spontaneous generation. In each of several trials using jars containing raw meat or dead fish, he left some jars open to air, others covered with fine gauze, and others covered with parchment. No matter how he did the experiment, the open jars developed maggots and flies, and the covered jars did not.

In 1750 John Needham, a Roman Catholic priest, published experimental results that seemed to show spontaneous generation—at least for animalcules. He put broth in a corked vial, heated it in hot ashes to kill any eggs or living creatures, set it aside for a few days, and then found it teeming with life. Did a "vegetative force" act on the broth to create animalcules?[4] Or did Needham fail to heat the vial long enough or hot enough? In 1769, Italian priest Lazzaro Spallanzani did a series of experiments showing no growth if the broth was boiled for over one hour and then kept hermetically sealed. He argued that animalcules move through the air and are killed by boiling. But Needham argued that Spallanzani's work proved nothing; his methods had killed the "vegetative force" or destroyed the "elasticity of the air." Spontaneous generation remained controversial,[5] and even Spallanzani did not connect the animalcules with disease.[6]

Then Louis Pasteur looked at yeast. Yeast is a living organism that feeds on the carbon in sugar, and where yeast doesn't grow, alcohol doesn't ferment. To demonstrate that yeast was not spontaneously generated but came from microbes in ordinary air, Pasteur in 1859 used a "swan neck" flask that trapped falling particles so they couldn't contaminate his boiled broths.[7] Broth stayed clear until he tipped the flask; then airborne microbes mingled with the liquid, and it clouded up. Pasteur's microscope was more powerful than Van Leeuwenhoek's, and he could see that specific microorganisms were responsible for normal and abnormal fermentations in wine, beer, and vinegar.

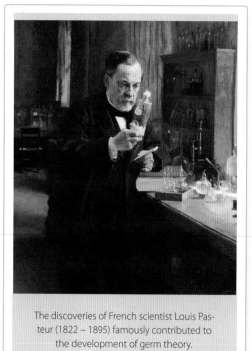

The discoveries of French scientist Louis Pasteur (1822 – 1895) famously contributed to the development of germ theory.

Musée d'Orsay

So yeast was not a product of spontaneous generation, but what about microbes isolated from wounds or diseased tissues? Did these microbes cause tissue to degenerate, or did they appear because tissue was degenerating?

In 1876, Robert Koch proved that microbes caused anthrax, an infectious disease that devastated livestock.[8] Pasteur did his own study of anthrax, and in 1878 announced "proof that the cause of transmissible, contagious and infectious diseases resides . . . in the presence of microorganisms."[9] Although the immune system was still a mystery, Pasteur developed vaccines against anthrax and chicken cholera, and in 1881 he published his germ theory of disease.[10]

When Pasteur and Koch injected healthy animals with microbes from the blood of sick animals, they transmitted the same disease, and microbes of the same species. Anthrax came from anthrax and cholera from cholera, with predictable effects on the bodies of their unlucky hosts. The

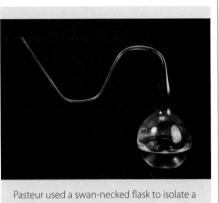

Pasteur used a swan-necked flask to isolate a boiled infusion from the air for months. Only after he tilted the flask to allow exposure to air did micro-organisms appear in the liquid.

Wellcome Images

discovery brought new hope: once the cause of a disease was identified, the disease might be conquered.

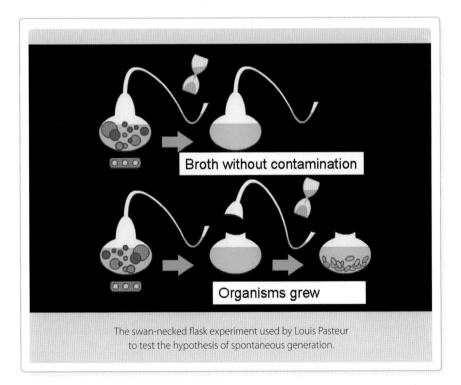

Broth without contamination

Organisms grew

The swan-necked flask experiment used by Louis Pasteur to test the hypothesis of spontaneous generation.

Joseph Lister Applies
Germ Theory to Surgery

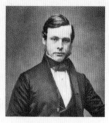

Joseph Lister in 1855, the year he looked at a wound healing without suppuration and told a friend, "The main object of my life is to find out how to procure this result in all wounds."

When Joseph Lister (1827–1912) became a surgeon, the "fetid, sickening odor" of hospitals was as much a part of life as their high mortality rates.[11] Wounds putrefied, suppurated (formed pus), and stank; patients suffered and often died of horrifying infections.[12] Anesthesia let surgeons do longer operations, so deeper wounds lay open to contaminants that included the surgeons' own unwashed hands and instruments.[13]

Lister examined damaged tissue through his microscope, looking for the causes of suppuration; his ambition was to prevent it in all wounds.[14] In 1865 he heard of Pasteur's finding that microbes in the air caused fermentation. Lister was inspired. He reasoned that suppuration was similar to fermentation and might also be caused by microbes. Open wounds almost always became septic (infected), while bones that fractured without breaking the skin did not. By protecting open wounds from airborne microbes, could he prevent putrefaction?

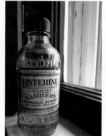

The antiseptic mouthwash named for Joseph Lister was developed in 1879 and is still in common use.

Britta Gustafson/Wikimedia Commons

He started covering wound dressings with tinfoil to keep the air out. Also, because carbolic acid was used to prevent smelly fermentation in sewage, Lister soaked the dressings in carbolic acid.[15] Over time he improved his carbolic acid solutions and introduced other antiseptic methods: shaving patients before surgery, disinfecting the skin, and sterilizing the material used for suturing. He was the first to apply the germ theory of disease to prevent surgical site infections. Later, others added more of the precautions we use today: surgical gloves,[16] masks, and modern ventilation systems. Unlike Semmelweis, who had developed similar theories about the spread of disease years earlier (Chapter 18), Lister got along with people and was persuasive. His publications and lectures won many converts to antiseptic procedures, and he always credited Pasteur.

Koch's Postulates

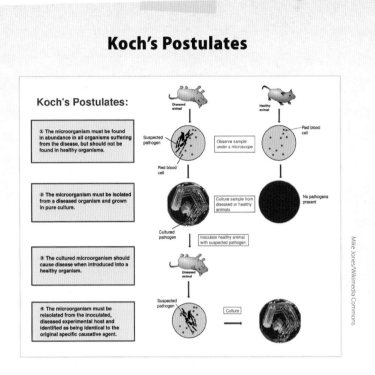

Mike Jones/Wikimedia Commons

In 1884, Robert Koch (1843–1910) outlined a set of guidelines, or postulates, for proving that a specific organism causes a disease. The proof is strong if the researcher can 1) find that organism in all cases of the disease; 2) grow the organism outside the body of a host—for instance, culture it in a test tube; and 3) use the cultured organism to infect a new host.[17]

Koch realized that these were not hard-and-fast rules. The first postulate originally said that the infectious microbe would not be found in healthy organisms; but later he discovered that seemingly healthy individuals might be harboring typhoid fever, tuberculosis, or some other disease. Not everyone who carries a germ will suffer the illness it could cause. But although Koch's postulates have been adapted to reflect new discoveries over the years, they remain a touchstone for disease investigators.[18]

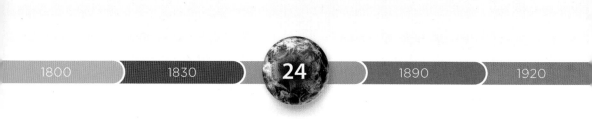

1882

Tuberculosis Emerges
from the Miasma

If you lived in London or Hamburg around 1800, and you knew people who were young or poor, you knew someone who was dying of tuberculosis. Now we call it TB; then it was consumption, or the White Death, and it killed up to 1,000 of every 100,000 city dwellers each year.[1] A century later it was still the leading cause of death in the U.S.[2]

People lived for years with tuberculosis, getting sicker over time. Hippocrates said the disease attacked the lungs "chiefly between the ages of eighteen and thirty-five,"[3] and in 1900 Romantics thought its pale young victims looked spiritual—beautiful and doomed. They coughed blood as death neared. Galen recommended fresh air, milk, and sea voyages,[4] but the Industrial Revolution packed workers into cities; some London neighborhoods averaged five residents to a room.[5] When anyone coughed, everyone inhaled the germs.

Since germs were unknown before the 1870s, TB's spread was a mystery. It can lurk in the body without causing symptoms for months or even years after exposure.[6] Thinkers in ancient Greece[7] and Renaissance Italy[8] may have guessed it was contagious, but there was room for doubt. In the nineteenth century, Southern Europeans generally thought it was infectious. Northern Europeans classified it as heritable[9]

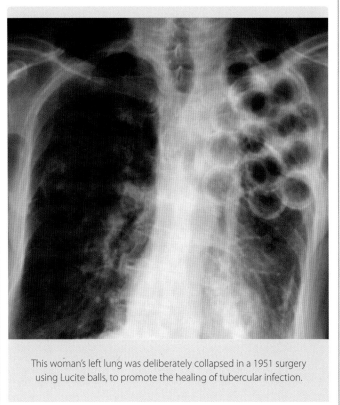

This woman's left lung was deliberately collapsed in a 1951 surgery using Lucite balls, to promote the healing of tubercular infection.

Department of Radiology, Military Teaching Hospital Clermont-Tonnerre, Brest, France

but thought lifestyle and environment affected the risk.[10] Sanitarians (including Florence Nightingale) emphasized the need for good ventilation and diet.

Gradually scientists learned more. In 1819, René Laennec clearly established that whether consumption's manifestations were pulmonary or extrapulmonary—in the lungs or outside them—it was the same disease. Sadly, his insight was possible because he had autopsied so many victims.[11] In 1865, Jean-Antoine Villemin's experiments demonstrated that tuberculosis was contagious. His findings were resisted on emotional as well as scientific grounds. Hermann Pidoux argued that if people believed Villemin, tuberculosis sufferers would be "sequestered like lepers."[12]

Those who could afford it were already being sequestered. In the 1850s a new kind of hospital evolved: the sanatorium, where patients with early signs of tuberculosis could hope to be cured with fresh dry air, exercise, rest, and good nutrition—just what Galen ordered.[13] Sanatoria were often in the mountains, where the altitude or the cold air was thought to help. In or out of the sanatorium, patients had to be compliant, accepting a "life of rules and regulations."[14] Some patients were cured or at least improved. Others were helped by plombage—a surgery that deliberately collapsed a lung with Lucite balls, about the size of ping-pong balls, to give it time for healing. Since every operation carries risks, the balls were sometimes left in place and removed only if they resulted in complications.[15]

Robert Koch identified the tubercle bacillus (*Mycobacterium tuberculosis*) as the cause of tuberculosis in 1882, but his discovery did not lead to a magic bullet. It did lead to laws against spitting,[16] as the emphasis of public health efforts shifted from infrastructure to individual behavior. It often led to stigmatizing disease victims (as Pidoux had feared)

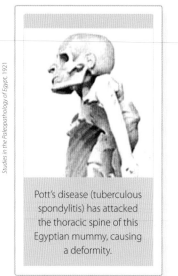

Studies in the Paleopathology of Egypt, 1921

Pott's disease (tuberculous spondylitis) has attacked the thoracic spine of this Egyptian mummy, causing a deformity.

or their social classes.[17] It led to a vaccine, developed by Albert Calmette and Camille Guérin in 1921, and to powerful antibiotics—streptomycin in 1944, isoniazid in 1952, and rifamycins in 1957.[18] Nothing yet has been completely effective. Worldwide, 9.6 million people fell ill with TB in 2014, and 1.5 million died from it.[19]

Yet even before 1882, TB mortality in Britain began to fall. Antibiotics helped, but in industrialized countries the epidemic was already on the wane.[20] Back in the 1500s Fracastoro guessed that TB was spread by unseen germs but preyed on victims whose resistance was weakened by constitutional or environmental factors. Was he right? Today, people infected with HIV are twenty or thirty times more susceptible to TB.[21] Koch won a 1905 Nobel Prize for his discovery, but we still have more to discover.

Desperate Cures: The Royal Touch and Burning the Vampire's Hearts

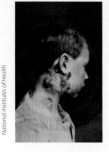

National Institutes of Health

Scrofula (Mycobacterial cervical lymphadenitis) is usually caused by tuberculosis or other mycobacterial organisms. In medieval England it was called the "King's Evil," and people believed that a divinely appointed king could relieve it by his touch.

How do you treat an incurable disease of unknown origins? In medieval Europe, you beg the king to touch it. In nineteenth-century Rhode Island, you find a vampire's heart, burn it, and drink the ashes.

The kings of medieval France and England were not considered gods in their own right, like Egyptian pharaohs and Roman emperors, but they did claim to be ordained by God. This gave them the supernatural power of healing scrofula—swollen lymph nodes on the neck, often caused by tuberculosis—by a touch. People flocked to be cured; Charles II of England touched 92,102 of them.[22]

Did it work? Possibly. Scrofula has been known to clear up on its own,[23] and the placebo effect could have played a role as well.

A New England folk remedy was less successful. After a series of tuberculosis deaths in a family, neighbors suspected vampire activity. One of the dead was returning at night, they thought, to drain life from the living. The solution was to dig up the dead, looking for a heart that still contained "fresh" blood. This happened as recently

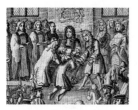

Charles II came to the throne in 1660, after England's Civil War; he touched 92,102 scrofulous subjects during his 22-year reign.

as March 1892, when neighbors pressured Rhode Islander George Brown to save his son Edwin's life by digging up his daughter Mercy and burning her heart. Edwin drank the ashes in water—but died two months later.[24]

Mercy Brown's heart was burned a decade after Koch's discovery of a bacillus more deadly than vampires. Hers may have been the last TB-related

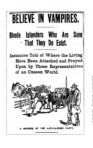

Boston Daily Globe

In 1896, the Boston Daily Globe reported on fears of vampirism in nearby Rhode Island: when TB felled one family member after another, could it be that one of the dead was sucking blood from the living?

exhumation. But where scientific discoveries offer no quick, clear-cut remedies, folk beliefs are likely to persist.

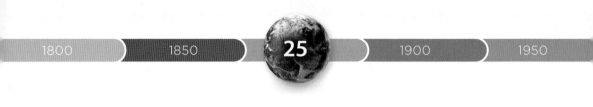

1894

A Barrel of Snakes and an Antitoxin

In 1891, young Albert Calmette (1863–1933) wrote to his parents in France with happy news. He had acquired a barrel of cobras— the species that killed 21,000 people a year in British India! Trying to escape a flood, the snakes had invaded homes in a Vietnamese village and bitten 40 people, killing four instantly. A mountain man, "part snake charmer and part wizard," captured 19 of the animals, and 14 reached Calmette. He extracted venom from their glands and looked forward to "very interesting experiments." No scientist ever before had such a fine supply of venom "under such favorable conditions."[1]

Calmette was just the type of doctor to welcome a barrel of snakes. In the Royal Navy he had studied malaria in Asia and sleeping sickness in Africa. In 1890 he had taken a course on bacteriology at the Pasteur Institute,[2] and now he was establishing a Pasteur outpost at Saigon to offer public health services and conduct research.[3] Since 1880, scientists had learned to make vaccines by weakening lethal pathogens that caused avian cholera, anthrax, tuberculosis, and rabies.[4] Humans were conquering germs. Why not snakebites?

Researchers had discovered that vipers were naturally immune to their own venom. Even non-venomous snakes had immunity, and pigeons injected with steadily increasing doses of venom could develop resistance—though not immunity.[5] Calmette himself had tried the increased dosage strategy, and he had tried to "neutralize" venom with chemicals. Nobody yet had created true immunity to venom.[6]

Then a new type of cure was conceived: therapeutic serum. Serum (plural, sera) is liquid that separates out when blood coagulates, and scientists were using it as the basis for vaccines. After an animal had been inoculated with diphtheria or tetanus, for instance, serum from its blood could be processed to make a vaccine against diphtheria or tetanus.

Calmette thought disease toxins and snake venom were similar. If a serum could work against one, couldn't it also work against the other? With help and advice from Emile Roux, Calmette managed to make animals immune to venom. Then he used serum from the immune animals to create immunity in other animals,[7] and in 1894 he announced the first antivenom seratherapy for humans.[8] Soon the Pasteur Institute was producing serum for use against cobra bites in India, and other

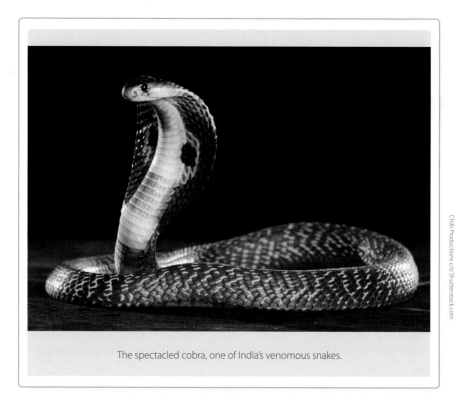

The spectacled cobra, one of India's venomous snakes.

Chilli Productions c/o Shutterstock.com

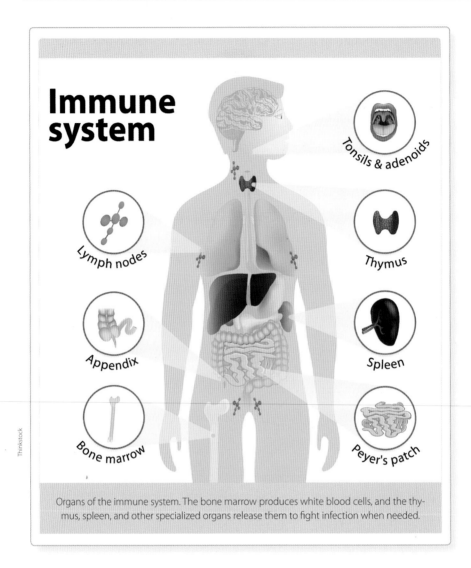

Organs of the immune system. The bone marrow produces white blood cells, and the thymus, spleen, and other specialized organs release them to fight infection when needed.

researchers around the world were developing specific antitoxins to combat the effects of specific snakebites.[9]

By this time, scientists were creating vaccines and antitoxins that worked, but they couldn't see the exact mechanisms at play. A new science, immunology, emerged as they developed and tested theories about immunization. Vaccines appeared to stimulate the body's own defenses against disease, infection, and even venom, but how did it all work? Calmette was one in a chain of discoverers who figured it out.

We now know the body has tissues and organs that produce, store, and carry white blood cells. When antigens such as bacteria and venoms invade, the white blood cells produce antibodies. Some antibodies destroy antigens; others make it easier for white blood cells to destroy them.[10]

But to be effective, every antibody must fit the antigen it's fighting. Each antigen has a unique shape, and to neutralize it the white blood cells produce antibodies matching that shape. Calmette's serum came from horses immunized against cobra venom. If it could be given quickly enough after a cobra bite, the horses' antibodies could help a human victim fight off the venom. Antitoxins are still used today for snake bites as well as rabies, botulism, hepatitis, and a few other diseases.

This of course is not the whole story. Nobel Prizes in 1908, 1919, 1972, 1984, 1987, and 2011 honored work in immunology, and we are still modifying our understanding of it. It's an understanding born of hands-on experimentation, a research process that saved lives as it went.

Resisting Poisons in Antiquity

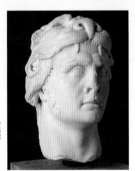

Louvre

Mithridates VI, portrayed here as Heracles, lived into his late nineties. Some believed it was regular doses of poison that kept him alive.

Mithridates VI (135–63 BC) was always on guard against assassins. He came to the throne of Pontus after his father's assassination and ruled for more than 80 years. Some said he owed his long life to cultivated immunity. He would regularly take a little of one poison, a little of another—not enough to kill him—and so he built up his resistance to all of them. Aulus Cornelius Celsus, Pliny the Elder, and various imperial Roman physicians all claimed to have the recipe for his "universal antidote" against poisoning, although their ingredients didn't necessarily match.[19]

Science as a Competition

Calmette was not the only one to discover antivenom in 1894. In Paris, the naturalist Césaire Phisalix (1852–1904) took another route to the same discovery.[12] Science is a cumulative endeavor, and each new discovery leads to new questions, so it shouldn't be surprising that discoveries are often made at the same time by different teams of researchers.

Scientists are often rivals. The rivalry between Louis Pasteur and Robert Koch was driven by nationalism: France and Germany had been at war. As the nineteenth century wore on, there were also prizes to spur competition. Calmette wanted to win a British government prize for a snake bite treatment.[13] National academies of science gave prestigious awards, and starting in 1901 there were Nobel Prizes. As competitive researchers raced to make the next great discovery, it

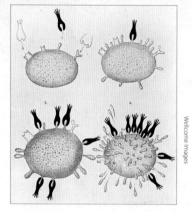

Wellcome Images

Paul Ehrlich drew these diagrams to illustrate his side-chain theory. Ehrlich thought blood cells could mistake toxins for nutrients and bind to them with chemical side-chains. When a toxin failed to satisfy its nutritional need, the cell would produce additional side-chains that were toxin-specific. The extra side-chains would break off, becoming antibodies and neutralizing toxins.[11]

became more important to track who published results first. Scientific etiquette dictated that the first to publish was the discoverer.

The 1908 Nobel Prize in Physiology or Medicine was shared between two rivals whose discoveries about the immune system appeared to conflict: Ilya Mechnikov (1845–1916) and Paul Ehrlich (1854–1915).[14] Mechnikov, a naturalist allied with the Pasteur Institute, first discovered "phagocytes" or "devouring cells" in starfish larvae.[15] In humans, the phagocytes are a type of white blood cell. Mechnikov thought they protected the body by engulfing and digesting infectious agents.[16] Meanwhile Ehrlich, a chemist who had worked with Robert Koch, hypothesized that there must be a close chemical relationship between antigens and specific antibodies, so they fit "like lock and key."[17] His theory was based on this physical match between invading cells and the body's own defending cells, the antibodies. Both sides were at least partly right,[18] and their rival insights made possible some of the major discoveries of twentieth- and twenty-first-century medicine.

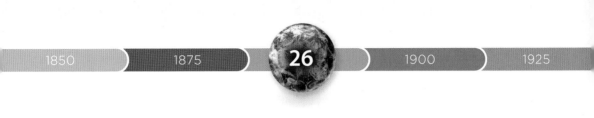
1896

The Discovery of X-rays

As a boy, Wilhelm Röntgen (1845–1923) was not a top student. In the early 1860s, he was kicked out of a Dutch technical school; he refused to identify the classmate who *really* caricatured their teacher on the board.[1] Yet he earned a Ph.D. in 1869, and went on to become a top scientist. In 1888, he was named director of a new physics institute at the University of Würzburg, where he made a discovery that catapulted him to celebrity: the X-ray. In 1901, he won the first ever Nobel Prize in Physics.[2]

The discovery of X-rays seemed to happen in a flash—an accidental flicker of light in a dark lab, and a flash of sudden realization. But, as Pasteur said, chance favors the prepared mind. Others had seen that fluorescence in their labs before Röntgen did, but hadn't pursued it. Röntgen investigated.

Scientists had been experimenting with Crookes tubes to observe cathode rays since 1869. A Crookes tube has two electrodes in a partial vacuum, and applying high voltage to it produces straight rays that can be bent by magnets. But what are they, exactly? Some nineteenth-century scientists theorized that they were electronically charged atoms, others that they were vibrations in a light-bearing medium called the "aether." Philipp Lenard had recently produced effects like darkened photographic plates up to an inch outside the tube, even in the absence of visible light. The cathode rays must be penetrating the glass. Did this prove they were composed of waves, not atoms?[3] Experiments gave conflicting results, and in fall 1895 Röntgen, gripped with curiosity, began his own investigations.[4]

On November 8, Röntgen's apparatus was swathed in black cardboard. He had small cardboard screens washed with a chemical, barium platinum-cyanide, that glowed with fluorescence if hit by cathode rays; he was using one screen to replicate Lenard's work. Then he spotted fluorescence on another screen, on a workbench a meter (3.3 feet) away—too far for the cathode ray to reach.[5]

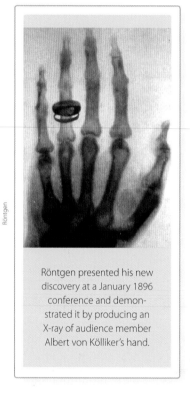

Röntgen

Röntgen presented his new discovery at a January 1896 conference and demonstrated it by producing an X-ray of audience member Albert von Kölliker's hand.

With growing excitement, Röntgen realized that the Crookes tube was emitting another kind of ray. He called it "X" because it was previously unknown, and he worked obsessively, day and night, to discover its properties. He held things between the Crookes tube and the screen—whatever he could pick up in the lab. The ray was hardly dimmed as it passed through books and papers, but metallic objects blocked more of it; it outlined them on the screen along with the bones of Röntgen's hand, holding them up.

Röntgen determined that the new rays travelled in straight lines, were not deflected by magnetic fields, and penetrated materials that blocked ordinary light. He documented secondary radiation and other X-ray phenomena. And on December 28, 1895, he submitted his thorough report "On a New Kind of Ray" to the Würzburg Physical Medical Society.[6]

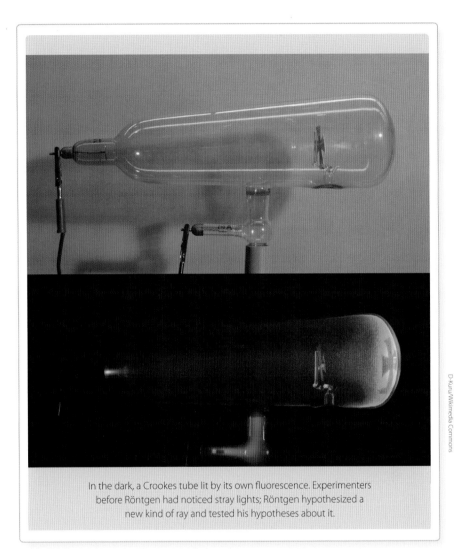

In the dark, a Crookes tube lit by its own fluorescence. Experimenters before Röntgen had noticed stray lights; Röntgen hypothesized a new kind of ray and tested his hypotheses about it.

Chemistry had revolutionized nineteenth-century medicine; now it was the turn of physics. Within months X-rays were used to locate foreign objects, diagnose broken or diseased bones, and look at unborn babies. Radiation therapy was tried on breast cancer. By 1898, patients were even swallowing bismuth subnitrate so X-rays could image their gastrointestinal tracts. X-rays were used in the early diagnosis and isolation of TB cases. As the process became cheaper, more and more people were X-rayed.[7]

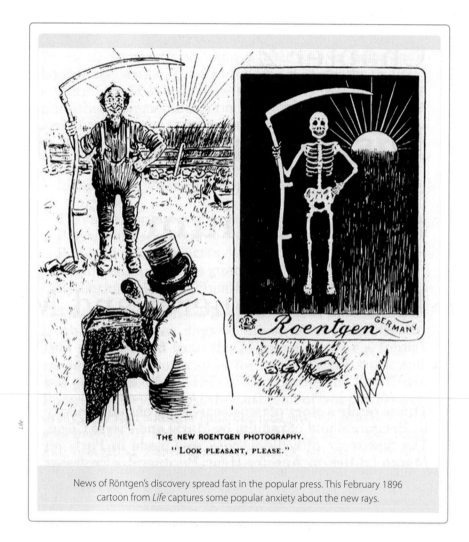

THE NEW ROENTGEN PHOTOGRAPHY.
"LOOK PLEASANT, PLEASE."

News of Röntgen's discovery spread fast in the popular press. This February 1896
cartoon from *Life* captures some popular anxiety about the new rays.

Nobody knew the dangers of radiation, but during 1896 cases of
hair loss and skin cancer raised concerns; Joseph Lister guessed that
X-rays passing through a body could affect internal organs, for good
or ill. As pioneers in radiation science and technology began to die of
various cancers, evidence for ill effects mounted.[8] Today, therapeutic
dosages are carefully limited, and medical personnel take precautions to
limit repeated exposure.

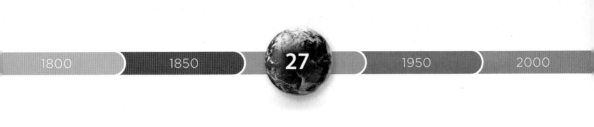
1898

A Small-Game Hunter Fights Bubonic Plague

In 1898, a French doctor working in Pakistan (then part of India) went hunting small game: rats and fleas. In a Karachi home he captured a sick rat, crawling with fleas. At his hotel he found a cat generous enough to give him some more fleas.[1] The hunt took courage. If Paul-Louis Simond (1858–1947) was right, those fleas could kill him. He picked up a rat with long forceps, tossed it into a paper bag, and dropped the bag into warm soapy water.[2] Cutting the bag open underwater to extract the fleas safely, he brought them under a microscope. There he found his real prey.

Simond was in Karachi to combat the plague. Like the Black Death that devastated Eurasia in the fourteenth century, a new epidemic had reached China's port cities in 1894. From there it could easily spread to every continent. The world shuddered, and scientists went from Austria, Egypt, England, Germany, Italy, and Russia to study the situation.[3] France's Pasteur Institute sent Alexandre Yersin to Hong Kong, where he isolated plague bacteria, a swarm of "microbes, all looking alike, with rounded ends."[4] Shibasaburo Kitasato, who had studied with Pasteur's rival Robert Koch, isolated the microbe independently.[5] But identifying the enemy was only the first step in a hard fight.

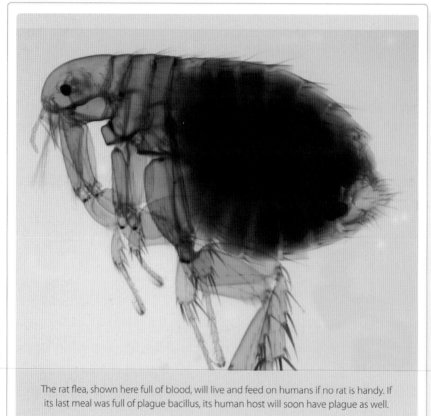

The rat flea, shown here full of blood, will live and feed on humans if no rat is handy. If its last meal was full of plague bacillus, its human host will soon have plague as well.

Katja ZSM/Wikimedia Commons

At least 12 million people died of plague in India, where in 1897 Pasteur Institute bacteriologist Waldemar Haffkine (1860–1930) developed the first vaccine and bravely tested it on himself.[6] Meanwhile, the Institute developed an experimental serum and sent it to Asia with Simond. Could he save those who were already ill?

While working to cure patients, Simond tried to figure out how the disease spread. Yersin had noticed that it affected rats,[7] and common folk had known this for centuries: piles of dead rats meant an epidemic was coming.[8] Scientists suspected plague was transmitted through air, food, or feces mixed with dust; maybe both rats and humans got it from infected soil.

Examining human victims, doctors had noticed that they often had small lesions on their feet and legs. Compared to other plague symptoms, these were hardly worth noticing. Patients often had huge swollen glands, the buboes that give "bubonic" plague its name. Some had septicemia, or blood poisoning; their fingers, toes, and noses turned black as their skin and other tissues died. Some developed pneumonia and couldn't breathe.[9] Small lesions were the least of their problems. But Simond found plague bacteria teeming in these lesions, which were just the right height for ankle-biting fleas. Could fleas be inoculating people with blood from sick rats? In his hotel room, Simond peered through a microscope at soapy drowned fleas. Sure enough, their intestines were full of plague.

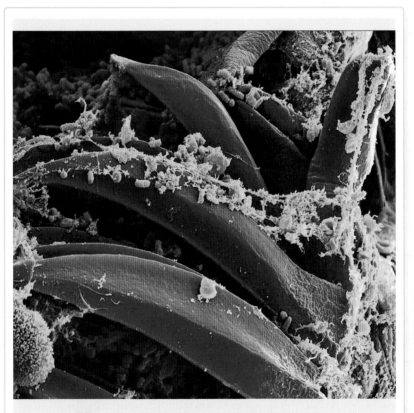

This scanning electron micrograph shows plague bacilli (green) clogging the spines (purple) between a flea's esophagus and its stomach. A plague-infected flea is always hungry because its digestive tract is blocked.

National Institutes of Health

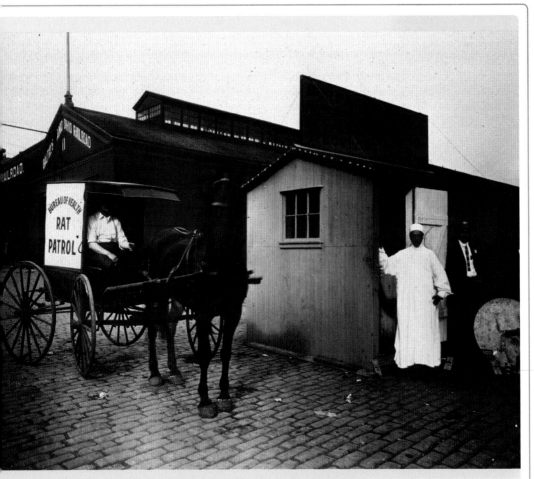

In 1914 a rat collector delivers corpses to a Bureau of Health Rat Receiving Station, where lab workers will test for the presence of plague.

So he experimented. First, he dangled a healthy young rat in a mesh cage above a dying rat in a tall glass jar. The rats could not touch, but when the first rat died, fleas in search of warm flesh jumped up to the healthy rat. Soon it, too, died of plague. When Simond repeated the experiment without fleas, his healthy rat stayed healthy. On June 2, 1898, Simond wrote, "I felt an emotion that was inexpressible in the face of the thought that I had uncovered a secret that had tortured man

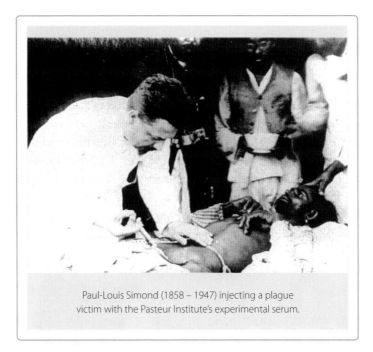

Paul-Louis Simond (1858 – 1947) injecting a plague victim with the Pasteur Institute's experimental serum.

since the appearance of plague in the world."[10] To stop plague, one had to stop fleas—which, practically speaking, meant rat control.

Scientists were skeptical at first. Simond had managed his experiment in an ill-equipped hotel room, and his controls weren't perfect. Had he ruled out the old miasma theory? If fleas could penetrate that mesh cage, so could air. The idea that insects could carry disease was still new and unproven. But in 1903 other experimenters replicated Simond's findings, and soon rat control joined vaccination as a weapon in humanity's war against plague.

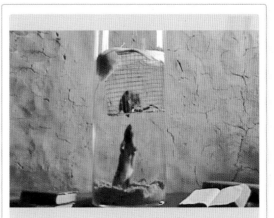

Simond hung a healthy rat over a plague-stricken one so the two could not touch, but infected fleas could leap through the mesh cage. Only when the sick rat had fleas did the healthy rat catch plague.

The Mystery of the Black Death, BBC documentary

Did *Yersinia Pestis* Really Cause the Black Death?

In AD 541, Justinian's Plague raged from Egypt through the Near East and across Europe. Whole regions were depopulated, food supplies failed for lack of farmers, and empires toppled. Epidemics recurred every few years until 750.[11]

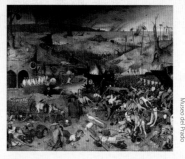

The Triumph of Death, by Pieter Brueghel the Elder (ca. 1562). The Black Death (1347–51) killed as much as a third of the population of Europe and Asia. A new plague pandemic reached Chinese ports in 1894, triggering global fears.

In the fourteenth century, the Black Death devastated Asia and swept into Europe, where by 1350 it had killed approximately one-third of the population.[12] It came back every few years until 1750.[13]

Historians have long thought Justinian's Plague and the Black Death were the same disease that broke out of China in the 1890s. Ancient and medieval witnesses described the buboes and other symptoms that seemed to match the modern plague. But could the historic epidemics, spreading like wildfire across Eurasia, really have been the same as the slower-moving bubonic plague of the 1890s? Those who doubt it find differences in historical descriptions.[14] They also ask if there were enough rats in medieval Europe to spread epidemics,[15] and if the temperature in Europe could have sustained the flea species that carries plague.[16]

A team of archaeologists and microbiologists from France looked for answers in mass graves from the fourteenth century. They found evidence: *Y. pestis* DNA in the dental pulp of presumed plague victims. Similar archeological evidence links *Y. pestis* to the Plague of Justinian[17] as well.

The DNA research suggests that *Y. pestis* evolved as it spread, and new strains caused differences among the reported symptoms of the three plagues.[18] Along with the *Y. pestis*, recent investigators have also found evidence of *Bartonella quintana* infection in those medieval French graves.[19] *B. quintana* is the agent of trench fever, a disease transmitted by lice. If plague victims were co-infected with trench fever and bubonic plague, could lice have carried both? Lice as vectors might explain some of the inconsistencies pointed out by plague skeptics, such as the scarcity of rats and fleas in medieval Europe, the apparent person-to-person transmission of plague, the speed of infections, and the high mortality rate.

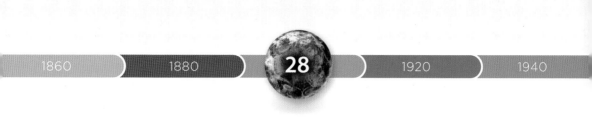
1898

Viruses Borrow Life Support from Tobacco Leaves and Humans

Koch's 1884 postulates (Chapter 23) quickly became the standard rules for proving a specific microbe caused a specific disease. Believing that "all infectious diseases are caused by protozoa, fungi, bacteria or spirochetes,"[1] scientists strained infected liquids through filters and examined the microbes left behind. Then in 1892 Dimitrii Ivanovsky reported that tobacco mosaic disease was caused by a "filterable agent," a pathogen too small to catch in the filtering process.[2]

In 1898, Martinus Willem Beijerinck suggested that the unseen agent might be something completely different. Material infected with it could be filtered and stored for three months, showing no sign of bacterial growth in that time—but still pass the infection on to healthy tobacco plants. The agent multiplied only in living cells. Whatever it was, it somehow had to become part of the plant's metabolism; it could not metabolize or reproduce on its own. Beijerinck was describing a virus. It was a "bold hypothesis," as Ivanovsky said, and at first not many accepted it.[3]

To study viruses, scientists had to adapt Koch's postulates.[4] Viruses could be cultured only in living cells, such as fertilized chicken eggs, and not all human viruses could infect lab animals.[5] Like bacteria, viruses did not always cause disease; some hosts became asymptomatic carriers. Scientists found new ways to prove a virus was not just associated with a disease, but was causing it.[6] Today, a good way to identify a virus is to sequence its DNA,[7] but DNA was not understood in the 1890s.

The first human virus identified was yellow fever, an incurable disease that kills up to half its victims.[8] Cuban physician Carlos Finlay reported in 1881 that it was spread by mosquitoes, and in 1901 Walter Reed confirmed this.[9] Insecticides, mosquito netting, and other public sanitation measures limited the epidemics, making possible the construction of the Panama Canal.[10] But creating a vaccine took years. Hideyo Noguchi's 1921 attempt was based on the wrong infectious agent. A team from the Rockefeller Institute isolated and cultured the real virus in 1927; several of them caught yellow fever in the process, and half a dozen died, including Noguchi.

In 1937, after years of effort, complications, and breakthroughs, Max Theiler finally developed an effective vaccine against yellow fever.[11] Even

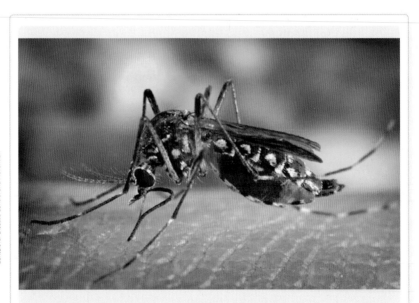

Centers for Disease Control and Prevention

Aedes aegypti mosquitoes breed around houses. To make yellow fever go viral, they only need to suck blood from one infected person, incubate the infection for a few days, and then feast on a susceptible population.

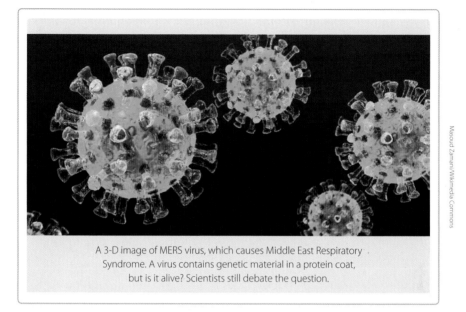

A 3-D image of MERS virus, which causes Middle East Respiratory Syndrome. A virus contains genetic material in a protein coat, but is it alive? Scientists still debate the question.

Masoud Zamani/Wikimedia Commons

then, problems continued. In 1941 and 1942, 7 million doses of vaccine were distributed to U.S. military recruits, and more than 25,000 men came down with jaundice months after vaccination. A small amount of human serum had been used in preparing vaccine, and another virus—hepatitis B—had infected it.[12]

At least 219 viruses are known to infect humans, with three or four more discovered each year.[13] Some cause epidemic diseases such as influenza, smallpox, polio, Ebola, and HIV; others seem benign. They evolve fast; new strains of influenza call for new flu vaccines every year. But from an evolutionary standpoint, the

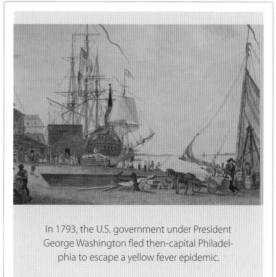

In 1793, the U.S. government under President George Washington fled then-capital Philadelphia to escape a yellow fever epidemic.

John Carter Brown Library, Brown University

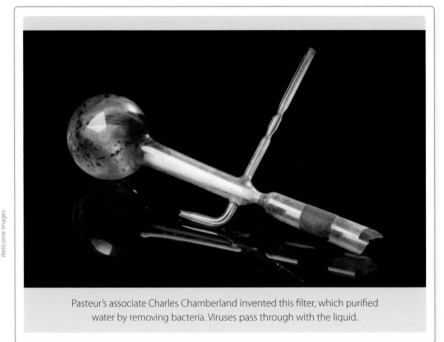

Pasteur's associate Charles Chamberland invented this filter, which purified water by removing bacteria. Viruses pass through with the liquid.

ideal virus should not kill its host too quickly, because the virus needs a host in order to survive.

A virus, after all, is just a package of DNA or RNA wrapped in a protein envelope. It cannot live, replicate, or perform any functions of a living organism unless it invades and commandeers the resources of a host cell. The host's best defense is to produce "antibodies" against the unique protein envelope, which it recognizes as foreign. The foreign identity of the protein envelope is often referred to as the "antigen" because it causes the host to produce "antibodies."

Except viruses, unlike bacteria, are not alive.[14] At least, that seemed undeniable in 1945: an agent that could not eat or reproduce independently could not be alive. Viral diseases have changed history more than once, but in the end, the viral challenge to our thinking about how we define life may be even more important.

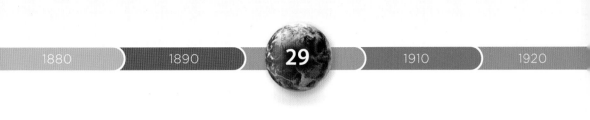
1900

Marie Curie's Lab Glows in the Dark

It was 1899, and Marie Sklodowska Curie (1867–1934) was happy. She was working long hours in France, stirring 45 pounds of boiling pitchblende at a time "with a heavy iron rod nearly as big as myself," and this wasn't even her day job. Her leaky workspace was hot in summer, cold in winter, and filled with poisonous fumes; a German chemist called it "a cross between a stable and a potato shed."[2] But she was married to Pierre Curie, and together they did great science. Now Marie was working on her doctoral thesis, using one of Pierre's inventions to measure observations.

Pierre Curie (1859–1906) was an outsider in the world of French science, but he had an international reputation for doing incisive research and making fine analytic instruments. In 1880 he and his brother Jacques had discovered piezoelectricity,[3] electricity resulting from pressure. Pierre invented an electrometer to measure it.

In 1896 Henri Becquerel left uranium salts in a dark drawer and found they made a photographic image. Uranium emitted energy rays! Using one of Pierre's electrometers, British scientist Lord Kelvin learned the rays produced electricity.[4] Now Marie showed that uranium radiation could be precisely measured, and that a given amount of uranium would always produce the same amount of radiation no matter what other elements it was compounded with. Radiation was "an atomic property of the element of uranium."[5] This was a revolutionary insight, and Marie invented the word *radioactivity* to describe the phenomenon.[6]

If one chemical element was radioactive, what about others? She gathered and tested samples of every known element, and found that thorium also emitted rays. But some ores were far more radioactive than the uranium and thorium they contained. Marie formed a new hypothesis: these ores must contain traces of "a substance much more strongly radioactive than either uranium or thorium." Her tests had already ruled out the other known elements, so this substance could only be "a new chemical element."[7]

In 1898 the Curies announced the existence of two new elements: polonium (named for Marie's homeland) and radium. Over the next two years they processed several tons of radioactive pitchblende ore, and in 1900 they isolated a few grains of radium. They found it emitted three types of rays: alpha rays with a positive charge, negative beta rays, and a third type—similar to light and to X-rays—that did not respond to magnets.[8]

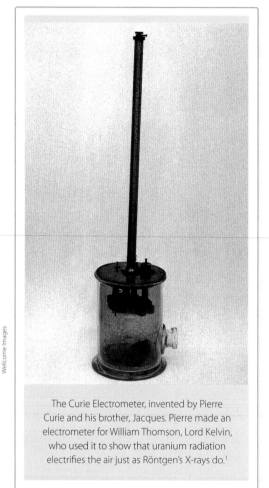

The Curie Electrometer, invented by Pierre Curie and his brother, Jacques. Pierre made an electrometer for William Thomson, Lord Kelvin, who used it to show that uranium radiation electrifies the air just as Röntgen's X-rays do.[1]

Radium earned Marie a doctorate and two Nobel Prizes, one in 1903 for physics and one in 1911 for chemistry. It also affected medicine. Becquerel tucked a bit of radium in his shirt pocket for about six hours in 1901, and ten days later got a radiation burn that took weeks to heal. Pierre Curie confirmed Becquerel's finding by applying radium powder on his forearm and leaving it for ten hours. The resulting dermatitis looked like X-ray burns,[9] and if X-rays were good medicine, why not radium?

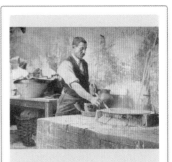

Extracting radium in the old shed. Marie herself extracted radium from tons and tons of pitchblende boiled in an open kettle.

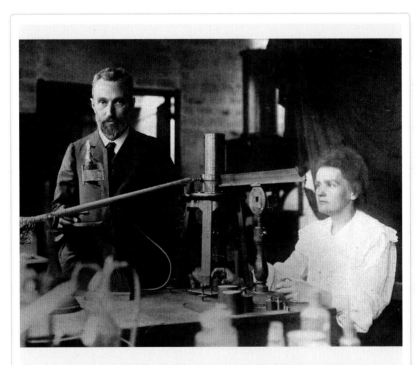

Pierre and Marie Curie worked long hours in a primitive laboratory adjacent to the shed where Marie kept several tons of pitchblende—a radioactive mineral rich in uranium. The shed had no electricity, but its contents glowed in the dark.

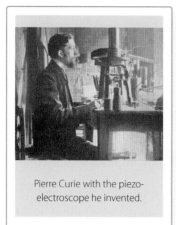

Pierre Curie with the piezoelectroscope he invented.

Radium was easier to use than X-rays. It could be injected, inhaled, swallowed, or applied directly to the skin—to targeted areas, such as tumors. Excited researchers hoped that carefully aimed radiation might burn away cancers while sparing healthy tissue. It might be safer than surgery, which until then was the only effective treatment for cancer.[10] Some even believed that radium could normalize cancer cells and heal X-ray burns.[11] Gradually doctors learned that radium worked best on easy-to-reach, localized cancers, and more gradually still they learned the serious dangers of radium. In 1976, France outlawed the medical use of radium.[12] After 1948, when effects on atomic bomb survivors became clear, there was a push for stronger safety regulations. Today, radiation therapy is only used for specific cancers in measured doses, and strict laws ensure medical personnel are protected from exposure. But safer radiation therapies have built steadily on what pioneers learned from radium.

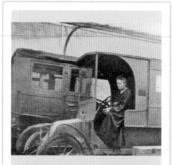

During World War I, Marie Curie organized 200 X-ray units in field hospitals and 20 mobile ones for battlefield use. She trained assistants, donated radium to sterilize tissue, and overall contributed to the care of more than a million soldiers

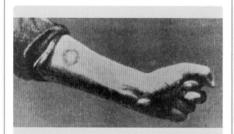

Pierre Curie was among the first to see that radium could be used in medicine. To observe how it affected the body, he deliberately burned his own arm with the substance.

Radiation Therapy: A Dangerous Panacea

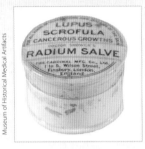

Around 1905, Doctor Shower's Radium Salve was sold as a cure for lupus, scrofula, and skin cancers.

Radiation is dangerous, and researchers now must wear protective clothing to handle Marie Curie's papers. Even her cookbook is radioactive.[13] In later life she suffered chronic ill health, and died at 66 of aplastic anemia; although she did not want to admit it, her years of unprotected work with radioactivity had almost certainly poisoned her.

In the first euphoric years of radiation therapy, however, it looked like a cure-all. It was used for cancer and for bumps that just looked cancerous. It was used to remove unwanted hairs and acne. It was tried against bacterial diseases such as rabies and syphilis.[14] Legitimate doctors worked with radiation, and so did hucksters and charlatans. Radium was added to everything from toothpaste to toys. Radioactive corsets supposedly eased low back pain,[15] and radium salts were marketed as both mental and physical stimulants. Who wouldn't want to swig "Radithor—the perpetual sunshine drink"?[16] But one athletic tycoon started drinking Radithor in 1927 to "improve his physique," and died of radium poisoning five years later, "a shriveled husk with multiple internal lesions."[17]

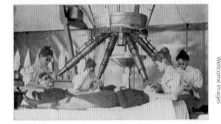

Treatment with the Finsen lamp in 1900. The lamp used quartz crystals to direct ultraviolet rays; nurses and patients protected their eyes with dark glasses. Inventor Niels Ryberg Finsen won a Nobel Prize in 1903 for his work on concentrated light radiation as a treatment for diseases such as lupus.

Meanwhile, young women at a New Jersey factory were painting watch dials with glow-in-the-dark radium paint. They sucked their brushes every so often to keep the tips sharp, and soon dentist Theodore Blum noticed his patients' jaws deteriorating. Nine of the dial painters died, and others struggled with serious illness, leading medical examiner Harrison Martland to conduct the first epidemiological study of radiation sickness.[18]

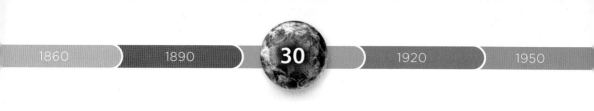
1901

Making Blood Transfusions Safe

What is blood? People have always known that blood keeps us alive. Warriors bled to death on the plains of Troy; early obstetricians saw women hemorrhage and die after childbirth. But what is blood made of, and how does it work to maintain life?

After William Harvey's 1628 book *On the Motion of the Heart and Blood*, doctors and scientists thought about the question anew. The heart pumped blood through a closed circulatory system, but maybe the system could be extended. Maybe blood could be moved from one individual to another.[1]

In 1665, Richard Lower demonstrated that a dog's life could be saved by a blood transfusion from a larger dog. But when scientists tried pumping the blood of lambs into human veins, patients went crazy. An English patient survived the treatment,[2] a Frenchman died, and transfusion was soon banned.[3]

Obstetrician James Blundell began experimenting with it again after 1817 while looking for a way to save new mothers. He found that animals could be revived by blood, but only blood from animals of their own species. Only human blood was safe for humans. In 1825, Blundell performed the first successful human-to-human transfusion.[4]

Yet some patients reacted badly to transfusion. Why? Blundell hypothesized that time outside veins could change blood, and he invented two devices—the *impellor* and the *gravitator*—to speed the process. Even so, he recommended transfusions only to save the dying,[5] and performed just ten in a decade.[6] Half his patients survived.

Some transfusions seemed to fail because of clotting, or agglutination. Did this happen because the blood moved too slowly, or because it lost contact with its own blood vessels, or because it reacted chemically to something in the air? In 1863, Joseph Lister (Chapter 23) tested all three hypotheses and ruled them out. In 1889, physiologist William Hunter mistakenly concluded that blood is a bodily tissue with neither nutritional nor respiratory function, and if patients suffered from too

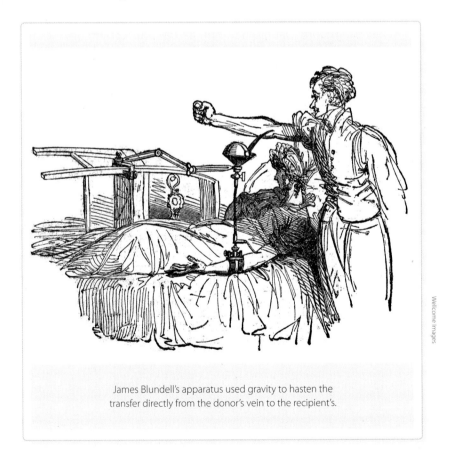

James Blundell's apparatus used gravity to hasten the transfer directly from the donor's vein to the recipient's.

Wellcome Images

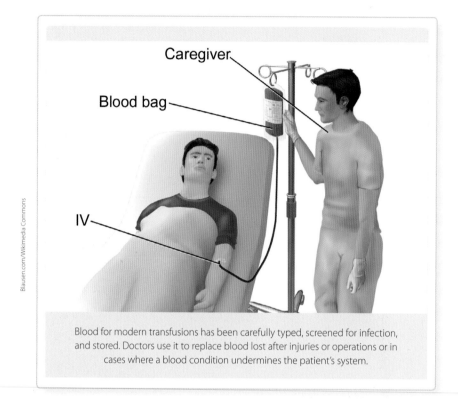

Caregiver

Blood bag

IV

Blausen.com/Wikimedia Commons

Blood for modern transfusions has been carefully typed, screened for infection, and stored. Doctors use it to replace blood lost after injuries or operations or in cases where a blood condition undermines the patient's system.

little fluid in their veins it was safer to infuse them with saline solution. Nobody knew what caused bad reactions to some transfusions, but practitioners stopped doing them.[7]

Then in 1901 Karl Landsteiner made a breakthrough that won him the 1930 Nobel Prize in medicine: he discovered human blood types. Biochemists had learned that individual plant and animal species have their own characteristic proteins. But did individuals within a species have "similar though smaller differences"?[8]

Landsteiner experimented. He knew that if blood serum from one species was transfused into another species, the recipient's red blood cells would agglutinate. He took blood serum and red blood cells from human subjects and cross-matched them in test tubes. Some matches showed no reaction—it was just as if the serum and the red blood cells came from the same individual. But in others, red blood cells agglutinated as if the serum came from another species.[9] He discovered three human blood groups: A, B, and O. In 1902, two of his colleagues discovered the fourth group, AB.

This was why so many transfusions had gone so tragically wrong: incompatibility. Red blood cells in groups A, B, and AB have patterns of proteins and sugars on their surface that act as antigens, triggering immune responses in the bodies of recipients whose red cells don't have the same patterns.[10] When a patient receives incompatible blood, the body identifies it as an alien substance, like the germ of a disease; the patient's own blood produces antibodies. Agglutination is a defense, clumping the "invading" cells for efficient disposal.

Landsteiner understood the implications of this discovery for skin grafts, organ transplants, and other operations.[11] Recognition was slow to come, but American surgeon George Washington Crile showed that saline was not an adequate substitute for blood. Trench warfare in World War I increased need, and with knowledge of the ABO system, blood transfusions improved.[12]

	Group A	Group B	Group AB	Group O
Red blood cell type	A	B	AB	O
Antibodies in Plasma	Anti-B	Anti-A	None	Anti-A and Anti-B
Antigens in Red Blood Cell	A antigen	B antigen	A and B antigens	None

The four main human blood types are distinguished by the antigens in their red blood cells and the antibodies in their plasma.

Blood Transfusions in War and Peace

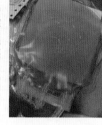

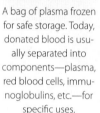

Diver Dave/Wikimedia Commons

A bag of plasma frozen for safe storage. Today, donated blood is usually separated into components—plasma, red blood cells, immunoglobulins, etc.—for specific uses.

War has often driven advances in medicine, and three twentieth-century wars—World War I (1914–1918), the Spanish Civil War (1936–1939), and World War II (1939–1945)—advanced blood transfusion. During World War I, doctors improved the storage of donated blood by adding sodium citrate, which kept it from clotting in the container.[13] They also learned to cross-match donor and recipient blood, preventing antibody reactions. In the Spanish Civil War, blood banks refrigerated blood for safe storage and registered blood donors and their blood types.[14]

Early in World War II, the English requested blood donations from the U.S. Between summer 1940 and February 1941, the Blood Plasma for Great Britain Project collected, processed, and shipped 15,000 pints of plasma in saline solution.[15] The American Red Cross used this urgent project to refine blood-bank procedures, and by December 1941, when the U.S. entered the war, they were well prepared to separate blood into components, freeze components, and keep everything anti-coagulated and sterile.[16] African-American surgeon Charles Drew, whose foundational work was key to the project's early success, resigned in protest against the unscientific practice of segregating donated blood by race, which the Red Cross finally discontinued in 1950.[17]

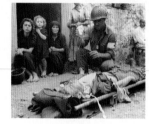

In wartime, emergency transfusions are given on the field or in makeshift facilities. Shown here is U.S. Private Roy Humphrey, wounded in Sicily during World War II.

Since then civilian blood banks have supported the progress of surgery, making open heart surgery and joint replacements possible, as well as long operations for cancer and trauma. Blood transfusions have saved many women who would otherwise have died in childbirth, and knowledge of incompatible blood type variants has saved many babies who did not match their mothers' types.

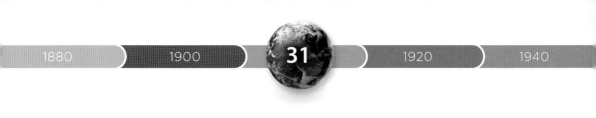
1905

Hormones and Endocrinology

At 17, Tanya Angus stood 5 feet 8 inches tall and looked beautiful on beaches and fashion runways. At 34 she would have stood 7 feet 2 inches tall if she hadn't been doubled over by pain, and she hated the mirror. Her jaw and forehead jutted, her voice was deep, and after two strokes her words came slowly. A "benign" tumor made her pituitary gland pump out human growth hormone (HGH), turning her into a giant.[1]

People joke about "hormone imbalance," but for Angus it was no joke. Too much HGH can cause you to outgrow clothes, furniture, and cars; you outgrow your own bones and circulatory system. Too little HGH can make you a pituitary dwarf, unable to reach ordinary household surfaces. Either way you lose your independence, having to depend on ordinary-sized people to function in a world that wasn't designed for you.

And HGH is just one of dozens of hormones released into the bloodstream by the thyroid, pancreas, and other glands in your endocrine system.[2] Hormones act throughout the body to regulate sleep, growth and development, metabolism, reproduction, and other biological functions. According to Ernest H. Starling—who coined the word "hormone" in 1905—they are "the chemical messengers which, speeding

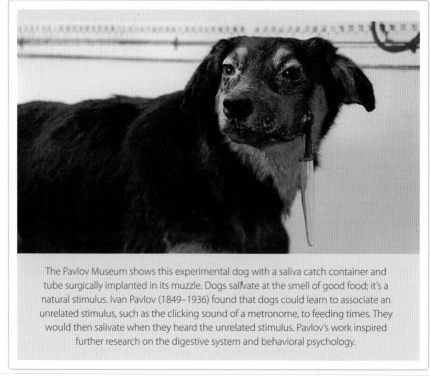

The Pavlov Museum shows this experimental dog with a saliva catch container and tube surgically implanted in its muzzle. Dogs salivate at the smell of good food; it's a natural stimulus. Ivan Pavlov (1849–1936) found that dogs could learn to associate an unrelated stimulus, such as the clicking sound of a metronome, to feeding times. They would then salivate when they heard the unrelated stimulus. Pavlov's work inspired further research on the digestive system and behavioral psychology.

from cell to cell along the blood stream, may coordinate the activities and growth of different parts of the body."[3]

Starling and William M. Bayliss discovered the first hormone on January 16, 1902. They were studying digestion—specifically, what makes the body secrete gastric juice and acid after eating. They knew saliva flowed in response to nerve impulses, and Pavlov's theory that other digestive processes were regulated by nerves was generally accepted. But in 1901, Leon Popielski ruled out most of the nerves that could have been responsible. So were pancreatic secretions controlled by local nerves in the gastrointestinal tract?[4]

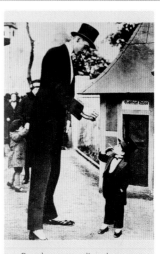

Rare hormone disorders can cause gigantism, dwarfism, and other conditions.

Bayliss observed that pancreatic secretion rose when partly digested food reached the small intestine. They experimented on an anesthetized dog, with a loop of its small intestine connected to the body only by its blood vessels. All the nerves had been severed. But even without nerves, when they introduced hydrochloric acid—an ingredient of that partly digested food—into the intestine, pancreatic secretion began. "Then it must be a chemical reflex," said Starling,[5] and they confirmed that hypothesis before the afternoon ended. They had discovered "secretin," the first hormone to be identified.

In 1905 John Sydney Edkins discovered another digestive hormone, gastrin. Starling announced that

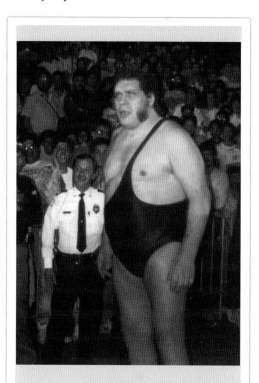

André the Giant was famous as a wrestler and actor, but like Tanya Angus and other pituitary giants, he suffered constant back pain.

"these so-called internal secretions" were regulated not by the central nervous system but by tiny amounts of "drug-like substances" released into the blood stream, where they evoked "an appropriate reaction in distant parts of the body."[6] Humoral regulation of bodily processes was a new theory that evoked an ancient one—"humoral" means "relating to the bodily fluids," including blood.

Pavlov held out for the nerve theory. He repeated Bayliss and Starling's work and got different results; they repeated his and got different results. When Pavlov's student Gleb V. Anrep met Bayliss and Starling in 1912, he found out why. The British dogs were anesthetized with morphine, and the Russian dogs had the acid in their stomach contents neutralized. Once these procedural differences were adjusted the researchers could replicate each other's results, and the discovery could be more widely accepted as legitimate.

A century later, scientists continue to research hormones. Although secretin was isolated in the 1960s and cloned in the 1990s, it still has secrets. More than 50 other hormones have been identified and studied, but their effects are subtle and their interactions complex, and there is much more to be learned.

La Mujer Barbuta

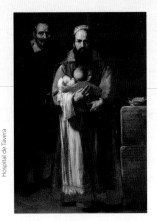

Hospital de Tavera

José de Ribera painted *Magdalena Ventura with Her Husband and Son* in 1631, when she was 52.

Magdalena Ventura was married and had three sons—and then, when she was 37, she sprouted a beard. Her hormone imbalance, called hyperandrogenism, was probably caused by a benign androgen-producing tumor in her ovary.[10] This portrait, painted 15 years after her unexpected development of male traits, raises questions. Was her beard that full from the very beginning? Did she actually have another child at the age of 51, or is the baby at her breast symbolic? But the image is a classic in endocrinology textbooks.

Female hyperandrogenism continues to be an issue to this day in the Olympics and other athletic competitions. Do women with higher than usual levels of male hormones have an unfair advantage against other female competitors? Should they be required to undergo testing to make sure they are truly female? The International Association of Athletics Federations suspended the policy of hormone and gender testing as of 2016 because there is not enough evidence to prove testosterone increases female athletic performance.[11]

The Pineal Gland

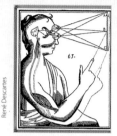

René Descartes

Philosopher René Descartes (1596–1650) was fascinated by anatomy but mostly wrong about it. He thought the pineal gland was the part of the brain where soul met body.

Philosophers and physicians alike have speculated about the pineal gland since ancient times. Could it be an inner "third eye," a sixth-chakra key to clairvoyance and meditation? Could it have something to do with medieval legends about the "stone of folly," something like a kidney stone that pressed on the brain and caused dementia? Could it truly be the physical seat of the human soul, as Descartes said?[7]

Almost every creature with a backbone also has some kind of pineal organ, which is almost invariably sensitive to light. Pineal organs help regulate seasonal migrations and breeding in birds and color changes and background adaptation in fish and amphibians.[8]

In humans the pineal gland appears to regulate wake-sleep cycles as well as daily and seasonal rhythms, largely through its secretion of a hormone called melatonin. Its potential usefulness in treating insomnia has made melatonin the most studied secretion of the pineal gland, but there are others. This gland may have important roles we don't yet understand in modulating different physiological processes.[9]

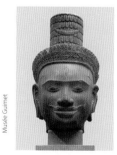

Musée Guimet

Madame Helena P. Blavatsky (1831–1891), founder of Theosophy, associated the pineal gland with the mystic "third eye."

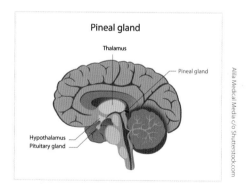

Allia Medical Media c/o Shutterstock.com

Tucked between the two hemispheres of the brain, the tiny pineal gland is shaped like a pine cone.

Serotonin: Not a Hormone

Hormones are not the body's only chemical messengers. Neurotransmitters also send messages from one part of the body to another; they help electricity flow between nerve cells. There are dozens of neurotransmitters—including amines, gases, peptides, amino acids, and purines—and we still have much to learn about them.

Probably the most famous one is serotonin. There's a popular belief that serotonin promotes well-being and prevents depression, but the real story is more complicated. It is true that many antidepressants work by preventing the re-uptake of serotonin that has been released by brain neurons, the result being that more serotonin is available. But does more serotonin in your brain make you happier? There's little or no evidence to prove this. The human brain is complex, with billions of neurons, and serotonin is only one neurotransmitter. There are more than one hundred which may or may not affect your feelings, moods, opinions, emotions, or imagination.

Some activities that increase serotonin do make people happier. Getting plenty of light boosts serotonin levels, and so does exercise. Do people feel happier when they have more serotonin, or do they produce more serotonin when they feel happy? It's an open question.[12]

But one popular myth can be exploded. Turkey and bananas contain tryptophan, and tryptophan helps produce serotonin—but tryptophan in your food does not produce serotonin in your brain. The evidence for turkey as an antidepressant is worse than sketchy. Could reports of well-being after turkey feasts be another example of the placebo effect?

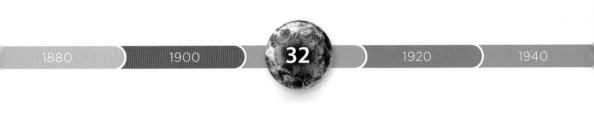
1907

Typhoid Mary Becomes the World's Most Notorious Cook

The cook did it. General Warren summered in Oyster Bay in 1907, and between August 27 and September 3, six of eleven people in his rented house caught typhoid fever. It wasn't the shellfish, the well, or the cesspool—but cook Mary Mallon had been newly hired on August 4. Sanitary engineer George Soper, arriving months later to investigate, immediately suspected her.[1]

She was long gone by then, but he traced her previous jobs and uncovered seven other household epidemics. Mallon was hired soon before each one and left soon afterward. Soper may have been the first to suspect her of causing the outbreaks; he had read the 1902 paper in which Robert Koch suggested that a "healthy carrier of infection" could spread typhoid fever.[2] He confronted Mallon in her latest kitchen and asked (diplomatically, he thought) for samples of her blood, urine, and feces. She took it badly and chased him out of the house with a carving fork. She was forcibly quarantined after Soper persuaded authorities at the New York City Health Department that she was "a living culture tube and chronic typhoid germ producer." She was held for three years, though she swore in court "that she had never had typhoid fever or caused it in others."[3] She was finally released after promising to stay out of kitchens, but soon she was cooking under a false name. It was how she made her living. Five years later she was identified when she caused another outbreak, recaptured, and quarantined for the rest of her life. How many typhoid cases did she cause? Soper counted fifty-three—three of them fatal. But if Mary knew she was a carrier, she never admitted it to the health authorities.

Typhoid fever is sneaky enough without adding the idea of a "healthy carrier." It's spread when food and beverages are contaminated by infected waste—even minute amounts from imperfectly washed hands. You wouldn't know when you were exposed, and a week or even three weeks later you would have a high fever, headache, and digestive symptoms.[4] How would you know what caused them?

In the 1840s, country doctor William Budd realized that typhoid disease was propagated through intestinal discharges; he said caregivers

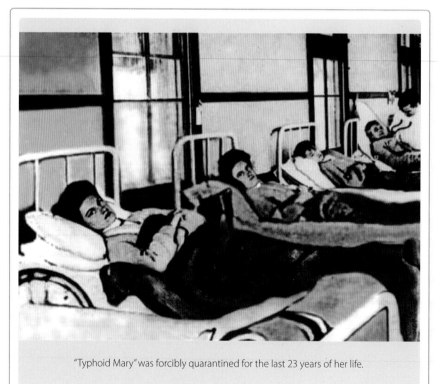

"Typhoid Mary" was forcibly quarantined for the last 23 years of her life.

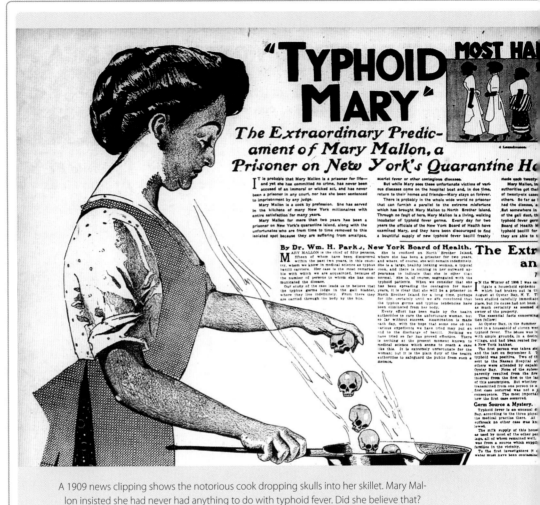

A 1909 news clipping shows the notorious cook dropping skulls into her skillet. Mary Mallon insisted she had never had anything to do with typhoid fever. Did she believe that?

The New York American

should not only wash their hands but flush drains frequently with powerful disinfectants.[5] In 1880, Karl Eberth described the bacillus we now call *Salmonella typhi*, and in 1884, Georg Gaffky was able to culture it.[6] Like cholera, typhoid fever became known as a "filth" disease, and the resulting stigma made it all the harder to trace. In a 1903 epidemic, doctors in Ithaca, New York, diagnosed middle- and upper-class patients with "grippe" instead of typhoid, even with positive tests for the lower-class disease.[7]

Meanwhile, systematic study of patients getting over typhoid confirmed Koch's 1902 concept of the healthy carrier. After acute typhoid, up to 5 percent of recovered patients excreted *S. typhi* for months or years. Moreover, "people with no history of typhoid" could also be carriers. In England, such a case was "Mr N.," who milked cows at five farms around Folkestone. Of 323 typhoid cases in the neighborhood between 1896 and 1909, 207 hit people who drank milk from a farm where Mr N was working at the time. In 1909, when he was finally tested, his stools did show *S. typhi*. He remembered an illness 30 years earlier, not bad enough to send him to bed, but involving "lassitude, loss of appetite, and general malaise"; could that have been typhoid?[8]

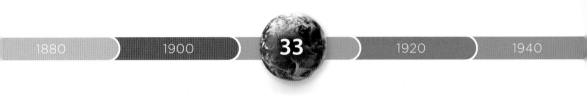
1909

Ehrlich's Magic Bullet and the Beginnings of Chemotherapy

Paul Ehrlich (1854–1915) had trouble passing examinations. The secondary school teachers who assigned an examination essay on "Life—a dream" may have expected poetic responses, but Ehrlich's ideas ran to science: dreams might simply be phosphorescence of the brain, he wrote. They let him pass,[1] and he got into medical school. "That is little Ehrlich," a professor told the great Robert Koch. "He is very good at staining, but he will never pass his examinations."[2] Yet of course he did complete medical school, and his 1878 dissertation was about histological staining—the dyeing of bodily tissues.

How did a medical student like Ehrlich come to experiment with fashionable new tints? Partly, it was timing. The first artificial dyes were developed in the 1850s, and they used coal tar, which Germany had in abundance. The German dye industry took off. Organic chemistry also got a boost, as the industry employed scientists to develop new dyes and scientists found new applications for both products and techniques. Researchers began staining tissues with coal tar dyes in the 1860s.[3] In 1873, an international recession pushed the big chemical companies toward diversification; some invested in medical research.[4]

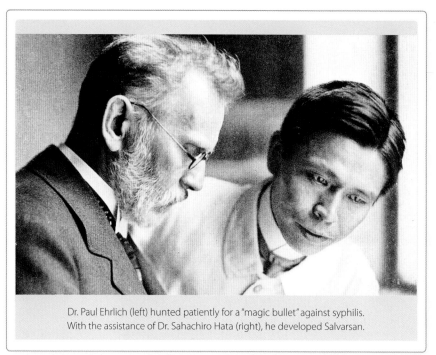

Hata Memorial Museum

Dr. Paul Ehrlich (left) hunted patiently for a "magic bullet" against syphilis. With the assistance of Dr. Sahachiro Hata (right), he developed Salvarsan.

Ehrlich first tried staining in 1873; he wanted a better view of how lead poisoning affected tissues.[5] In 1882, he put his skills in the service of Robert Koch. After hearing the master speak on the discovery of the tuberculosis bacillus, Ehrlich worked all night and presented Koch with a better staining process the very next day.[6]

Stains interested Ehrlich as more than visibility enhancers. Good dyes stuck to wool, silk, and other organic materials, but the same dye might color one fabric (or cell) and not another. There were different chemical reactions between dyes and textiles, Ehrlich thought, and similarly there must be different chemical reactions between medications and living organisms. The ideal drug would be a magic bullet. It would poison one organism—a pathogen—while not harming the pathogen's infected host. Drugs don't work if they aren't bound, he said.[7] He wanted a drug that would bind only to the pathogen. A British team had come close with "atoxyl," an arsenic compound that fought sleeping sickness. Unfortunately, while saving lives, atoxyl sometimes caused blindness.[8]

So Ehrlich and his team looked systematically for a drug that would cure sleeping sickness without major side effects. Ehrlich's ties to the pharmaceutical industry gave him essential resources. First the team synthesized hundreds of chemical structures, arsenic compounds more or less closely related to atoxyl. Then they screened them to see if they worked and were safe. This systematic approach was exemplary; it became standard for twentieth-century drug development.[9] But only Compound 418 worked against sleeping sickness, and it was less powerful than atoxyl.

Then Fritz Schaudinn and Erich Hoffmann discovered that syphilis was caused by the spirochete *Treponema pallidum*, a kind of bacteria much like the one that caused sleeping sickness. This discovery made it possible to detect asymptomatic syphilis with a blood test, but not to cure it. Hoffmann suggested that Ehrlich should try his arsenic compounds on it, and Ehrlich assigned the task to Sahachiro Hata, a new student and colleague who had worked with syphilis. Reassessing their compounds, they found that Compound 606 worked.[10]

Ehrlich was as systematic and careful about clinical trials as he had been about developing and screening the compounds. By the end of 1910, 65,000 doses of the drug had been given to more than 20,000 patients—an unprecedented trial.[11] Marketed as Salvarsan, it was not perfect. It had to be carefully manufactured to avoid explosions and carefully packaged to avoid oxidation and toxicity. Neosalvarsan (Compound 914) was more convenient and less toxic, but still not perfect. The drugs brought about

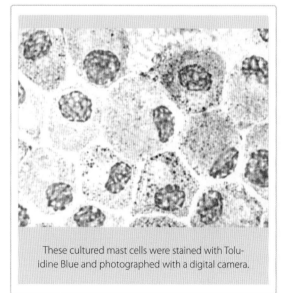

These cultured mast cells were stained with Toluidine Blue and photographed with a digital camera.

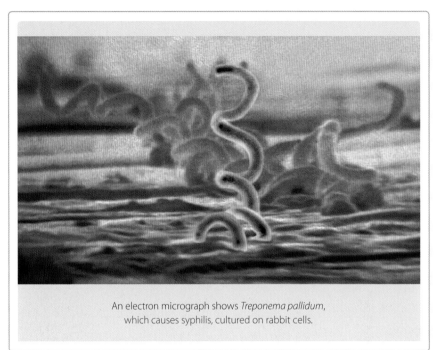

Centers for Disease Control and Prevention/Dr. David Cox

An electron micrograph shows *Treponema pallidum*,
which causes syphilis, cultured on rabbit cells.

some miraculous cures in the early stages of the disease, but could not touch late-stage syphilis. Demand was high until something better came along: antibiotics.[12]

Medicine and Artificial Dyes

Medicine and the dye industry have been connected for centuries. The alchemists sought the elixir of life—and on the side, they worked with dyers to make better colors for textiles.[13] Most colors were based on plants, insects, or shellfish.

Alchemy had given way to chemistry by 1856, when an 18-year-old chemist named William Henry Perkin invented the first synthetic dye. It was an accident. He was trying to synthesize quinine, an anti-malarial medication derived from a tree bark. One of his experiments yielded a black coal-tar precipitate, and when he tried dissolving it in alcohol, he got an amazing purple color. Perkin failed to make artificial quinine, but jump-starting the artificial dye industry made him rich.[14]

Syphilis: Somebody Else's Disease

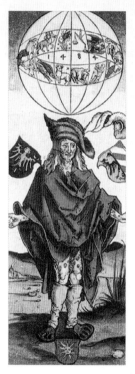

Illustration from a 1496 medical text. This ill-starred young man is pocked with what was then called the "French disease" or the "Great Pox."

When Europeans discovered the New World, they exposed Native Americans to smallpox and other lethal diseases (Chapter 11). In exchange, America may have given Europe syphilis, a sexually transmitted disease that the Old World quickly learned to dread.[15] The first European epidemic struck after France occupied Naples in 1495, so Italians called it the "French Disease." The French, however, called it the Spanish disease, the Russians called it Polish, and the Poles called it German.[16] They all knew foreign soldiers and sailors gave it to prostitutes, who gave it to new clients. They soon found there was no cure.

Its name comes from a 1530 poem by Girolamo Fracastoro (Chapter 10) in which a shepherd boy named Syphilus defies the god Apollo and falls victim to a spotted disease.[17] Fracastoro's poem described the symptoms and recommended treatment with guaiacum or mercury. Paracelsus (1493–1541) knew guaiacum was ineffective, and although he recommended mercury as a salve or a fumigant, he warned against inhaling it; mercury is poison.[18] Despite his warnings, it remained a popular treatment until the early twentieth century, along with many other quack remedies, tonics, and patent medicines.[19]

Only in the twentieth century did syphilis begin to yield, first to Salvarsan, and after World War II to a more convenient drug with fewer side effects: penicillin.[20] Today it infects millions worldwide, but it can be cured.

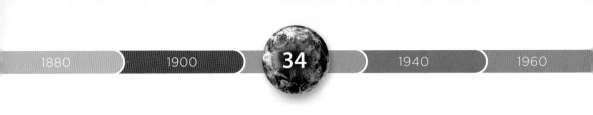
1922

Controlling Diabetes

Leonard Thompson was dying. He was only fourteen, but he had been diabetic for three years, and in 1922 diabetes was a death sentence.[1] Egyptian doctors could diagnose it in 1500 BC[2]; shamans and Vedic physicians knew that the sweet urine of diabetics would attract ants.[3] By 1889, scientists were zeroing in on what caused it: Oskar Minkowski and Joseph von Mering found that removing a dog's pancreas left it with diabetes,[4] but removing only part of the pancreas just gave it indigestion.

The pancreas is a gland that releases digestive enzymes.[5] Scientists already understood the role of these juices, the "external secretions" of the pancreas. After 1889 they hypothesized that the pancreas also emitted an "internal secretion" to keep the body's sugar levels normal. Maybe this mysterious substance came from the islets of Langerhans,[6] clumps of cells described in 1869 by Paul Langerhans.

Guessing the substance existed was easier than using it in treatment. While hundreds of researchers struggled to develop a diabetes therapy using pancreatic secretions,[7] doctors and drug manufacturers tried everything from java plums, whortleberries, and opium to arsenic.[8] A Chicago researcher, Ernest Lyman Scott, achieved promising results in 1912 by injecting diabetic dogs with pancreatic extract, but there were side effects; Scott's mentors advised him to abandon that line of research.[9]

A decade later, Leonard Thompson's doctors still had no better treatment for him than a starvation diet. Skeletal at 65 pounds, the teen was slipping into a diabetic coma when his desperate father allowed researchers from the University of Toronto to try one more therapy. Leonard was the first human to be saved by insulin injections; he lived 13 more years.

Leonard's diabetes was not cured; even now, diabetes is not cured. But insulin controlled the disease much better than starvation, so Leonard and many patients after him were restored to active life. Word of this breakthrough spread, and diabetics flocked to Toronto for healing. Lead researchers J.R.R. Macleod (1876–1935) and Frederick Banting (1891–1941) were

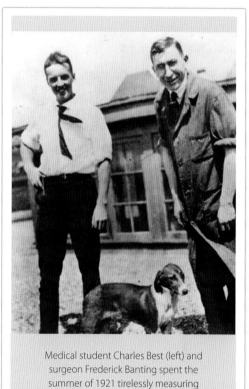

Medical student Charles Best (left) and surgeon Frederick Banting spent the summer of 1921 tirelessly measuring sugar in the blood and urine of dogs as they tested antidiabetic substances.

Library and Archives Canada

jointly awarded the Nobel Prize in Physiology or Medicine the very next year—although they didn't go to Oslo to accept their honor.[10] The two disliked being in the same room with each other.[11]

It seems remarkable that such ill-assorted colleagues accomplished so much. The impetus came from Banting, a farm boy whose medical education had been interrupted by World War I. After serving in the Canadian Army Medical Corps (1915–19) and doing his surgical residency,[12] he set up a very slow practice.

One night, a journal article gave him an idea: maybe the reason nobody had isolated the internal secretion of the pancreas was that its powerful digestive juices were getting in the way. Maybe he could ligate the ducts—tie them off—so most of the pancreas would atrophy, leaving the islets of Langerhans. Maybe he could find an effective treatment for diabetes.[13]

The project required lab resources. In November 1920, Banting introduced himself to Macleod, a physiology professor with an international reputation. Macleod knew the work of Scott and others who had tried what Banting proposed; he saw Banting as naive and ill-prepared.

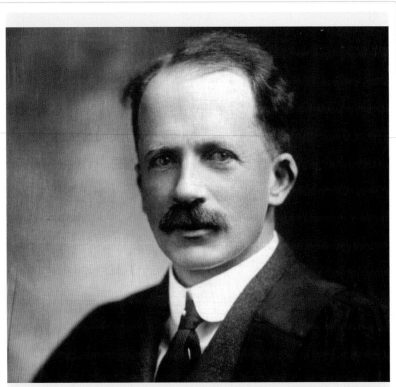

University of Toronto

Professor J.R.R. Macleod was skeptical when Frederick Banting, brash and naive, demanded his support for a research project others had tried unsuccessfully. In the end Macleod's knowledge, administrative assistance, and support were as necessary as Banting's inspiration and stubborn energy to their success.

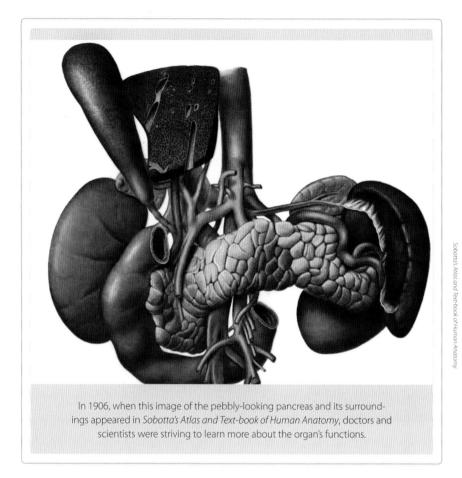

In 1906, when this image of the pebbly-looking pancreas and its surroundings appeared in *Sobotta's Atlas and Text-book of Human Anatomy*, doctors and scientists were striving to learn more about the organ's functions.

Sobotta's Atlas and Text-book of Human Anatomy

On the other hand, Banting was a surgeon, and techniques for measuring blood sugar had improved since Scott's experiments.

Macleod supported Banting's research with expert advice, experimental facilities, and the assistance of medical student Charles Best. Later John Collip joined the team, adding "only" what "any well-trained biochemist could be expected to contribute."[14] Though he came to blows with Collip at least once,[15] Banting needed that expertise.

Banting, who thought Macleod stole credit for work that wasn't his, gave half his Nobel money to Best; Macleod gave half of his to Collip. The four gave their patent money to the University of Toronto, to support research. The enemies' legacy was a gift to humanity.

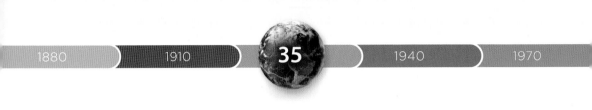
1929

Fleming's Dirty Dishes
Give Us Penicillin

A tidier man than Scottish bacteriologist Alexander Fleming (1881–1955) would never have discovered penicillin. He would have hustled petri dishes off to be sterilized after use.[1] But after a 1928 vacation, Fleming looked at mold in a petri dish and did a double-take. The mold was a common nuisance.[2] It could have wafted upstairs from the lab of a fungus expert, who called it *Penicillium rubrum*.[3] What interested Fleming was the clear zone around the mold, where his staphylococcus culture was dying off. Anything that could kill staph deserved attention.

Fleming worked with bacteriologist Almroth Wright, whose fierce insistence on typhoid inoculation had reduced British deaths in World War I (1914–1918). Wright believed in prevention; once disease struck, doctors had too few resources. Endocarditis, meningitis, and pneumonia were commonly fatal, and women still died of puerperal fever.[4] Even prevention could backfire. Wounds infected with staph could force amputations, but irrigating wounds with antiseptics might actually kill the body's protective white cells along with invading germs.[5] Wright preferred to boost what we now call the immune system.

Others were looking for drugs that could be injected or swallowed, to fight disease systemically throughout the body. Pasteur reported "microbial antagonism" as early as 1877, raising hopes that benign microbes could be harnessed to fight disease. The idea seemed promising, and investigators achieved modest success with drugs based on bacteria and fungi, applied to localized infections.[6] In 1921 Fleming himself discovered lysozyme, a bacteria-inhibiting substance in snot, tears, and other body fluids—a natural defense against illness. But Fleming and Wright found that bacteria could potentially evolve into deadly killers that resisted lysozyme.[7]

Now Fleming tested his new discovery on different microbes. It didn't affect influenza or typhoid fever germs, but it blocked streptococcus, staphylococcus, and others.[8] Yet it wasn't toxic to rabbits or human blood cells. Fleming had never found a substance that would attack infection without sapping the body's own defenses. He was excited.

But his 1929 report on penicillin didn't lead straight to the Antibiotic Revolution. The mold was hard to isolate and purify; biochemist Harold Raistrick said in 1935 that "the production of penicillin for therapeutic purposes" was "almost impossible."[9] Meanwhile a German team announced Prontosil, which worked inside the body to treat bacterial infections. A sulfa drug made from coal-tar dye, it turned researchers' attention to sulfonomides.

During World War II (1939–1945) a team

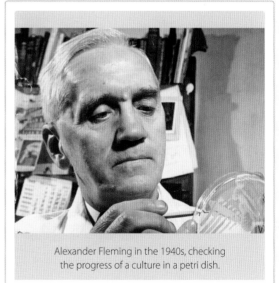

Alexander Fleming in the 1940s, checking the progress of a culture in a petri dish.

Ministry of Information

at Oxford, headed by Howard Walter Florey (1898–1968) and Ernst Boris Chain (1906–1979), succeeded in purifying a sample of Fleming's original mold and found it protected lab mice against fatal infections by staph, strep, and *Clostridium septique*.[10] Clinical trials in early

1941 saved the lives of three out of six dying humans as well. Sadly, the Oxford group learned that treatment had to be continued after apparent recovery,[11] and they could not mass-produce penicillin in their small research lab.

They needed help from government and industry, but Britain was under siege. Florey visited the U.S. and rallied support for mass production of penicillin, helped by hundreds of researchers in 39 major academic and industrial laboratories in both countries.[12] In 1941, the U.S. lacked enough penicillin to treat a single patient; by September 1943, there was enough for the U.S. armed forces and their allies.

Fleming took this photograph of his mold-infested petri dish. Did the large *Penicillium* mold colony at the top of this dish just keep colonies of staphylococci from growing in the surrounding clear zone, or did it actively kill them?

Penicillin was terrific for war morale; nations that could beat staph, strep, and gangrene could surely beat the Germans. Fleming, more available to the press than Florey and Chain, became a celebrity. In 1945, the three men shared the Nobel Prize in Physiology or Medicine. But Fleming kept warning against overusing antibiotics. If you need them, he said, take them until any microbial infection is gone. Do not let a strain of germs acquire resistance and then escape. A cautious Scot, he foresaw a messy future.

Molds and Folk Medicine

Fleming was not the first to have discovered that molds could be good treatments for infection. The ancients reportedly used them on wounds and skin diseases, and they show up as ingredients in folk medicine throughout the world. Thousands of years ago the Egyptians used moldy bread, and the Chinese used moldy soy beans.[13] The Talmud used kutach bavli or chamka, a mash of moldy corn soaked in water or date wine. English and Irish herbalists grew therapeutic molds on bread, oranges, ham, potatoes, and even shoe leather, and Australian aboriginals used molds taken from eucalyptus trees.[14] The British surgeon Joseph Lister noted that samples of urine contaminated with mold didn't allow bacteria to grow.[15] And a French medical student named Ernest Duchesne successfully tested a substance from mold that inhibited bacterial growth in animals, but he died at an early age in 1912 and was never credited with this important discovery.[16]

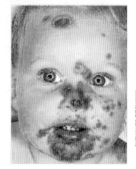

Wikimedia Commons

This little boy's face is marred by impetigo, a skin infection that English herbalists used to treat with mold poultices.

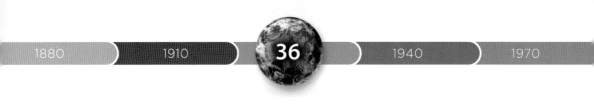
1930

Psychosurgery

Not every discovery looks good in hindsight. The prefrontal lobotomy, once hailed as a medical breakthrough, is remembered as a brutal mistake. A "surgical operation involving an incision into the prefrontal lobe to mitigate severe symptoms of serious mental illnesses,"[1] it was developed in the 1930s by Portuguese neurologist António Egas Moniz and earned him a Nobel Prize in 1949. He recommended it only as a last resort.

But lobotomy was an option Lou Dully chose for her 12-year-old stepson Howard. "He objects to going to bed," she told Dr. Walter Freeman. "He does a good deal of daydreaming and when asked about it he says 'I don't know.' He turns the room's lights on when there is broad sunlight outside."[2] So in 1960, Howard became one of Freeman's youngest patients.

Dully survived, though he struggled in life. He was luckier than patients who died or were severely disabled like President John F. Kennedy's sister Rosemary.[3] A Canadian researcher followed up 119 lobotomy patients and found that some were helped after drugs and talk therapy failed. On the other hand, 39 percent did not recover enough to live outside an institution. And 91 percent had "personality defects,"

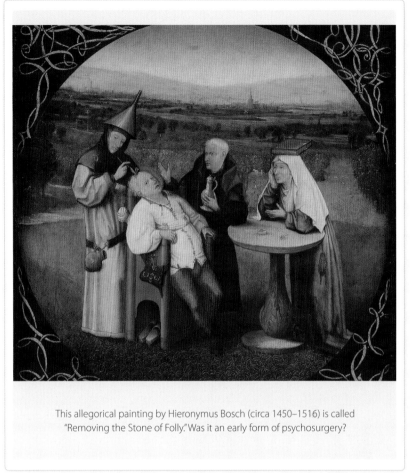

This allegorical painting by Hieronymus Bosch (circa 1450–1516) is called "Removing the Stone of Folly." Was it an early form of psychosurgery?

Prado Museum

although it was impossible to tell if those defects were because of the operation.[4] Moniz was right: lobotomy should have been a last resort.

He conceived of the prefrontal lobotomy in 1935 after hearing a conference presentation about a raging chimpanzee calmed by brain surgery.[5] Moniz hypothesized that insane humans had abnormal neural connections originating from the frontal lobes, and severing them would relieve obsessions and depression.[6] The operation involved drilling burr holes in the skull[7] to access the frontal lobe. Moniz had discovered a location in the brain where his operation could ease personality disorder without blocking vital functions. As a neuroanatomist, Moniz knew which areas of the brain were responsible for particular cerebral functions, like the famous Broca's area of the temporal lobe, which was known to be responsible for speech. He knew that the frontal lobe did not control any vital functions.

How could this have seemed like a good idea? Insanity was looking more and more like a disease of the body. Three illnesses (dementia, neurosyphilis, and thyroid deficiency) were associated with abnormal brain anatomy,[8] suggesting a physical cause, but no drugs had been found to cure them. And cures were needed. In 1937 an estimated 450,000 patients were institutionalized in 477 U.S. asylums, and nearly half the stays lasted at least five years. Neurosyphilis victims, traumatized World War I veterans, and schizophrenics crowded together in often substandard placements.[9] To keep the violent from harming themselves or others, institutions typically resorted to straightjackets, padded rooms, and harsh restraints.[10] Families struggled to pay.

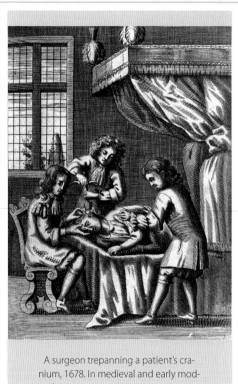

Wellcome Images

A surgeon trepanning a patient's cranium, 1678. In medieval and early modern Europe, trepanation was used to treat skull injuries, seizures, and other ailments.

Lobotomy was a risky proposition—even now we know all too little about the structure of the brain—but it could make inmates more manageable. By 1950 lobotomies had been performed on about 20,000 Americans, many by Freeman, who considered the operation successful if it left patients functioning at "the level of a domestic invalid or household pet."[11]

Freeman was more interested in social function than mental health. His goal was to "apply a simple operation to as many patients as possible in order to get them out of the hospital," and he was proud to be called the "Henry Ford of Psychiatry."[12] In 1946 he introduced the transorbital icepick lobotomy, using an ordinary household tool to reach the brain through the eye socket without drilling burr holes. Knocking out the patient with an electric shock instead of anesthesia and gently tapping the instrument through the bone with a hammer,[13] Freeman operated on 22 patients in 135 minutes.[14]

Frontal lobotomies fell out of favor with the introduction of new antipsychotic drugs in the 1950s, and neurosurgery developed new techniques such as deep brain stimulation.[15] Even if mental illnesses are indeed caused by malfunctions of the brain, lobotomy is too crude a treatment. Today's neuroscientists continue to search for better answers.

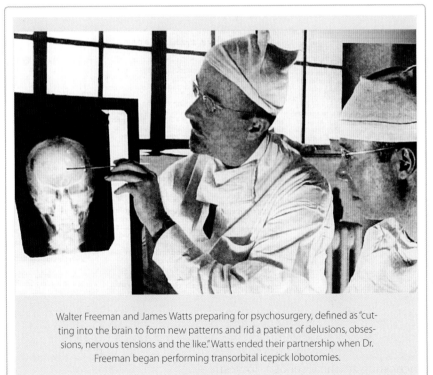

Walter Freeman and James Watts preparing for psychosurgery, defined as "cutting into the brain to form new patterns and rid a patient of delusions, obsessions, nervous tensions and the like." Watts ended their partnership when Dr. Freeman began performing transorbital icepick lobotomies.

Harris A. Ewing

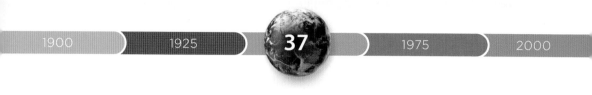
1939 – 1955

Rat Poison for a U.S. President

In February 1933, Ed Carlson drove 190 miles through a howling blizzard, with the temperature near zero, from his farm to the University of Wisconsin. He was desperate. Five of his cows had bled to death since December; now blood was oozing from his bull's nose. The veterinarian diagnosed "sweet clover disease," but Carlson hoped the vet was wrong. Sweet clover had never bothered his cattle before, and it was all he had to feed them now.

He arrived at the Wisconsin Agricultural Experiment Station with a can of blood that wouldn't clot, 100 pounds of spoiled sweet clover, and a dead heifer—only to find the state veterinarian's office closed. Looking for help, he stumbled into a biochemistry lab where Dr. Karl Paul Link was working on a related project.[1] Coumarin, which causes that sweet clover smell, actually tastes bitter. Link and his team were assigned to breed a clover with less coumarin and more cow appeal.[2]

Carlson's visit gave them a new focus. They agreed with the vet: Carlson's cattle needed fresh hay and blood transfusions. They felt terrible about it. People couldn't afford such things in the depths of the Depression. "Vat vill he find ven he gets home?" raged a German lab worker after Carlson left. "MORE DEAD COWS!!"[3] It was a tragedy worth preventing. From February 1933 to June 1939 the lab worked to identify the anticoagulant—the component of sweet clover that kept blood from clotting.

Veterinarians had been studying the problem for years. In the winter of 1921–1922, cattle in the upper Midwest and Canada had succumbed to a mysterious new disease with mortality rates of 80 percent or more.[4] Healthy cows would suddenly develop hemorrhages under the skin and in the muscles, dying all too quickly. The cattle showed no signs of infection. They had no fevers; their swellings were not inflamed. Researchers could find no bacteria, nor could they transfer the disease from sick to healthy animals under controlled conditions. But the affected cattle had eaten sweet clover hay, and the 1921 harvest season had been wet. Was the disease caused by moldy clover?[5] After hand-sorting moldy and mold-free plants from a haystack of sweet clover, they found that only moldy plants caused the disease. In 1929 L.M. Roderick found that moldy clover destroyed a blood clotting

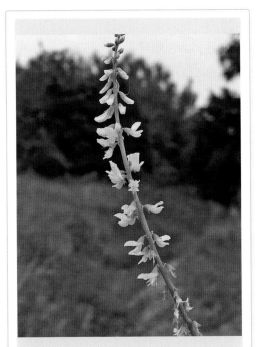

Sweet clover does well on dry soil, and early twentieth-century farmers were urged to use it for building soil and feeding cattle. But in the winter of 1921–22, farmers went bankrupt as cattle began bleeding to death.

H. Zell/Wikimedia Commons

factor called prothrombin, but not all molded hay was dangerous; the same mold would cause hemorrhagic disease when grown on certain clovers but not on other plants.

In 1939 Link's Ph.D. student Harold Campbell found the anticoagulant, dicoumarol. By 1940 the team discovered its chemical structure and synthesized it in the lab. The puzzle was finally solved: sweet

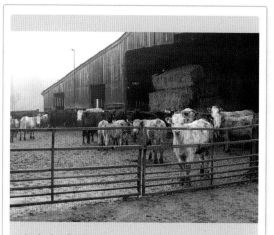

In the harsh Wisconsin winter of 1933, Ed Carlson had to give his cattle stored feed—but the sweet clover hay had gone bad, and the cattle started to die.

Richard Webb/Wikimedia Commons

clover became poisonous when some of its coumarin content reacted with certain fungi that grew on the hay in wet weather.[6]

This discovery was useful in ways Ed Carlson never could have imagined. The anticoagulant that killed his cows would be used to treat humans at risk for thrombosis— blood clotting in the wrong places.[7] Thrombosis can cause heart attacks and strokes, so a good blood thinner saves lives.

The Mayo Clinic reported promising trials in 1941,[8] but in practice dicoumarol had safety issues. To keep clotting times within normal ranges, labs had to standardize prothrombin activity assays. Also, though Link concluded that Vitamin K was a reliable antidote to dicoumarol in case of overdose, others were initially skeptical.[9]

Link changed course and developed a more potent coumarin compound that he called warfarin (for Wisconsin Alumni Research Foundation) for use as a rat poison. Clinicians concluded that warfarin might be safe for humans in 1951, when an attempted warfarin suicide was saved

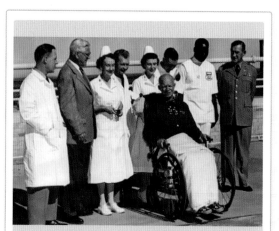

President Dwight D. Eisenhower's 1955 heart attack did not prevent his reelection in 1956. He was treated with warfarin.

Dwight D. Eisenhower Presidential Library

by Vitamin K.[10] By 1955, the rat poison was considered safe enough to treat President Dwight D. Eisenhower after his massive heart attack. As Link put it, discovery meant "breaking the bonds of the usual patterns of thought."[11]

Vitamin K

While Link and his collaborators were developing coumarin-based blood thinners, researchers on both sides of the Atlantic were studying the other side of the problem: what helps blood clot or coagulate? In Denmark, Henrik Dam found that chicks on a very low-fat diet began to hemorrhage easily, and their blood clotted slowly. At first he suspected scurvy, caused by a vitamin C deficiency (Chapter 12), but continued experimentation showed that there was another vitamin at play. By 1938 Dam was calling it the coagulation vitamin, or Vitamin K. In 1939, American investigator E.

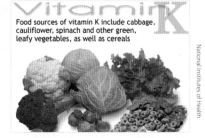

Food sources of vitamin K include cabbage, cauliflower, spinach and other green, leafy vegetables, as well as cereals

National Institutes of Health

Link and his fellow researchers found that nutrition influenced the effects of dicoumarol. Rats that got enough Vitamin K in their diets were harder to kill.

A. Doisy successfully prepared two different K vitamins—K_1 from lucerne seed and K_2 from fish meal—and determined the vitamin's chemical structure, which he was able to synthesize in his lab. The 1943 Nobel Prize in Physiology or Medicine was awarded jointly to Dam and Doisy.[12]

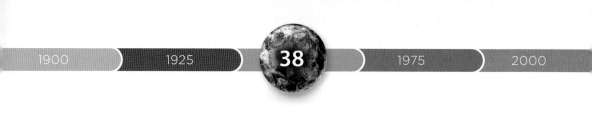
1944

Discovering DNA

Oswald Avery (1877–1955), sometimes called the most deserving researcher never to win a Nobel Prize, had a long attention span. He was hired in 1913 for pneumonia research at the Rockefeller Institute for Medical Research and officially retired in 1943, but kept right on working there until 1948.[3] He was pulled away from the task only once, to help investigate the great influenza pandemic of 1918.[4] Yet he is remembered today not for pneumonia research but for his discovery that DNA carries genes—a finding so controversial in the 1940s that it may have prevented his winning a Nobel Prize.[5]

Pneumonia was a leading cause of death in the early twentieth century, and Avery and his colleagues were expected to develop more effective serum treatments for it. They needed to type the invading organisms, create rapid diagnostic tests, and work out reliable methods of producing serum in horses and standardizing it so all doses would be the same.[6] But the pneumococcus bacteria that presumably caused pneumonia were hard to pin down. They could not be found in every case of the disease, but showed up in some apparently healthy individuals. And there were different strains of pneumococcus, and the team tried to develop a serum for each.

"Smooth" strains had capsules that helped them slide past the body's immune defenses; "rough" strains lacked capsules and were more easily caught by antibodies.[7] Smooth strains made people sicker, and it was harder to develop sera for them because typical lab preparations could change the shape of those capsules, making them impossible for the immune system to recognize.[8] The team's study of these capsules was interrupted by World War I.[9]

In 1928, British scientist Frederick Griffith (1879–1941) exploded a bombshell. Lab manipulations could make pneumococcus bacteria *change* their immunological characteristics![10] Working on a vaccine, Griffith injected mice with two strains. Smooth III-S bacteria were virulent, but could be made harmless by boiling; rough II-R bacteria were not virulent. But when Griffith mixed heat-killed III-S with live II-R bacteria, the mixture was virulent enough to kill mice. In their blood he found living III-S. Could the II-R bacteria have been transformed by something in the heat-killed III-S bacteria?[11]

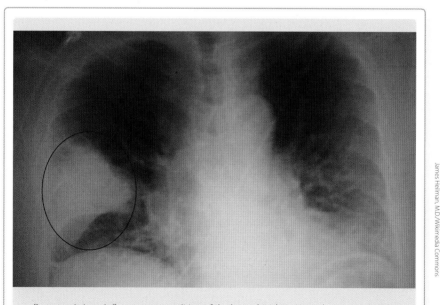

Pneumonia is an inflammatory condition of the lung; this chest X-ray shows a case in the middle lobe of the right lung. Bacterial infection is one possible cause of pneumonia.

Avery was reluctant to believe that pneumococci could undergo transmissible hereditary changes, but other scientists—including a Rockefeller Institute colleague—reproduced Griffith's results. So Avery investigated. He went a step beyond Griffith's results and discovered the substance responsible for the hereditary alteration.[12] It was not a protein, as scientists had expected. It was deoxyribonucleic acid, or DNA.

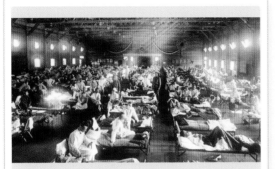

Army hospitals took in dozens of patients daily at the height of the 1918–19 influenza pandemic.[1] Camp hospitals in the U.S., like this one at Camp Funston, Kansas, were overwhelmed. Most deaths were caused by bacterial pneumonia invading the lungs along pathways cleared by the flu virus.[2]

Scientists knew DNA existed, but nobody recognized its importance. Friedrich Miescher discovered it in 1871 while studying pus,[13] and in the 1880s it was called nucleic acid.[14] In the 1890s, researchers established that chromosomes, made up of nucleic acids and proteins, play a major role in the growth and replacement of living cells. Interest in Mendel's work on hereditary traits (Chapter 21) revived, and in 1902 Walter Sutton observed that the behavior of chromosomes during cell division could explain Mendel's laws.[15]

Excitement built through the first half of the twentieth century, as scientists learned more about chromosomes, began to map the locations of genes relative to one another, and tested theories on carefully bred sea urchins, maize, and microbial fungi. Some even irradiated fruit flies,

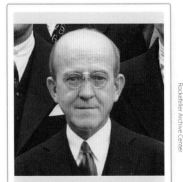

Oswald Avery (1877–1955) skipped medical conferences and award ceremonies to spend most of his time in the laboratory, studying the lifecycle of pneumococcus bacteria.

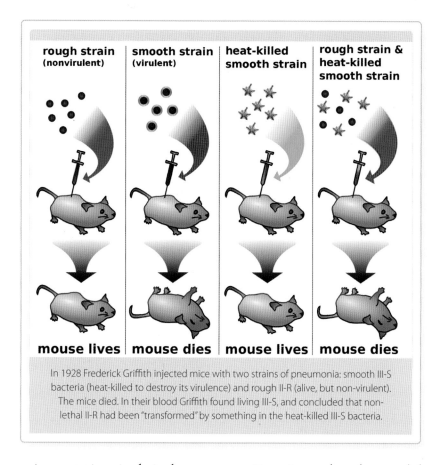

rough strain (nonvirulent)	smooth strain (virulent)	heat-killed smooth strain	rough strain & heat-killed smooth strain
mouse lives	mouse dies	mouse lives	mouse dies

In 1928 Frederick Griffith injected mice with two strains of pneumonia: smooth III-S bacteria (heat-killed to destroy its virulence) and rough II-R (alive, but non-virulent). The mice died. In their blood Griffith found living III-S, and concluded that non-lethal II-R had been "transformed" by something in the heat-killed III-S bacteria.

causing mutations in their chromosomes. Experimental work around the world proved it: something about chromosomes governed heredity.[16]

But surely not DNA. The scientific community was as reluctant to accept Avery's findings as he had been to accept Griffith's. Many still thought proteins must carry the genetic information, since they were larger and more complex than DNA; it was even suggested that Avery's DNA preparations must have been contaminated by protein. It took years of cumulative experimentation by many investigators to persuade the skeptics. Avery was nominated for a Nobel 44 times, but was never awarded one.[17]

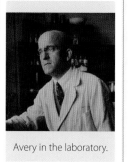

Avery in the laboratory.

Watson and Crick Discover the Structure of DNA

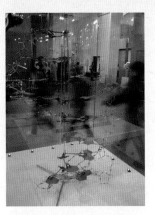

Watson and Crick built this model of the DNA molecule, shown in the National Science Museum of London.

By the early 1950s, interest in DNA was intense. American James D. Watson felt that he and his partner, Briton Francis H.C. Crick, were in a race to discover the structure of the DNA molecule before Linus Pauling or Rosalind E. Franklin and their teams. Franklin, an X-ray crystallographer, made useful images of the molecule; her colleague Maurice Wilson showed the images to Watson and Crick, and Max Perutz passed them Franklin's interpretation of the images without her knowledge. Did their unauthorized access to Franklin's work help Watson and Crick beat her to the discovery? The question is still debated.

The model they proposed was a double helix—two long molecules with backbones of phosphate and sugar residues, wound around each. Ribbed along the backbones were four nucleobases: adenine (A), cytosine (C), guanine (G), and thymine (T). Adenine from one molecule pairs with thymine from the other, and guanine pairs with cytosine.[18] Coded in the order of these four bases are the genetic instructions that tell an organism how to grow, by encoding blueprints for proteins—the molecular machinery of the cell.

Watson and Crick published their model in 1953. "We wish to propose a structure for . . . D.N.A.," they wrote. "This structure has novel features which are of considerable biological

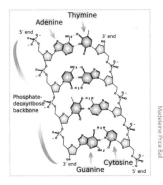

The four nucleobases in DNA encode genetic instructions.

interest."[19] This was a famous understatement. In a letter to his son, Crick wrote, "We think we have found the basic copying mechanism by which life comes from life. You can understand that we are very excited."[20]

(Continued on next page)

(Continued from previous page)

The model explains at least four essential questions: how genetic material is replicated, how specific traits are preserved, how genes can mutate, and how information is coded in the DNA molecule.[21] Not everyone accepted it right away, but Watson and Crick, along with Franklin's colleague Maurice Wilkins, were awarded the 1962 Nobel Prize in Physiology or Medicine for their discovery. Franklin died in 1958, of cancer.

Since 1953, scientists have learned more about the mechanism of DNA replication, developed a theory of the genetic code, and made strides in gene technology and biochemical gene analysis. Discovery is an ongoing process.

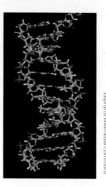

Zephyris/Wikimedia Commons

This image of a DNA segment shows the bases as horizontal links between the spiraling backbones.

The Human Genome Project

Human cells normally have 23 pairs of chromosomes. Each human gets 23 chromosomes from each parent, and each chromosome contains tens of millions of nucleic acid pairs. Even the smallest human chromosome, #21, contains almost 47 million nucleic acid pairs.

The Human Genome Project was an international scientific project that began in 1984 and was completed in 2003.[22] The object of the project was to "map" all 23 human chromosomes by deciphering the sequence of nucleic acids in human DNA strands. This was an enormous undertaking, because more than 3 billion pairs of nucleic acids had to be sequenced using methods capable of reading only a thousand or so bases at a time from random segments of the genome, meaning that after sequencing there was a computational mapping effort akin to assembling 23 giant DNA jigsaw puzzles. The potential benefits of the project are profound. It is already enabling researchers to develop highly effective diagnostic tools, to understand a patient's health needs based on his genetic make-up, and to design genetically customized treatments for disease.

Genetic Counseling

Now doctors can have patients' DNA tested to see if they carry genetic disorders that predispose them to getting certain diseases. One of the more popular genetic tests offered is the test for mutations in the BRCA1 and BRCA2 genes.[23] This test is performed for women who have a family history of breast cancer and ovarian cancer in several close female relatives. If a woman has a mutant BRCA1 allele, she carries a 55 to 65 percent chance of developing breast cancer by age 70, compared with a 12 percent chance in the general population. If she carries a BRCA2 allele, her chance of breast cancer by age 70 is 45 percent. BRCA1 and BRCA2 mutations also elevate risk for ovarian cancer from 1.3 to 39 percent and approximately 14 percent, respectively.[24] Based on information from genetic testing, some women choose surgery to prevent disease before it occurs.

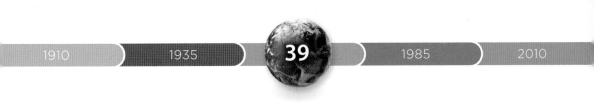
1945

A Miracle Drug in the Sewage

"I had that cure before he had!" cried an 82-year-old Irish woman, reading about Fleming's discovery of penicillin.[1] She was well known for her cures, and she grew a greenish mold on oranges to mix in a salve for skin lesions or administer orally. How had she learned to do this? It was probably a folk remedy, handed down through generations, like the purple foxglove Dr. Withering (Chapter 13) heard about in 1775.

The development of modern pharmaceuticals, however, is beyond the resources of folk healers. It was beyond the resources of Fleming, who ran a laboratory in a research hospital; and it was beyond the resources of Giuseppe Brotzu (1895–1976), who ran the three-century-old University of Cagliari during World War II. Brotzu made Cagliari the first Italian university to give its students free health care, and he built up its schools of medicine and mining. But when he personally made a discovery to rival Fleming's, he could not get support for its development.[2]

The war had ended in defeat for Italy and its allies, Germany and Japan. Cagliari, heavily bombed, had been half deserted; now it was struggling to recover. Maybe 1945 was not the ideal time to request help developing a new antibiotic.

Yet Brotzu, a good epidemiologist and hygienist before he was made head of the university, found time to investigate a public health

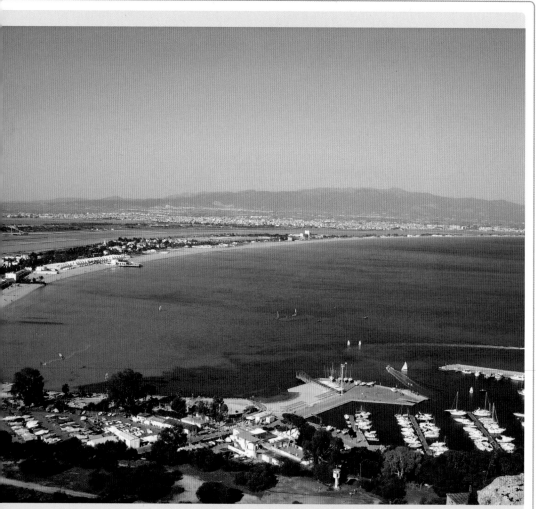

Cagliari, capital of Sardinia. In the 1930s, the island's coasts were breeding grounds for malaria. Giuseppe Brotzu, as a hygienist and a politician, spearheaded public health initiatives.

question. He had mapped the flow of *Salmonella typhi* through Cagliari's sewer system, which emptied into the ocean at Su Siccu.[3] Mussel fishing was forbidden there,[4] yet students swam nearby. Why weren't they coming down with typhoid fever? Brotzu knew how Fleming had discovered penicillin, and he hypothesized that a similar antibiotic organism might be inhibiting typhoid around the sewer outlet.[5] And on a sultry July day, he and his assistant, Professor Antonio Spanedda, found it: an "ochre-colored colony with shades of pink," suppressing typhoid and several other germs.[6]

Brotzu was able to seed colonies from the sewage area on agar plates, incubate them at room temperature, and test them against typhoid and other bacteria. He determined that the *Cephalosporium acremonium* fungus had great antibiotic potential. When he tested it directly on bacterial skin infections, sores and infections healed without side effects; it also cured fevers, including typhoid.[7]

Without funding or resources to develop the drug further in Italy, Brotzu self-published his results, "in the hope that other better-equipped institutes may be able to

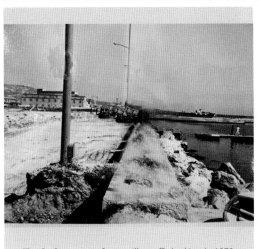

The Su Siccu waterfront, still scruffy-looking in 1970.

make greater progress in the selection of the fungus and in the culture preparation and extraction of the antibiotic."[8] At the same time, he practiced international scientific networking, inviting British medical officer Blythe Brooke to use university resources in his off hours.[9] Brooke helped get Brotzu's paper and a fungus sample to Sir Howard Florey's Oxford group, the team that had developed Fleming's penicillin.

Sir Edward Abraham, who spent years developing the fungus, later asked Brotzu about his journal article. How often was *Works of the Institute of Hygiene of Cagliari* published? Brotzu smiled. There had been only one issue, but there would be a second "if he made another discovery of comparable importance."[10] But if discovery was ever fully accomplished in one flash of insight, that was no longer true in the 1940s. It took

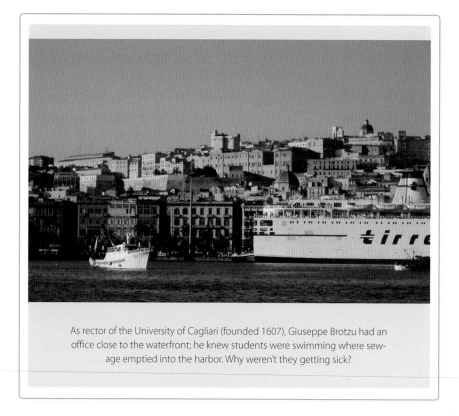

As rector of the University of Cagliari (founded 1607), Giuseppe Brotzu had an office close to the waterfront; he knew students were swimming where sewage emptied into the harbor. Why weren't they getting sick?

Abraham and his team until 1962 to develop *Cephalosporin* C, the parent molecule of a new generation of antibiotics based on Brotzu's C. *acremonium* fungus.[11]

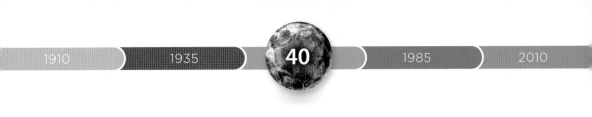

1945

Saving Lives with Sausage Casings, Washing Machines, and Juice Cans

Willem Kolff's patient was coming out of her coma. "Can you hear me?" he asked.

"I am going to divorce my husband!" she announced.[1]

Amazing! Kolff (1911–2009) had invented the rolling drum artificial kidney, and since 1943 he had used it on sixteen other patients. Some had survived for hours or even days. One revived enough to ask for a newspaper. But this one, the seventeenth patient, was going to survive long enough to divorce her husband. The artificial kidney had saved its first life.

Kolff had been working on the problem of dialysis for years. As a hospital resident in 1938, he witnessed a slow death from kidney failure. The patient was young and "could have been saved," said a senior physician, "if only 20 g of urea could have been removed from his blood every day."[2] Urea is a waste material that leaves the body in urine—but when kidneys fail, it builds up in the patient's system.[3]

Could there be a substitute for the kidneys? Kolff plunged into the medical literature. Dialysis—the clinical purification of blood—was something researchers had long hoped to achieve. An 1861 study of the way liquids pass through membranes made it seem possible, and other researchers had tried dialysis with animals as early as 1914.[4]

Kolff and a collaborator, biochemist Robert Brinkman, began work on an artificial kidney, or dialysis machine, in the town of Kampen, in the Netherlands. In some ways, 1938 was a good time. They would need a good blood thinner, and the anticoagulant heparin was newly available. They would need a membrane to filter waste from the blood, and cellophane, patented in 1912, was ideal; it was being used for sau-sage casings. Kolff filled a length of sausage cas-ing with blood and urea; when he shook it in a saline bath for a few minutes, almost all the urea passed through the cellophane, leav-ing purified blood.[5] By 1939, Kolff and Brink-man had developed pro-totypes that worked in the laboratory, although they were not ready for human trials.[6]

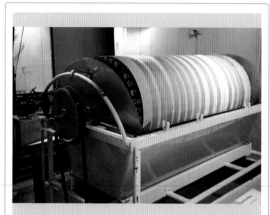

Rob Koopman/Wikimedia Commons

Willem Kolff developed this rotating-drum "artificial kidney," or dialysis machine, during World War II. Eight were made, and four were stored in different parts of town to avoid losing them all in the bombing.

But 1939 was a bad time. Research slowed when Germany invaded the Netherlands in 1940. Kolff worked with the Dutch resistance; he hid Jews from the Nazis.[7] But he also continued work on the artificial kidney. Eight of them were built, and four were scattered around town so that not all would be lost in a bomb attack. It was 1945 by the time one of those machines saved Patient Seventeen.

During the Korean War (1950 – 1953), dialysis reduced Ameri-can deaths from kidney problems by 40 percent. But Kolff, who moved to America in 1950, was troubled to see the cost of dialysis rising with its popularity. Would only the rich be able to afford it? In 1955, with

Austrian researcher Bruno Watschinger, he developed a disposable "twin-coil" kidney for the mass market,[8] using cheap materials: cellophane tubing, juice cans, and window screening. The whole thing fit in a gallon-sized can. In the 1960s, he and his team developed a "washing machine artificial kidney" for home use,[9] and in 1967 he came up with a protective sleeve to guard home patients against infection and trauma where shunts connected their arms or legs to the dialysis machine. The sleeve could be made for about $1.50.[10] In 1970, the team developed a wearable artificial kidney—a vest unit that allowed patients in need of regular dialysis to live more active lives.[11]Kolff's work on kidney dialysis prepared him to make other advances. He and his teams worked on kidney transplants; on the heart and lung bypass machines that make many surgeries possible; and on the first transplantable artificial heart (TAH). He succeeded in giving millions of patients extra years of independent, productive life—and he wasn't above using sausage casings to do it.

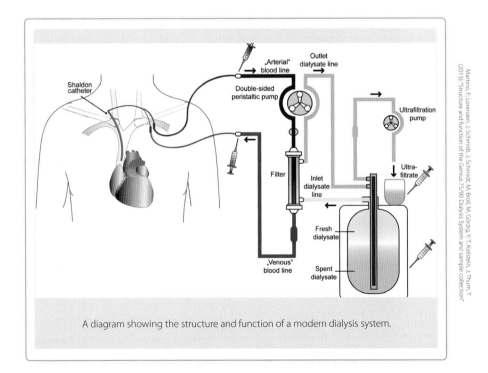

A diagram showing the structure and function of a modern dialysis system.

Martino, F, Lorenzen, J, Schmidt, J, Schmidt, M, Broll, M, Görzig, Y, T, Kielstein, J, Thum, T (2013): "Structure and function of the Genius 75/90 Dialysis System and sample collection".

The Iron Lung

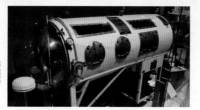

Until the 1950s, patients unable to breathe on their own were commonly placed in negative pressure ventilators, or "iron lungs," with only their heads outside. When air pressure inside the sealed tank was reduced, the patient's chest would rise, and air from the room would be pulled into the lungs.

The artificial kidney moved an essential bodily function outside the body, but it wasn't the only large, clunky machine to do that. In the 1950s, at the height of the polio epidemic, rows of iron lungs lined big city polio wards. Nurses sometimes called them "yellow caskets,"[13] but they held life, not death. Victims too paralyzed to breathe lay there with only their heads sticking out. When the air pressure inside was reduced, a patient's chest rose, pulling air into the lungs; when air pressure was increased, the chest dropped and air flowed back into the room.

The machines, imagined in the seventeenth century and built in the nineteenth, had been improved by the 1950s. A bed slid in and out of the cylinder, and portholes let nurses reach in as needed.[14] Most of the helpless and inaccessible patients were children. Nurses did their best to liven things up; one brought in peashooters so patients could build vital capacity by trying to hit the ceiling.[15] Happily, most patients did escape in a week or so, but at least two lived sixty years in iron lungs.[16]

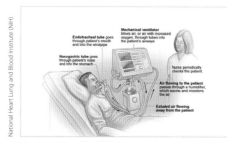

Medical ventilators developed since the 1950s make it easier for patients to move and caregivers to attend to their needs. The ventilator pushes warm, moist air (or air with increased oxygen) to the patient.

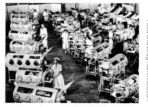

In a ward at Rancho Los Amigos Hospital, dozens of polio victims lie in iron lungs. Motor-powered bellows generate heat as they pump air, making a rhythmic "whoosh-whoosh-whoosh" sound that comforts patients; nurses swelter.[12]

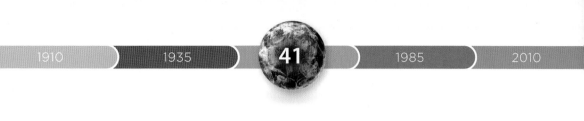
1951

Frankenstein and the Heart Machines

Outside, crazy weather batters the tower; thunder rolls. Inside, mysterious electrical devices spark and sizzle. The mad scientist and his assistant uncover a monstrous form and hoist it, strapped to a gurney, to an opening in the ceiling. Lightning sheets over it. As they winch it back to the floor, its hand flexes. "It's alive!" cries Dr. Frankenstein.[1]

Deliciously terrified children watched all this in darkened movie theaters. The 1931 film was in black and white and its special effects were amateurish by today's standards, but it starred marquee actor Boris Karloff and made a creative impact on at least two boys: Jean Rosenbaum and Earl Bakken.[2] Rosenbaum nearly dropped out of medical school after seeing a young woman die; her heart stopped beating and she could not be revived. But recalling the old film, he wondered— could an electric current revive a stopped heart?[3] In 1951, he invented a device to prevent such untimely deaths: a cardiac pacemaker.

What does a pacemaker do? Its most basic function is to monitor the heart's electrical rhythm from beat to beat. If the beat falters, the pacemaker will send a short low-voltage pulse to stimulate the heart and restore its rhythm so it can continue to pump blood.

Rosenbaum was not the first to invent such a thing. In 1928, Australian Mark Lidwell stimulated the heart of a stillborn infant for ten

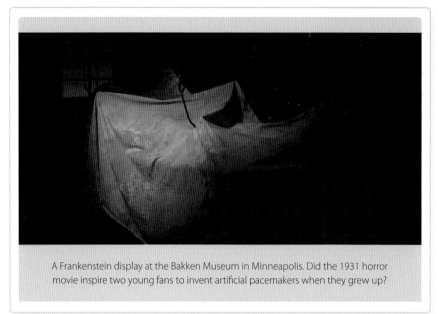

J. Bizzie

A Frankenstein display at the Bakken Museum in Minneapolis. Did the 1931 horror movie inspire two young fans to invent artificial pacemakers when they grew up?

minutes; the heart began beating, and the baby lived. Lidwell's machine plugged into a wall socket. In 1932, American physiologist Albert Hyman invented a pacemaker "powered by a spring-wound hand-cranked motor,"[4] but got bad press for it. People thought he was interfering with nature, like Frankenstein.

Rosenbaum, with colleague Darwood Hansen, worked for two years to make his "cardiac stimulator" portable, affordable, easy to operate and repair, quick to apply in emergencies, and safe "for both patient and physician."[5] Still, they had trouble getting permission for clinical trials before finally being granted the opportunity to demonstrate the device on a patient whose heart had stopped for three minutes. They revived the patient, making medical history. Rosenbaum went on to become a psychiatrist, prolific author, and aerobics instructor.[6]

Meanwhile, young engineer Earl Bakken helped found a repair business called Medtronic; he specialized in fixing hospital equipment. Hospitals kept hearts going with large machines plugged into the walls, and when a 1957 power outage caused a baby's death, surgeon Walton Lillehei asked Bakken to find a better solution. Bakken dug out a 1956 *Popular Electronics* article about a transistorized metronome—a device for measuring musical rhythms—and quickly adapted it to monitor and maintain heartbeats instead. Bakken's pacemaker—the first partly implantable electrical device in the history of medicine—went into production in 1958.[7]

Partial implantation increases risk of infection, so one innovation led to others. In October 1958, Swedish doctors gave 43-year-old Arne Larsson the first-ever implanted pacemaker. It worked for only a few hours; the second lasted about a week. But the team persisted, and by the time Larsson died—at the age of 86—he had used more than 20 pacemakers.[8]

An accidental 1958 discovery by Buffalo engineer Wilson Greatbatch led to better implantable devices. While working on an oscillator, he grabbed a wrong-size resistor, and his machine began to oscillate atypically. Normally that's bad, but Greatbatch recognized the rhythm of this oscillation—just right for a human pulse. Soon he had patented a new pacemaker and licensed it to Medtronic. He went on to found his own company and develop an improved battery.

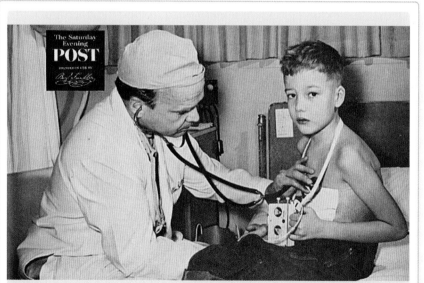

Dr. C. Walton Lillehei inspects a patient's Medtronic pacemaker. Earl Bakken developed the device in 1957, just weeks after Lillehei asked for it.

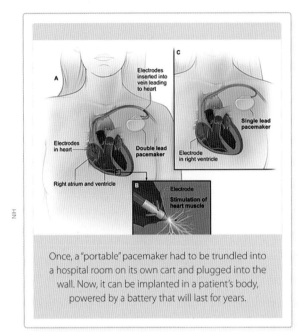

Once, a "portable" pacemaker had to be trundled into a hospital room on its own cart and plugged into the wall. Now, it can be implanted in a patient's body, powered by a battery that will last for years.

NIH

Millions of pacemakers have been implanted since 1960, and the devices continue to develop. New tweaks aim not just to keep patients alive, but to improve their health and quality of life. Pacemakers with microprocessors can record and store events, helping physicians with diagnoses. Tied to the internet, they can deliver powerfully flexible therapy[9] and raise questions about privacy.

Alas, Poor Yorick!

What good does a cardiac pacemaker do in a plastic skeleton without a heart? At best, it's a teaching device. Yorick, the bionic skeleton created by FDA engineer Ed Mueller, used to make guest appearances at schools to show off all his implants: "a cranial plate, silicone nose, carbon tooth root, inter-ocular lens, cochlear implant, heart valve, artificial heart, cardiac pacemaker, infusion port, vascular grafts, urinary sphincter prosthesis, artificial patella, bone plate, artificial tendons, bone growth stimulator, and artificial hip, knee, elbow, and finger joints."[12] Since his 2003 retirement, Yorick hangs out in the Smithsonian's Museum of American history.

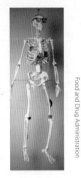

Food and Drug Administration

Yorick, the FDA's mascot skeleton until 2003, wore devices tested and approved by the agency.

Before Pacemakers: "I Sing the Body Electric!"

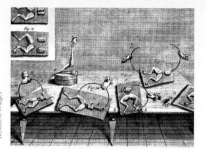

In 1791, Luigi Galvani published the results of many experiments showing the effects of electricity on dead frogs.

Pacemakers, defibrillators, and other devices work because our tissues—and especially our hearts—respond to electrical signals from our nerves. Luigi Galvani discovered that touching their nerves with an electric arc would make dead frog legs jump; his 1791 publication told the world that electricity was an inherent part of organic tissue. The French Revolution (1789–99) produced many human cadavers, enabling scientists to establish that electricity ran through humans as well as frogs.[10] Mary Shelley was aware of the science when she wrote *Frankenstein* in 1816. It made her nervous.

But instead of patching together corpses to make a monster, nineteenth-century researchers invented things like the electrocardiogram (EKG). Physiologist August Desiré Waller, who demonstrated it in 1887, thought the EKG was unlikely "to find any very extensive use in the hospital."[11] Why would anybody want a moment-by-moment electronic record of the heart's action? But from 1892 on, Willem Einthoven developed and refined the tool. It measures weak electrical signals from the heart and traces the pattern of heart waves onto a monitor or a strip of paper. EKG information tells hospital personnel when to use an emergency defibrillator, which interrupts the random twitching and restarts the normal heartbeat with a brief electric shock. By 1924 the invention's usefulness was clear, and Einthoven won a Nobel Prize.

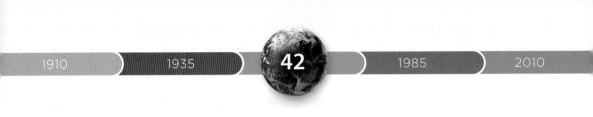
1967

Baruch Blumberg Discovers a Cancer-Causing Virus

D r. Baruch S. Blumberg (1925–2011) modeled his life of science and adventure on the careers of nineteenth-century naturalists.[1] Charles Darwin traveled the world, observed nature, and arrived at a new understanding of evolution. Blumberg traveled the world, observed diverse human populations, and discovered a cancer-causing virus, hepatitis B. By getting it removed from blood supplies and helping to develop a vaccine against it, he saved millions of lives.[2]

Blumberg did not set out to discover the cause of viral hepatitis, or liver inflammation. Working at the National Institutes of Health until 1964 and then at the Institute for Cancer Research in Philadelphia, he and his team were researching the inherited differences reflected in people's serum proteins.[3] They were checking samples from patients who had received many transfusions, looking for antibodies acquired with blood, when in 1963 they discovered the Australia antigen (Au)—so called because the only match they found for it at first was in the blood of an Australian aborigine. (An antigen is an infectious agent that causes an immune response when introduced into a person or other organism.)

From that discovery they followed an unexpected path, hypothesis by hypothesis, to a destination Blumberg couldn't have predicted.

As a medical student Blumberg had worked for a few months in Surinam, where he saw that people from diverse ethnic groups responded very differently to infectious agents.[4] Later, as a Ph.D. student at Oxford, he met Anthony Allison, discoverer of the link between sickle-cell genes and malaria resistance (Chapter 21). Allison introduced Blumberg to the concept of polymorphisms, genetic variations that can affect how populations respond to disease. On a trip to Nigeria, they collected blood specimens and studied inherited polymorphisms of the serum proteins of milk and hemoglobin. Blumberg loved the people and the research. He was hooked.

Blumberg collected more than 300,000 blood samples[5] in his travels and systematically catalogued them for use in the study of polymorphisms and inherited susceptibility to

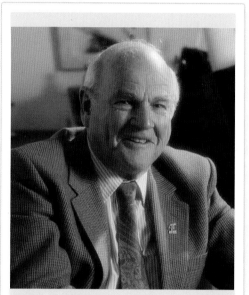

Dr. Baruch Blumberg in 1999, when he was named the first director of NASA's Astrobiology Institute, founded to study the origins, evolution, distribution, and future of life in the universe—a good mission for a curious scientist with a taste for adventure.

NASA/Tom Trower

disease. With this resource, the 1963 team soon found that Au was common in Micronesia, Vietnam, and Taiwan as well as Australia. In the U.S. it was rare, but showed up more often in patients with leukemia.[6] Blumberg looked at several hypotheses. Were Au and a susceptibility to leukemia both inherited? Did leukemia cause Au? Was Au related to a virus that caused leukemia?

Au did seem to run in families, but it also turned up in the blood of a patient with acute hepatitis and in others who had received blood transfusions. Blumberg hypothesized that Au was associated with liver disease. In 1966 this hypothesis was strengthened when a repeat test of one of their own patients showed a change from Au negative to positive—just as he developed hepatitis. In 1967 the team's first laboratory technician also developed hepatitis and tested her own blood. She too had become Au positive.[7]

It had been suggested in the 1950s that viral hepatitis might cause cirrhosis and cancer of the liver, but there was no test available then to identify the viral agent.[8] Could Au be the agent that caused viral hepatitis? Blumberg's hypotheses were independently confirmed by researchers in other parts of the world, and using electron microscopy, Blumberg's team localized the Au particle in the liver cells of hepatitis patients.[9] They warned the hospitals they worked with not to use donor blood with Au, and the rate of hepatitis after transfusions fell.[10]

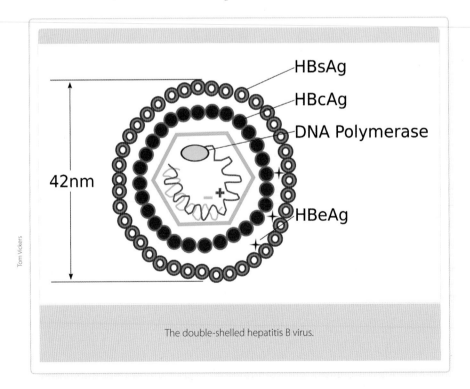

The double-shelled hepatitis B virus.

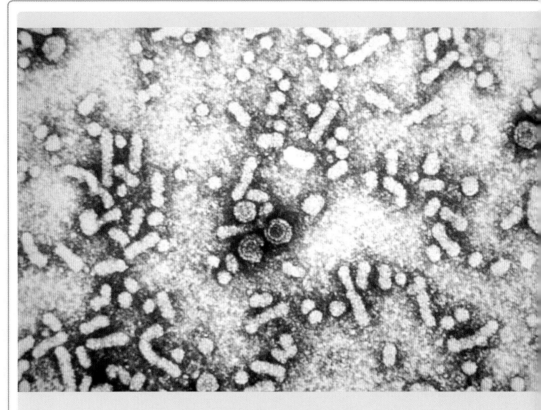

Centers for Disease Control and Prevention

Hepatitis B virions (also called Dane particles) are the circular, double-ringed objects in this electron micrograph image.

We now know Blumberg's Australia antigen as hepatitis B or HBV, one of several viruses that attack the liver. It can be carried by apparently healthy people and is often passed from mothers to children around the time of birth.[11] More than 80 percent of primary liver cancers are caused by chronic hepatitis.[12] Blumberg worked with colleague Irving Millman to develop a vaccine, and in 1981 the FDA approved it, the first cancer prevention vaccine to be successfully developed and marketed.[13] Blumberg won a Nobel Prize in Physiology or Medicine in 1976, and kept reminding scientists that basic research—just asking questions and following clues—can lead to useful if unexpected results.

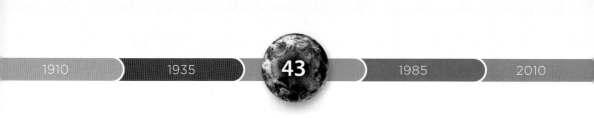
1967

The First Heart Transplant

On December 3, 1967, South African surgeon Christiaan Barnard became an international celebrity when he successfully transplanted the heart of a traffic victim into a 55-year-old man.[3] The man survived 18 days with heavy doses of drugs and radiation to suppress his immune system and prevent his body from rejecting its new heart. Unfortunately, this left him open to infection, and he died of double pneumonia.[4]

An 18-day survival after the first human heart transplant seemed hopeful. Dogs lived an average seven to thirty days with donor hearts.[5] Human kidney transplants had worked in identical and fraternal twins, but as of 1963 only five non-twins had survived more than six months with transplanted kidneys.[6] But Barnard's second patient lived more than nineteen months,[7] and hopes soared. By December 1968, 100 heart transplants had been made—some of them to recipients whose first transplants failed.[8]

Physicians had tried to transplant human tissue since the early 1800s with little success; even skin grafts were rejected. To help World War II burn victims, Peter Medawar studied the problem.[9] He and his colleagues found that after rejecting a donor's skin graft, a patient would reject later grafts from the same donor even faster. They demonstrated

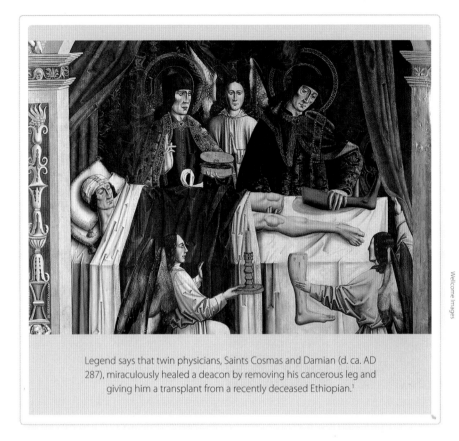

Legend says that twin physicians, Saints Cosmas and Damian (d. ca. AD 287), miraculously healed a deacon by removing his cancerous leg and giving him a transplant from a recently deceased Ethiopian.[1]

Wellcome Images

that rejection was an immune response, a host versus graft (HVG) reaction.[10] Like transfused blood (Chapter 30) and snake venom (Chapter 25), almost all cells transplanted from another individual can act as antigens. The recipient's immune system makes antibodies to fight off the donor's foreign antigens.

Given these findings, doctors hoped to prevent transplant rejection by turning off the immune system. They experimented with various techniques on animals and tried the more promising ones on clinical patients. One approach was total body X-ray treatment[11] to shut off the bone marrow, where immune cells are formed, but this did not boost patient survival rates much.[12]

Then immunologists tried using drugs along with or instead of radiation. Both dogs and humans were better able to accept kidney transplants after receiving anti-rejection drugs. Clinicians found they could reverse kidney rejection with high-dose steroid injections.[13] Steroids, like radiation, shut down the recipients' immune systems, and patients developed tolerance to their donated kidneys.

It turned out that immunological tolerance can be acquired. In 1953, Medawar and his colleagues Rupert Billingham and Leslie Brent brought it about in unborn or newborn lab mice.[14] They inoculated white blood cells from one strain of mouse (the donor strain) into another strain near the time of birth. As recipient mice matured, their immune systems accepted skin and tissue from the donor strain, although they rejected all other strains but their own. In 1960 Medawar and Macfarlane Burnet shared the Nobel Prize in Physiology or Medicine for discovering acquired immunological tolerance.[15]

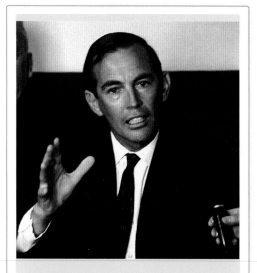

Mario De Biasi/Mondadori Publishers

Celebrity surgeon Christiaan Barnard. After his first human heart transplant, Barnard felt media coverage damaged professional friendships, inspired copycat transplants by ill-prepared teams, exploited morbid public interest, and undermined trust in hospitals' confidentiality procedures.[2]

Successful transplants still depend on close tissue matches. Much as blood is typed by its ABO factors (Chapter 30), organs and other tissues are typed by the human leukocyte antigen (HLA) system.[16]

Today, tens of thousands of patients worldwide are living with donated organs, and many more are on waiting lists to receive compatible hearts, kidneys, livers, lungs, and pancreases.[17] Damaged bones, tendons, corneas, and skin are frequently replaced by grafted tissue from donors. Transplants extend life and improve its quality, but we still have much to learn.

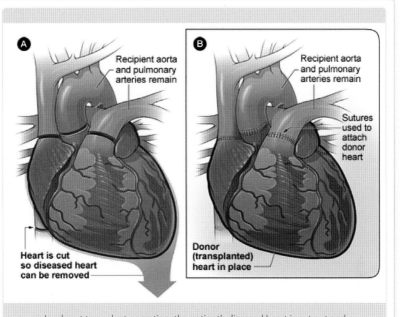

In a heart transplant operation, the patient's diseased heart is cut out and removed; a donor's healthy heart is then sutured to the patient's arteries and veins.

Ethical Issues in Transplantation

Media coverage of the early heart transplants raised serious moral, ethical, and religious issues. *Newsweek* quoted the first recipient as saying, "I am a new Frankenstein," and went on to speculate about how doctors would play God in an era of transplantation.[18]

To start with, the moment of death had to be redefined. It was not necessarily the moment a heart stopped beating; even without defibrillators, pacemakers, and heart-lung machines, patients were often resuscitated.[19] The ideal organ donor would be very recently dead, from some cause that wouldn't affect the health of the donated organ. In 1971, Finland adopted brain death—the complete and irreversible loss of brain function—as its legal definition of death.[20]

Decisions had to be made about who would receive transplants. There could never be enough organs to save all the patients with end-stage organ failure. In the beginning, selection was a matter of luck: Dr. Barnard had a brain-dead woman with a healthy heart, a dying man with no other hope, and resources to keep both heart and recipient alive through surgery.

(Continued on next page)

(Continued from previous page)

Now there are criteria for both donors and recipients; not everybody is eligible. But who should decide, and how?

The cost of a transplant is enormous. In 2011, the average ranged from $262,000 for a single kidney to more than $1,148,000 for a heart-lung transplant.[21] Who should pay for transplants, and how? Are the costs justified when many more lives could be saved at less expense? The cost of oral rehydration therapy, for instance, is about 10 cents per packet, and ORT could save 90 percent of the children who die of diarrhea each year. Is saving one kidney transplant patient more important than giving ORT to over 2.6 million children?

And who owns a transplanted organ? After Dr. Barnard's second heart transplant, the donor's wife asked to have the heart back once the recipient was done with it. A spiritualist said her late husband needed it; he wasn't resting peacefully without it.[22]

Microchimerism and Transplant Surgery

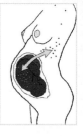

In 1992, Dr. Thomas Starzl discovered that white blood cells from donors were still found in the blood and tissues of humans who had undergone successful transplant surgery three to twenty-nine years before.[23] The presence of two types of white blood cells in organ recipients is called microchimerism. Microchimerism also occurs during pregnancy, when cells from the baby cross over into the mother's circulation.

Microchimerism is frequently found in transplant recipients who develop tolerance to their transplanted organs. It shows that there is a dynamic equilibrium between the resident immune system of the host and the imported immune cells that

There is two-way traffic of immune cells between the mother and fetus.

came with the donor transplant. This phenomenon is most common in liver transplant patients, perhaps because the liver contains many immune cells that can migrate from the organ to the recipient's lymphatic tissue. Understanding this dynamic equilibrium between donor and recipient has allowed doctors to use less toxic doses of anti-rejection medication once the recipient has developed tolerance to the transplant.

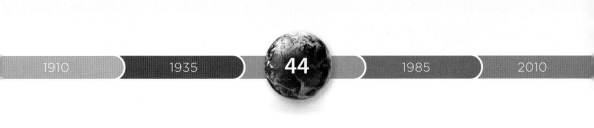
1972

A Magic Bullet from Ancient Chinese Medicine

In 1969, 38-year-old Tu Youyou was asked to head a secret research group, part of Project 523. The honor brought hardship; her husband had been banished, and now Tu had to travel, leaving her four-year-old child in a nursery.[1] But the work she did at such personal cost has saved millions of lives.

The 1960s were hard in China. During the Cultural Revolution (1966–1976) many intellectuals were accused of capitalist sympathies and sent to detention camps for "re-education." At the same time, scientists were needed. China was backing North Vietnam in its war against capitalist America, and the Vietnamese needed Chinese help against disease. Drug-resistant malaria was killing as many troops as enemy gunfire.[2]

Project 523 was a military secret. It involved more than 500 scientists in about 60 Chinese laboratories, and the short-term goal was to treat malaria on the battlefield. Looking farther ahead, project scientists searched for new antimalarial drugs from traditional Chinese medicine.[3] This was consistent with Chinese leader Mao Zedong's public health strategy, which called for the "complete unification of Chinese

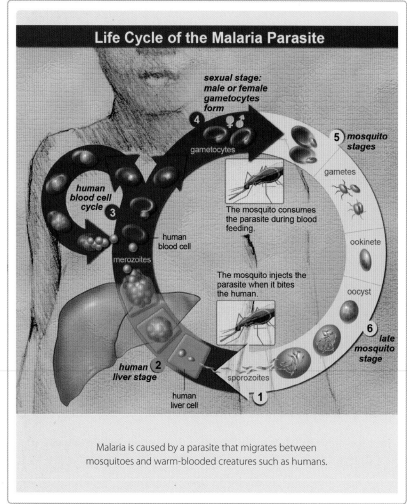

Malaria is caused by a parasite that migrates between mosquitoes and warm-blooded creatures such as humans.

medicine."[4] Using the best of modern science and ancient recipes, Mao hoped to impress the world and meet China's medical needs.

With training in both Western and Chinese medicine,[5] Tu Youyou was well qualified to help. Her team investigated more than 2,000 herb preparations and picked 640 for further study. They made more than 380 extracts from about 200 promising herbs. Finally, they tried artemisia. Known as wormwood or mugwort in English and qinghao in Chinese, artemisia had been used in folk medicine for centuries. It had been used against fever, and malaria causes desperate fevers. Artemisia seemed promising.

The team got an artemisia extract to inhibit the malaria parasite in mice, but then they had trouble repeating the experiment. Tu combed the literature for clues, and found only one reference to qinghao as a malaria treatment. Ge Hong (283–343) advised, "A handful of qinghao immersed with 2 liters of water, wring out the juice and drink it all."[6] Tu had a sudden insight: maybe, by boiling artemisia to make an extract, the team had destroyed its antimalarial components. She switched to a lower-temperature extraction method using ether.[7]

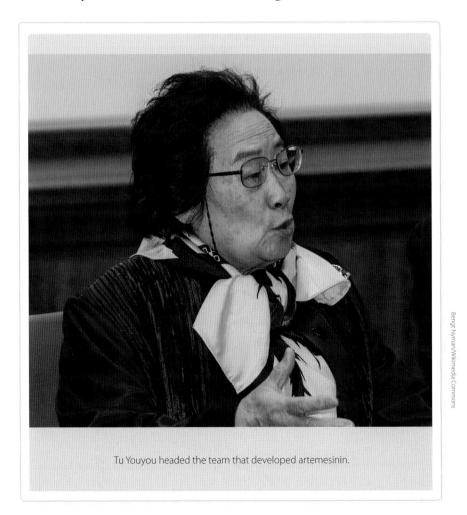

Tu Youyou headed the team that developed artemesinin.

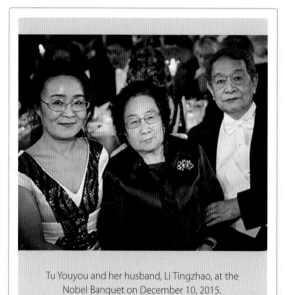

Tu Youyou and her husband, Li Tingzhao, at the Nobel Banquet on December 10, 2015.

This resulted in an extract that was antimalarial but toxic. Tu kept working, removing toxic ingredients, until extract number 191 proved 100 percent effective against mouse malaria—without killing the mice. In March 1972 she presented her findings at a 523 meeting in Nanjing, and although her own team was struggling, two other teams soon made progress.[8] One problem: there are many species of *Artemisia*, and Tu's group used the one common to Beijing. To get enough of the antimalarial compound artemisinin, they needed the fresh leaves of a Sichuan species, *Artemisia annua*. Step by step, the collaborators arrived at an effective antimalarial drug. Another problem: during the Cultural Revolution, facilities for clinical trials were scarce. Tu and her colleagues volunteered to be human guinea pigs, testing the drug's safety on themselves.[9]

Artemesinin makes malaria patients feel better within hours—and all too often, they stop treatment when they feel better. Some of

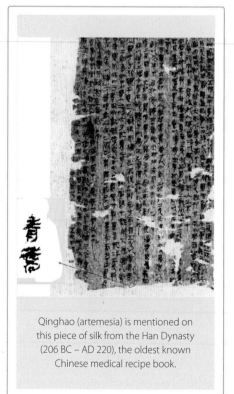

Qinghao (artemesia) is mentioned on this piece of silk from the Han Dynasty (206 BC – AD 220), the oldest known Chinese medical recipe book.

the parasites survive, and malaria can develop resistance to artemesinin as it did to the previous drug of choice, chloroquine. To prevent this, artemesinin is now used in combination with partner drugs.[10]

The malaria death rate has fallen by 60 percent since the year 2000,[11] largely because of artemesinin. Who discovered it? American malaria researcher Louis Miller asked at a 2005 meeting in Shanghai. Nobody knew; Miller investigated.[12] Tu, a researcher with no M.D., no Ph.D., no foreign study, and few publications, suddenly became prominent. For work that saved millions of lives, she received the 2011 Lasker-DeBakey Clinical Medical Research Award and shared in the 2015 Nobel Prize in Physiology or Medicine.

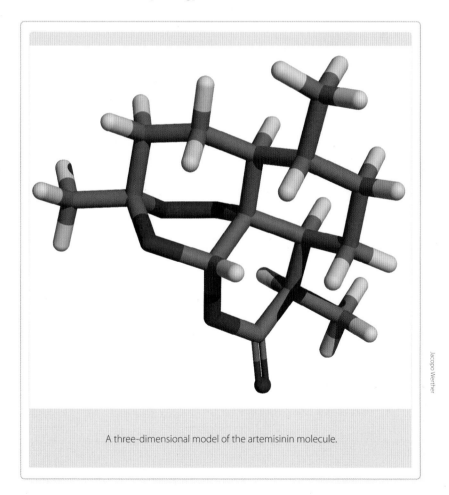

A three-dimensional model of the artemisinin molecule.

Jacopo Werther

Chairman Mao, Biomedicine, and Traditional Chinese Medicine

When Fleming (Chapter 35) and Brotzu (Chapter 39) discovered molds with antibiotic properties, researchers around the world began looking into old folk remedies. Interest was especially high in China, where there were too few West-ern-trained physicians to care for the nation's vast population. Previous govern-ments had tried to abolish the old medical practices, called *yi*, which were "seen as old-fashioned, irrational, superstitious, and based on unprovable theories and principles."[13] Communist Chairman Mao Zedong (1893–1976), who came to power in 1950, responded differently: he proposed a unification of Western and Chinese practices. The new term "Traditional Chinese Medicine," or TCM, sounded like a validation of China's age-old folk practices,[14] but Mao said in 1956, "we must use modern Western science to research the regulation of traditional *yi* learning, and develop a Chinese version of new medicine."[15]

Mao himself used Western doctors. With half a billion Chinese depending on the old *yi*, he did not move to abolish it, but clearly expected that practices not validated by Western science would fade away. Meanwhile he supported the establishment of Institutes for the Study of Chinese Medicine, where he hoped researchers would find new miracle drugs in ancient texts.

The era of government-sponsored TCM did not last long. The Cultural Rev-olution worsened the doctor shortage, and Mao recruited a half-million work-ers to serve as "barefoot doctors" or medics in the countryside. With three to six months' training, they worked mainly on sanitation and hygiene campaigns. They taught hygiene and contraception, but also administered immunizations and first aid.[16]

Forty years after the death of Mao, a new era of integration of TCM with Western biomedicine has begun in China. For instance, the "Herbalome Project" uses modern experimental methods to test for active compounds and toxic con-taminants in TCM remedies.[17] Meanwhile, like Chinese food, traditional Chinese medicine has migrated to America, with changes. Many Americans seek health through Chinese herbal medicine, acupuncture, massage, exercise, diet, and other practices—the same rich assortment that Mao planned to evaluate and rationalize with the techniques of Western medicine.

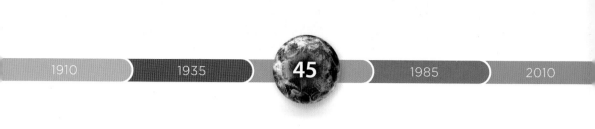

1978

The First Test Tube Baby

In 1978, a truck driver's wife was admitted to the hospital under a false name. Her gynecologist wanted to monitor her high blood pressure—a danger in late pregnancy, but not rare enough to justify a media circus. Yet reporters disguised as plumbers, window-washers, and priests invaded the hospital to see Lesley Brown.[1]

The Browns had been trying to conceive for nine years before they tried in vitro fertilization (IVF), and finally Lesley was giving birth—to the world's first test-tube baby. Some expected a monster, but baby Louise emerged pink and healthy on July 25. By 2012, IVF technology had resulted in over 5 million births worldwide.[2]

Human pregnancy usually begins in a woman's fallopian tubes, when a man's sperm cell fuses with a mature egg and forms a zygote, or fertilized egg. But approximately one in seven couples has difficulty conceiving a child,[3] and if medical treatments fail, the IVF procedure is now an alternative. The woman's egg is removed from her body, fertilized by the man's sperm in a glass container, and transferred back into the mother's womb.

The process was developed by physiologist Robert Edwards and gynecologist Patrick Steptoe.[4] Others had done it with animals; a transfer of rabbit embryos was reported as early as 1891.[5] But in the 1950s,

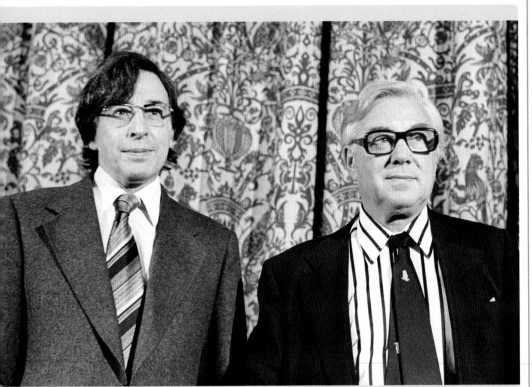

Robert Edwards (left) was excited by new discoveries in both reproduction and immunology; he teamed with Patrick Steptoe (right), whose skill with laparascopy made human IVF possible.

new findings on human genetics attracted Edwards's attention. It was agreed that humans normally have 46 chromosomes, 23 from each parent, and that different numbers of chromosomes underlie developmental abnormalities. Edwards had seen that the timing of chromosomal events was important for maturing mouse eggs, and he wondered if anomalies in human development were caused by missteps in the same kind of timed sequence. By studying the question, he hoped to prevent genetic and chromosomal illnesses.[6]

Patrick Steptoe directed a fertility clinic. Using laparoscopy, a minimally invasive procedure sometimes called "keyhole surgery," he was able to gather eggs from infertile volunteers at the clinic. By 1969 he and Edwards were collaborating, refining their techniques and publishing landmark papers.[7] Solving both scientific and technical problems, they finally achieved success.

Today, before an IVF procedure, a woman is medicated to suppress her own menstrual cycle. Then she receives fertility drugs to make her ovaries produce more eggs than normal. Ten or twenty eggs are incubated with sperm from the man, usually creating far more embryos than necessary. Parents must decide how many embryos to implant in the womb, and what to do with the others.[8] Should they be donated for research, given to another infertile couple, frozen for possible future use, or destroyed? And what about embryos with anomalies—embryos that would grow up with congenital disorders? The legal, ethical, and moral complexities are daunting.

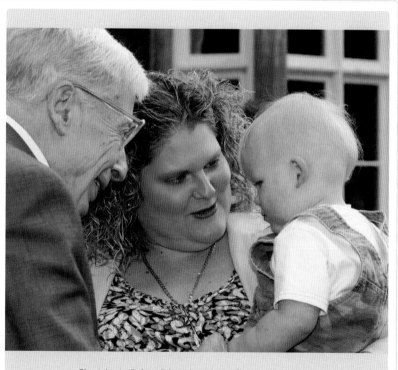

Physiologist Robert Edwards with the first test-tube baby, Louise Brown, and her son Cameron.

PA Images/Alamy Images

People sent hate mail to Lesley Brown in 1978, "menacing and scary," splattered with fake blood.[9] IVF is a flash point for ethical dispute because—like other medical breakthroughs—it allows humans some control over what used to be considered fate. It allows infertile couples to have children, but also same-sex couples, single parents, and transgendered individuals. Eggs and sperm can be donated by outsiders, and when a woman is unable to carry her own embryos, they may be implanted in the uterus of a surrogate mother.

Edwards and Steptoe faced opposition for years, and unresolved questions still multiply. But in 2010, Edwards—the surviving partner—was awarded the Nobel Prize in Physiology or Medicine.

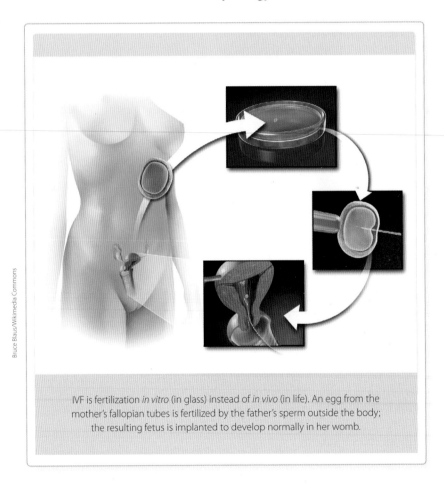

Bruce Blaus/Wikimedia Commons

IVF is fertilization *in vitro* (in glass) instead of *in vivo* (in life). An egg from the mother's fallopian tubes is fertilized by the father's sperm outside the body; the resulting fetus is implanted to develop normally in her womb.

Whose Baby Is It?

Assisted reproductive technology (ART)—including fertility medication, artificial insemination, IVF, and surrogacy—challenges traditional ideas of maternity and paternity, the status of women in society and in the family, and the definition of personhood.[10] The questions of parental rights are often poignant:

- Melanie Boivin donated her eggs for IVF so that her daughter, who was sterile because of a genetic disorder, could have children.[11] Who is the mother?

- Diane Blood extracted and preserved sperm from her dying husband, making him the biological father of two children conceived after his death.[12] Who is the father?

- Anna Johnson was a surrogate mother; she had a contract with the biological parents of a child conceived by IVF. After she gave birth, she wanted to keep the baby. Who is the mother?[13]

- After an IVF mix-up, a white couple delivered black twins. Both the white couple and the black couple wanted the twins. Who are their legal parents?[14]

- Cynthia Daily used a sperm donor to conceive a baby. Seven years later, on a Web-based registry, she found that her child had at least 150 half-siblings from the same donor.[15] What is a family?

The issues seem endless. If a sperm donor leaves his estate to "progeny" rather than to named individuals, does his unknown biological child have a claim? What if unknown siblings fall in love and marry? And what about those frozen embryos—are they legal property, or persons?

Robert Edwards hoped his study of human embryos would help prevent genetic diseases. Now it is possible to diagnose anomalies in developing embryos and simply refuse to implant those that are flawed. But is that the same, morally, as abortion? And if prospective parents can choose to have only healthy children, can they also choose to have only males?

(Continued on next page)

(Continued from previous page)

Civilization struggles with these and other questions. Laws are passed; a U.K. law established the Human Fertilization and Embryology Authority to oversee policy. Case law is hammered out in court. Philosophers, religious leaders, and professional organizations debate the ramifications; Robert Edwards, as chair of an international advisory board, was first signatory to the 1984 "Helsinki Statement on Human *in Vitro* Fertilization."

Contraception

As much as some people long to conceive children, others want to prevent conception. Women over the ages tried contraceptives ranging from crocodile dung (probably ineffective) to lead, arsenic, and mercury (often fatal). Nineteenth-century birth control methods included condoms, sponges, douches, and suppositories, some of which may have worked some of the time. And even if physicians had known a foolproof way to prevent conception, they weren't allowed to tell.[18]

In 1873, Anthony Comstock and his Society for the Suppression of Vice advocated passage of a federal law against obscenity; many states passed similar laws.[19] Around the same time, the states outlawed abortion on the basis of public safety; too many women died of infection after the procedure.[20] Margaret Sanger and others established birth control clinics in defiance of the law, facing jail as a result.[21] In 1965 the United States Supreme Court ruled that married couples could use birth control to prevent pregnancy.[22] In 1972 the Court extended this right to unmarried couples,[23] and with *Roe v. Wade* in 1973 it struck down Texas laws against abortion.[24]

Meanwhile, Dr. Gregory Goodwin Pincus had developed a better contraceptive. In 1957 the U.S. Food and Drug Administration approved Enovid to treat menstrual disorders; in 1960, it was approved as a contraceptive. A generation of newly liberated women called it "the pill," and, like IVF, it changed society.

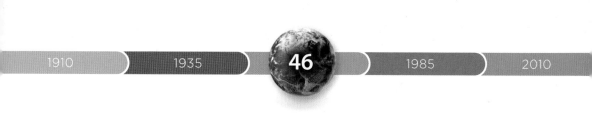

1983

Preventing Cancers

Immigrant George Papanicolaou arrived in New York City in 1913 with a Greek medical degree and a German doctorate in zoology,[1] and after a difficult job search (for a while he sold carpets[2]) he landed a position in the Anatomy Department of the Cornell University Medical Center. In 1917 he discovered a way to tell when guinea pig eggs were ripe for experiment by taking smears from the animals' vaginas and watching the cells change from day to day. This was very useful in studying reproduction.

In the 1920s, Papanicolaou found that some vaginal smears included cancer cells along with the body's own cells. Instead of a needle biopsy to tell if a woman had cervical cancer, her physician could simply use a vaginal swab.[3] It would be so cheap and non-invasive that women could be tested routinely, before they showed any symptoms, and the disease could be nipped in the bud.

This discovery was not well received, and for years Papanicolaou's career stalled. Then in 1939 Joseph C. Hinsey became head of the Anatomy Department. Soon Papanicolaou had research partners, access to gynecological patients, and grant funding. Nowadays American women get routine Pap smears (named for Papanicolaou) to detect cancer before it is too far advanced to stop. Papanicolaou's simple test

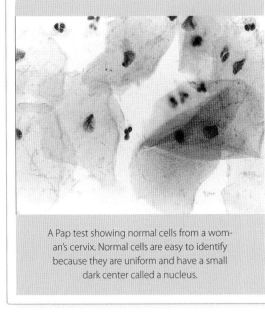

A Pap test showing normal cells from a woman's cervix. Normal cells are easy to identify because they are uniform and have a small dark center called a nucleus.

prevents up to 91 percent of all invasive cervical cancers in countries where national mass screening programs have been implemented.[4]

The Pap test is an example of "secondary" prevention; early detection saves lives by catching small cancers or even precancerous conditions before they spread. "Primary" prevention means preventing cancers from occurring. Since some cancers are caused by chronic infections, vaccines could be a possible source of primary prevention.

Researchers long suspected that cervical cancer had something to do with sex. In 1842 Rigoni-Stern studied 80 years of Verona records and found that nuns and virgins didn't get cervical cancer, but prostitutes did.[5] Epidemiological studies in the 1950s found it was most common in women who became sexually active at a young age and had multiple partners.[6]

And there were hints of a connection to genital warts. Studies in the 1930s linked rabbit papilloma (wart) virus to cancer,[7] and anecdotal reports described genital warts becoming cancerous in humans.[8]

But tracing the relationship between a cancer and a pathogen is not easy. HPV and other cancer-causing agents are widespread in many populations, and people who carry them do not always develop cancer. When cancers do develop, it is typically decades after the original infection, so the causal link is not obvious.[9]

In the 1970s, Harald zur Hausen and colleagues studied wart biopsies and found that human papillomavirus (HPV) is a large family, comprising many types. HPV-16 DNA was present in about 50 percent of cervical cancers, and HPV-18 in another 20 percent.[10] There are over 100 strains of HPV, but vaccines against HPV-16 and HPV-18 have been developed.[11] Gardasil, approved by the FDA in 2006, is recommended for young women from 9 to 26 years old.

Other viruses (including Epstein-Barr, HIV, and hepatitis B and C) and pathogens (including *H. pylori* bacteria and at least two flatworms) have been conclusively linked to different cancers.[12] As these agents are identified and isolated, researchers develop vaccines against them. So for cancers that begin with infectious agents, primary cancer prevention is already a reality.

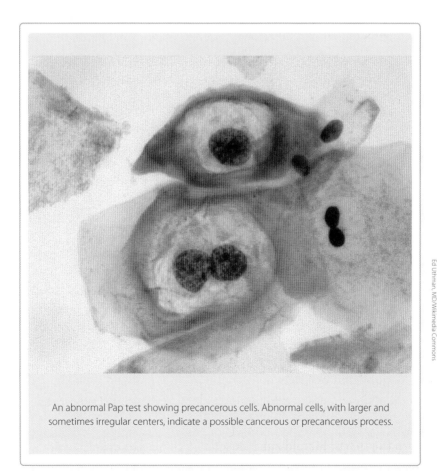

An abnormal Pap test showing precancerous cells. Abnormal cells, with larger and sometimes irregular centers, indicate a possible cancerous or precancerous process.

Ed Uthman, MD/Wikimedia Commons

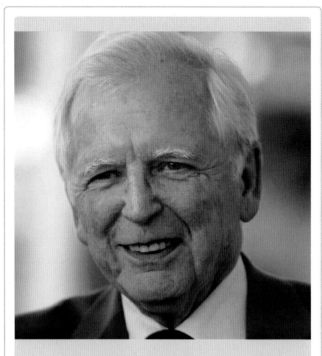

Harald zur Hausen won a Nobel Prize in 2008 for his discovery that human papilloma viruses (HPV) cause cancer, a discovery that has led to widespread vaccinations.

The Ethics of Discovery: Informed Consent

How could you find out if a human cancer is contagious? See if you can give people cancer by injecting them with living cancer cells. Chester Southam and his colleagues did this in the 1950s, saying, "Such studies are of fundamental importance to our knowledge of tissue transplantation and host defense mechanism."[13] They took material from seven cancer cell lines—cells that had been isolated from cancer tissues and kept alive in the lab—and implanted that material into prison inmates. Some of the volunteers developed cancer; those who already had other cancers were at greater risk.

(Continued on next page)

(Continued from previous page)

Such studies raise obvious ethical questions. Traditional medical ethics warn doctors not to harm patients,[14] but do researchers have the same obligation to subjects? Medical discoveries and innovations may save countless lives, but first they must be tested. Some early researchers experimented on themselves. A few, like Walter Reed, used contracts to make sure volunteers knew the risks and benefits involved.[15]

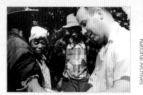

Subjects in the Tuskegee Study of Untreated Syphilis were not told they had syphilis, but they were given placebo treatments for "bad blood."

But many researchers used subjects who could not give free, informed consent. Prison inmates and soldiers had to accept orders; asylum inmates and children might not understand the risks. Did the potential benefits of research justify overriding the rights of such vulnerable subjects? In 1900, German law required full disclosure of risks and patient consent for treatment,[16] but physicians worldwide were slow to internalize the principle.

After World War II, Nazi concentration camp doctors were tried for atrocities they had inflicted on inmates in the name of medical research. The Doctors' Trials shocked the world,[17] and in their 1947 verdict, judges included the 10-point Nuremberg Code of Medical Ethics. The first point: "Required is the voluntary, well-informed, understanding consent of the human subject in a full legal capacity."[18]

Scandal broke in 1972 when news media exposed the Tuskegee Study of Untreated Syphilis, supported by the U.S. Public Health Service. The study began in 1932, when Salvarsan and other available treatments were far from ideal; the object was to discover the rate of spontaneous cure.[19] It was horribly unethical by today's standards. Over 400 African-American men with syphilis were observed for four decades. They were not told they had syphilis, so they could not give informed consent; they received deceptive placebo "treatments"; and the study did not terminate when the introduction of penicillin made it pointless.

The Tuskegee scandal led to passage of the 1974 National Research Act. Ethical oversight is now stricter, and to obtain federal funding, research proposals must first be approved by Institutional Review Boards, independent ethics committees which typically include non-scientists, humanists, and lay individuals.[20]

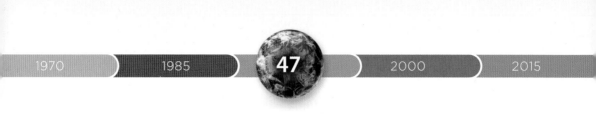

1998

MMR Vaccine, Autism, Discovery, and Fraud

Kieran is a cheerful little soul, and his loving mother follows her doctor's recommendations. At 12 months he gets the MMR vaccine against measles, mumps, and rubella. Suddenly he has a fever. He arches his back, goes rigid, and screams—an endless high-pitched scream. Worse, he withdraws. He refuses food, play, and hugs. He goes mute. At 20 months he gets a diagnosis: autism.[1]

Autism, or ASD (autism spectrum disorder), affects learning, thinking, and especially social interactions.[2] Although 44 percent of autistic people have average IQs or are gifted, most need special help in their lives. Kieran will not have a normal childhood; much of life will be a struggle for him and his family. They will not be alone. In 2000, an estimated one child in 150 had ASD; by 2012, the estimate was one in 68.[3] Many believe the MMR vaccine causes this scourge. They are wrong.[4]

And their mistake may cost lives. Before the MMR vaccine, almost every child caught measles, mumps, and rubella; this was considered good, saving them from more severe cases as adults.[5] But measles is still a leading cause of children's death worldwide.[6] While it typically just brings a miserable fever, runny eyes and nose, a cough, and a full-body rash, one in 20 victims may get pneumonia and one in 1,000 may develop encephalitis, leaving some blind, deaf, or intellectually disabled.[7] Rubella, or "German measles," seems milder, but when women catch it early in pregnancy their children risk congenital rubella,[8] leading to deafness, growth retardation, seizures, or developmental delays—including autism.

Measles was eradicated in the U.S. by 2000, after two centuries of work and discoveries. People had always known that measles, like smallpox, leaves survivors with lifelong immunity. And since inoculation worked against smallpox, in 1758 it was tried for measles, with only partial success.[9]

Germ theory and the discovery of viruses paved the way for more effective vaccines. John Enders and his colleagues cultivated the measles virus in 1954, and by 1960 they had a strain that stimulated antibody production. In

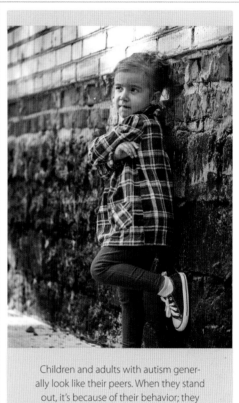

Children and adults with autism generally look like their peers. When they stand out, it's because of their behavior; they tend to be socially awkward and have trouble picking up social cues.

Thinkstock

1963, two vaccines were approved for the U.S. One used live virus; it produced an immune response in more than 95 percent of susceptible children, and its side effects (fever and rash) could be controlled. The other vaccine, using "killed" virus, had less severe side effects but proved less effective. Scientists in Sweden and the Netherlands initially favored the killed vaccine, but its drawbacks emerged over time.

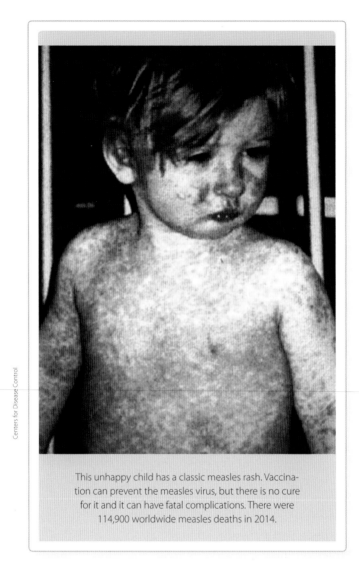

This unhappy child has a classic measles rash. Vaccination can prevent the measles virus, but there is no cure for it and it can have fatal complications. There were 114,900 worldwide measles deaths in 2014.

Besides effectiveness and side effects, vaccine developers considered ease of use. If parents had to bring their children for too many vaccinations and booster shots, could they keep the schedules straight? Combining several antigens in a single vaccine simplified things, and in 1971, Merck licensed the MMR vaccine.[10] It was the creation of microbiologist Maurice Hilleman, who may have saved more lives than any other medical scientist of the twentieth century.

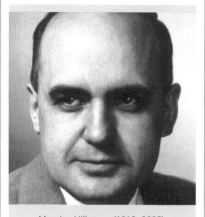

Maurice Hilleman (1919–2005), whose measles vaccine prevents an estimated million deaths each year.

In 1998, 91 percent of children in England got the MMR vaccine, and only 56 got measles. That year, Dr. Andrew Wakefield published a paper claiming a link between MMR vaccine and autism in 12 children. In 2000 he did a televised interview that alarmed parents. In 2008, fewer than 80 percent of English children were vaccinated, and 1,370 caught measles.[11]

Other scientists found no link between autism and the vaccine—even in a study reviewing the records

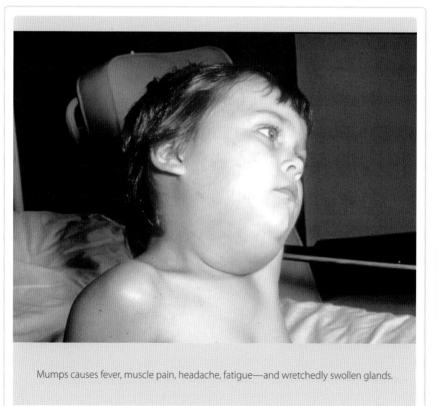

Mumps causes fever, muscle pain, headache, fatigue—and wretchedly swollen glands.

227

of 95,727 children.[12] Investigators discovered that Wakefield had been paid $670,000 to consult in lawsuits against vaccine manufacturers and that he got his results by biased sampling and misrepresentation. Guilty of medical and scientific misconduct, he had published a fraudulent paper.[13] But although his work has been debunked, too many parents still believe him. Travelers from abroad can be contagious before they show symptoms, and in December 2014, measles infected dozens of unvaccinated victims in a place children love: Disneyland.

Herd Immunity

Vaccinations protect the people who get them—and they protect others as well. Infectious diseases spread from person to person as long as they can find susceptible new hosts. But not everybody is susceptible; those who have already survived the disease or been successfully vaccinated against it are immune. The more people in a population are immune, the more likely it is that the chain of infection will be broken and the disease will stop spreading. Those who are not immune themselves will be spared if immune members of their community block the infection so it doesn't reach them.

For measles, the most transmissible human disease known, 96 percent of the population must be immune for herd immunity to work.[14]

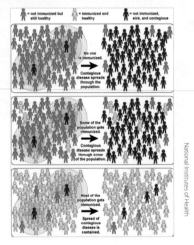

National Institutes of Health

When nobody is immune to an infectious disease, it can quickly become an epidemic. But if only a few people lack immunity, they may be protected from infection by the immune population around them.

Scientific Discovery and Fraud

Scientific discovery is a cumulative process, and sometimes its pace is frustratingly slow. To develop an effective measles vaccine took years—even centuries, if you count from the 1758 attempt. Research on autism, a condition first defined in 1943,[15] may take even longer.

Andrew Wakefield's 1998 paper seemed like a breakthrough, linking a "regressive" form of autism to enterocolitis and suggesting that both were caused by the MMR vaccine. His sample size was small, with just 12 children, but Leo Kenner's groundbreaking 1943 paper analyzed autism in just 11. A small study can be good, if it is honestly done.

Unfortunately, Wakefield's study was a sham. He had concealed major conflicts of interest: the $670,000 he earned as an expert consultant to attorneys suing vaccine makers, and his own patent interest in an alternative

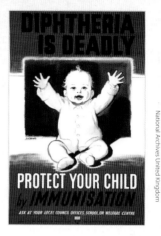

National Archives United Kingdom

Public health poster promoting diphtheria vaccination. Because of gastroenterologist Andrew Wakefield's 1998 paper wrongly linking autism to the MMR vaccine, many parents refuse to have their children vaccinated.

vaccine. He had biased his subject selection, looking only at children whose parents believed the vaccine had caused their problems. Even then, he had to misrepresent their cases: three of the children had no diagnosis of autism, and another five had developmental concerns before they were vaccinated.[16]

Scientists in several countries searched for evidence linking the MMR vaccine to autism, and they reviewed Wakefield's data carefully before declaring it fraudulent. But meanwhile, celebrities adopted Wakefield's ideas and became anti-vaccine activists. Many still do not realize that his work has been debunked. Science is slow, cautious, and difficult. A fraudulent piece of pseudoscience can be flashy, easy to understand, and all too believable. But one scientific virtue is self-correction. Dubious methods and fake findings are caught and renounced in the end, and legitimate research goes on.

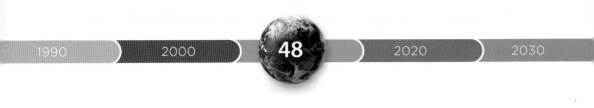
2011

Bionic Parts

Brooke Hayes was still in her twenties, and there was so much to enjoy—concerts, motorcycles, water sports—but by 2011 she was "living like an 80-year-old," hobbled by pain. Born with spondyloepiphyseal dysplasia congenita (SEDC), a bone growth disorder, Hayes was under four feet tall but had always been unstoppable. Now her bones ground together when she moved. Yoga and injections didn't help; she needed hip replacements, and they wouldn't be easy. Standard models wouldn't fit her small, unusually shaped frame. It took a combination of advanced technologies to give Brooke her life back.[1]

Every year, surgeons implant millions of artificial devices to replace body parts that aren't working. Cataracts, clouding the eyes, typically lead to blindness—but intraocular lenses replace the clouded ones, giving people back their sight.[2] Teeth are lost—and titanium pegs capped with porcelain crowns replace them. Heart valves fail—and artificial ones are implanted to control blood flow. And when knees, shoulders, and other joints are worn away, artificial joints replace them.

Osteoarthritis is the leading cause of joint failure. It wears away protective cartilage until uncushioned bones rub against each other. The hip is a ball-and-socket joint. In Brooke Hayes's osteoarthritic hips, the balls—the tops of her thighbones—scraped against their sockets in her

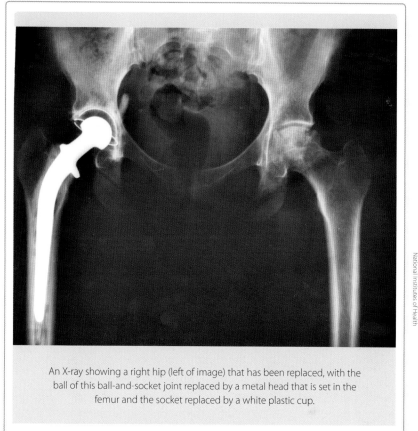

National Institutes of Health

An X-ray showing a right hip (left of image) that has been replaced, with the ball of this ball-and-socket joint replaced by a metal head that is set in the femur and the socket replaced by a white plastic cup.

pelvic bones every time she took a step or struggled out of a chair. In hip implants a ball made of ceramic, polyethylene, or metal fits into a cup, making an artificial joint with the same range of motion as a biological hip. Typically, implants give patients fifteen years of normal activity before replacements are needed.[3]

Every implant is the product of many discoveries and inventions—starting with the selection or development of the substances it's made of. Artificial lenses of acrylic or silicone do not trigger rejection or foreign body reactions.[4] Titanium in dental implants and hip joints bonds with bone. A layer of hard plastic in the implanted hip socket prevents metal from scraping metal, releasing high levels of ions into the blood.[5]

New devices are constantly evaluated. For instance, a transcatheter aortic valve implantation (TAVI) may offer hope to people too old or sick for open-heart surgery. It is introduced through a leg artery in a folded state, threaded up the body to the heart, and deployed like an umbrella inside the patient's non-functioning valve. Tens of thousands of people have had this operation, but it is expensive, and investigators for the Belgian health care system found that it places patients at greater risk of stroke.[6] Procedures designed to solve one problem can often cause others, and assessments of a flawed invention drive new research to improve it.

Brooke Hayes was helped by a combination of CT scans and 3D printing. A computed tomography (CT) scan takes X-rays from many angles and combines them to produce cross-sectional images. Brooke's surgeons at the Mayo Clinic fed CT data into a 3D program to print models of her bones, allowing them to plot and practice her surgeries in advance.[7]

3D printing was invented in the 1980s, and has been used since the early 2000s to create dental implants and custom prosthetics, from

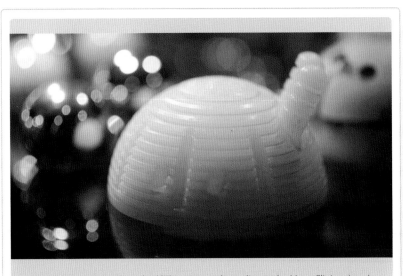

Using computer tomography (CT) images, orthopedists at the Mayo Clinic printed 3D models of Brooke Hayes's hips and plotted her operations in advance.

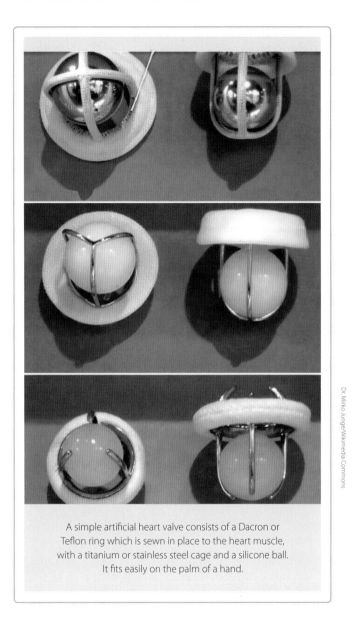

A simple artificial heart valve consists of a Dacron or
Teflon ring which is sewn in place to the heart muscle,
with a titanium or stainless steel cage and a silicone ball.
It fits easily on the palm of a hand.

Dr. Mirko Junge/Wikimedia Commons

bones to ears;[8] in 2015 China approved 3D hip implants.[9] Other recent medical uses include tissue and organ fabrication (windpipes, cell cultures, stem cells, and vascular networks) and pharmaceutical research (drug discovery, delivery, and dosage forms).[10] In the future, printed stem cells may scaffold artificial bladders and other hollow organs,[11] or regenerate organs like the pancreas, eliminating the need for diabetics to take insulin.[12] This will take time, and many concerns must be addressed first.[13] Around the world, collaborating and competing, researchers will be weaving together major insights and modest innovations to make workable solutions for the future.

Drug-eluting Implants

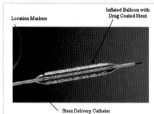

Food and Drug Administration

A stent is a tube that can be implanted into a blood vessel or other passageway to keep it open; this could be done while a patient heals after an operation. A drug-eluting stent is one that slowly releases a needed drug into the patient's system.

A drug-eluting implant is an implantable drug delivery system. It is made of materials that do not harm living tissues,[14] and it contains medicines to be slowly absorbed at body temperature. For instance, drug-eluting stents in blocked coronary arteries can deliver blood thinners directly at the site of blockages so that new clots do not form.[15]

Some implants require a surgical incision to be placed under the skin. Others, like long-acting contraceptive or hormone-containing rings, are worn for one to three months inside a body cavity without need for surgery. Birth control implants inserted into the womb are also gaining favor because they work for three to five years.[16] A new intravaginal device is being developed for both birth control and HIV prevention.[17,18]

Some drug-eluting devices deliver targeted chemotherapy for cancers of the lung,[19] bowel,[20] or pancreas.[21] Others are used to deliver pain relief for one to three months[22] or to treat drug addiction by delivering addiction medication in a long-acting form.[23]

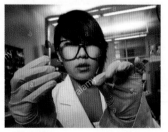

Reuters/Alamy Stock Photo

Assembling a stent that is used to test how a drug is released inside a human body from an implanted medical device.

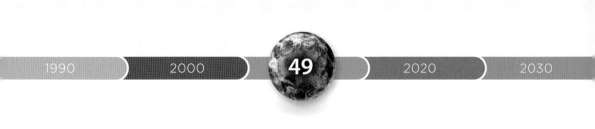

2013

Poop Therapy for the Human Microbiome

The intestinal tract is full of bacteria. That is to say, we are all full of—microbes? For every cell in our bodies we're probably carrying at least ten microbes.[1] Most of them don't make us sick; many even help keep us healthy. Like the ecosystem that surrounds us, our personal collections of microbiota—the tiny ecosystems or microbiomes we lug around with us—are astoundingly diverse. We are just beginning to discover how our colonies of bacteria, viruses, and other microorganisms interact with each other and with us.

But if their balance is upset, trouble can result. Take *Clostridium difficile*, first described as a cause of diarrhea back in 1978. Many people acquire it in hospitals and nursing homes, making it the top healthcare-acquired pathogen in the U.S.[2] It has evolved; it makes people sicker than it used to and resists more antibiotics. As of 2015, nearly half a million Americans get *C. difficile* infections (CDI) each year, and about 29,000 die within a month of diagnosis.[3]

One big risk factor for getting CDI is being treated with antibiotics for something else. It's a case of friendly fire. The antibiotic fighting your case of pneumonia or strep throat is your ally, but it also wipes

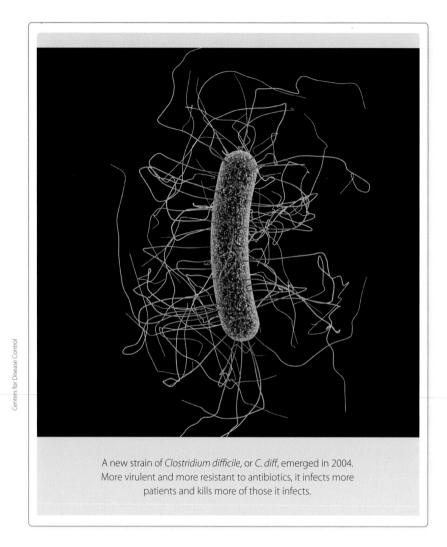

Centers for Disease Control

A new strain of *Clostridium difficile*, or *C. diff*, emerged in 2004. More virulent and more resistant to antibiotics, it infects more patients and kills more of those it infects.

out useful microbes in your gut. Colonies of C. *difficile* may resist the antibiotic and invade the vacated habitat. Soon you are running a fever, doubled over with cramps and diarrhea.

So you need another antibiotic, such as metronidazole or vancomycin. Most patients recover quickly the first time this happens, but 15 to 35 percent suffer relapses. With every round of treatment, patients are more likely to get diarrhea that just won't go away. Hospital stays and IVs don't cure them. Soon after they go off antibiotics they are back in the ICU.

What do we try when antibiotics fail? Why not a poop transplant? To overcome the "ick" factor, medical journals often call it fecal microbiota therapy, or FMT. The idea is to get carefully filtered healthy stools into the gut of a patient suffering from CDI or some other intractable bowel condition. Ge Hong (283–343) described fecal therapies back in China's Jin Dynasty, Li Shizhen (1518–1593) used them in the Ming Dynasty, and during World War II German soldiers tried camel stools, a Bedouin cure for dysentery. In 1958 Colorado surgeon Ben Eiseman reported four colitis cures using fecal enemas.[4]

Does FMT really work? It's worth researching. One review turned up 59 reports of fecal transplants for *C. difficile* infection (CDI) and other bowel disorders. Only two were randomized controlled trials; most were studies of single cases or small series of cases.[5] In the larger randomized trial, 16 patients with recurrent CDI received donor feces after four days of vancomycin; 26 patients in control groups received 14 days of vancomycin treatment. The study was terminated early because the feces were so much more effective than vancomycin: 15 of the 16 experimental patients recovered, compared to 7 of 26 in the two control groups.[6] In a more recent study, doctors at the Mayo Clinic treated 30 *C. difficile* patients with pills containing spores from about 50 species of bacteria found in healthy stools; 29 of the patients recovered.[7]

These studies are promising, but too small to guarantee that FMT is safe and effective. The results have to be taken with caution.[8] But FMT seems to work by restoring healthy levels of microbiota diversity to patient guts.[9]

Progress in FMT research and treatment may require new federal policies; some argue that fecal material should be classified as human tissue, not an experimental drug.[10] But new discoveries also need new ways of looking at things. Over the centuries we have imagined health problems caused by angry gods, humoral imbalances, miasmas, attacking swarms of microbes, or genetic mutations. The human microbiome may turn out to be a more complicated explanation than any of these.

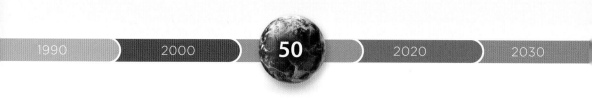
2016

Researching the Zika Virus

In French Polynesia a man in his forties drove his daughter to school, then went home and lay down. In two minutes he was paralyzed. He spent eight months in intensive care and more than a year in rehabilitation. Larry Ly had the country's worst case of Guillain-Barré Syndrome, but there were others. In fall 2013 an epidemic began, bringing 42 cases of GBS—about ten times the annual average.[1] Nine victims, including Ly, had to be put on ventilators;[2] none died, but some were left with job loss and family upheavals.

Two years later, shocked mothers lined hospital corridors in Brazil. One looked up from the baby on her lap to ask everybody's question: "Doctor? His head is going to grow, right?"[3] Mothers could see their infants' low foreheads and tiny skulls; scans showed small brains dotted with calcification and lacking the complex folds of normally developing brains. Brazil normally had about 150 annual cases of microcephaly (MC),[4] but between October 2015 and July 2016, 8,571 cases were reported.[5]

The GBS cases in French Polynesia and the MC cases in Brazil were both associated with the Zika virus, long thought harmless. Zika was first isolated in the blood of a feverish monkey in 1947 and infected humans in 1952.[6] It seemed milder than its cousins yellow fever and dengue,

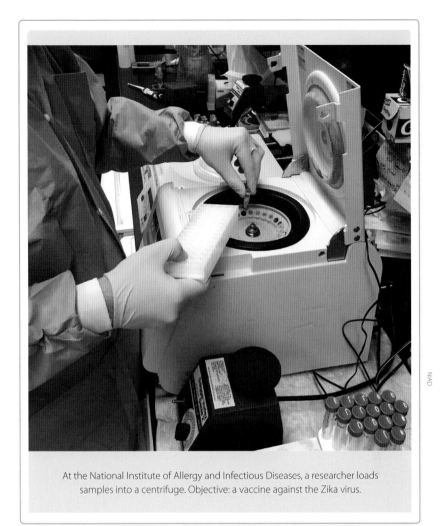

At the National Institute of Allergy and Infectious Diseases, a researcher loads samples into a centrifuge. Objective: a vaccine against the Zika virus.

nasty mosquito-borne viruses that have been known to cause encephalitis. In 2007, when Zika broke out on Yap Island in the Pacific, only about 20 percent of those infected experienced symptoms: mild fevers, slight rashes, achy joints and muscles, headaches and itchy eyes—those flu-like symptoms we typically ignore. Most recovered without hospital care. The world paid little attention until 2015, when GBS cases spiked in the Brazilian state of Bahia. Then came the microcephalic babies.

Suddenly everyone wanted answers from the World Health Organization (WHO) and the Centers for Disease Control. If Zika caused

GBS and MC, was it safe to travel to affected countries? What precautions should people take? What was being done to protect the public?

Researchers went into overdrive. As of this writing, there is no effective vaccine against Zika or drug to cure it. The best approach is to stop its transmission by avoiding mosquito bites, unprotected sex, and pregnancy during Zika outbreaks.[7] But although even the pope suggested using condoms to prevent spreading Zika, avoidance is not always possible. The WHO is prioritizing mosquito control tools, diagnostic tests, and vaccines.[8] What if the Zika virus couldn't replicate in mosquitoes? Some pragmatic investigators hope to induce mosquito

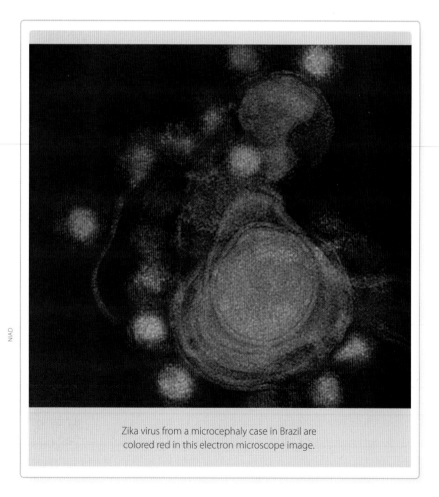

NIAD

Zika virus from a microcephaly case in Brazil are colored red in this electron microscope image.

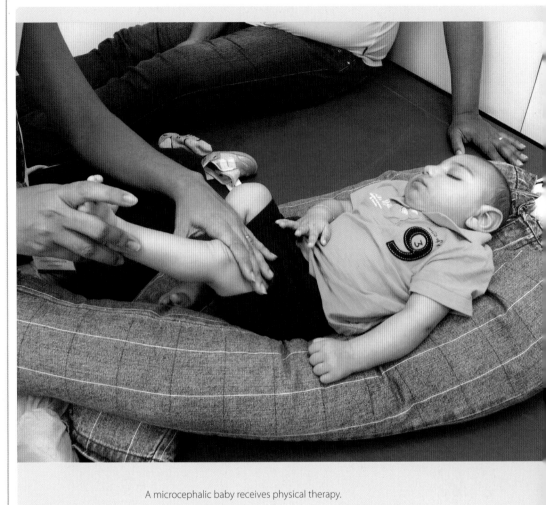

Sumaia Villela/Agência Brasil/Wikimedia Commons

A microcephalic baby receives physical therapy.

sterility by gene modification; others hope to infect mosquitoes with *Wolbachia* bacteria, which could interfere with the virus's own opportunities to multiply.[9]

Authorities were reluctant to say that Zika caused MC.[10] It can be caused by other viruses, by environmental factors, or by mutated genes, but Zika looked like the culprit because of a higher incidence of MC births after Zika outbreaks; virus detected in amniotic fluid and tissues of some

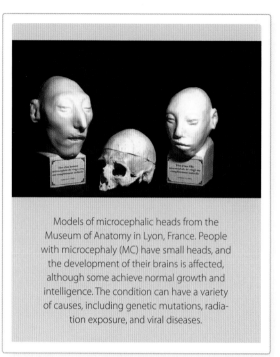

Oguedel/Wikimedia Commons

Models of microcephalic heads from the Museum of Anatomy in Lyon, France. People with microcephaly (MC) have small heads, and the development of their brains is affected, although some achieve normal growth and intelligence. The condition can have a variety of causes, including genetic mutations, radiation exposure, and viral diseases.

affected newborns; and higher rates of birth defects in the fetuses of women who knew they had Zika while pregnant. One study identified fetal abnormalities in 29 out of 42 Zika-affected pregnancies.[11] By July 2016, Brazil's Ministry of Health had confirmed that 1,709 diagnoses of microcephaly in live births and 102 stillbirths and miscarriages were linked to Zika; hundreds of cases remained to investigate.[12]

So the causal link is now generally accepted, but how does it work? How does the Zika virus cross the placental barrier? Why does it attack the brain and nervous system? Whatever we learn about Zika is likely to give us unexpected new insights into other diseases and our own bodies.

Conclusion

Ötzi the Iceman (Chapter 1) carried a pouch of medicinal herbs on his belt to treat whipworms in his intestines. Ötzi used *Piptoporus betulinus,* a fungus that causes diarrhea when ingested. This mushroom has been used for thousands of years to expel intestinal worms, which are estimated to affect over one billion people worldwide.[1] But *P. betulinus* doesn't kill the worms; it just expels them.

By a curious coincidence, our story of medical adventures and discoveries brings us full circle to the 2015 Nobel Prize in Physiology or Medicine, which honored two discoveries. The first, by a team of researchers, was a novel treatment to eradicate intestinal worms by using an antibiotic that interferes with the metabolism of the worms so they become paralyzed and die. This antibiotic is derived from a soil bacteria of the *Streptomyces* species.[2] The discovery has enormous worldwide importance, because some intestinal worms are not just a nuisance. Some cause blindness, and others cause chronic disfiguring and debilitating infection of the lymphatic system. The new antibiotic is called Ivermectin, and it works in animals as well as humans. It has low toxicity and only needs to be administered once or twice a year. If Ötzi had had Ivermectin, he would not have needed to purge himself in an effort to eliminate his worms. Who knows, maybe the dehydration caused by purging contributed to his death. Maybe if he'd had Ivermectin, he wouldn't have been entombed by an alpine glacier for discovery thousands of years later.

But that is only half the story. The other half of the 2015 Nobel Prize in Physiology or Medicine was awarded to Tu Youyou for her work with Artemesia and the discovery of its antimalarial properties (Chapter 44).

Artemesia, also called wormwood, is an herbal remedy used in many cultures to repel insects, expel parasitic worms, kill fungi, and bring down fevers. It is mentioned in the *Ebers Papyrus*, the Hebrew Bible, and in the *Materia Medica* of Dioscorides, Pliny, and Galen, confirming its use for millennia all around the globe. In China it was listed in an ancient text called the *Fifty-two Remedies* as an anti-fever remedy.[3]

There are over 400 species of the genus *Artemesia,* and they all share a bitter taste and a reputation for being poisonous. In North and South America the plant is known as sagebrush, a sacred herb often used in Native American remedies. In some Native American cultures it is also burned in spiritual purification ceremonies known as "smudging." In traditional Chinese moxibustion therapy, it is mugwort (Artemisia) that is made into cones and burned over particular points on the body. Artemesia's reputation as an antimalarial agent in the West led to its use by the French troops in Algeria in the early 1800s to prevent malaria and get rid of worms.

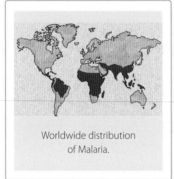

Worldwide distribution of Malaria.

Centers for Disease Control

Unfortunately, Youyou Tu's research could only be published in Chinese journals, so her work went unnoticed by the outside world until 1981, when she presented her findings at an international conference on the chemotherapy of malaria in Beijing, where she was the keynote speaker. Project 523 was disbanded by the Chinese government in 1981, but Tu's research had sparked interest on the part of the World Health Organization (WHO) and the World Bank.

Funding for further research came from the multinational pharmaceutical company Novartis and many other international non-governmental organizations seeking a medication that would have worldwide impact. The result was ACT (Artemisinin-based combination therapy), which, together with vector control by means of insecticide-treated mosquito nets and indoor spraying, reduced the mortality rate of malaria by 60 percent globally (and by 65 percent among children under 5) between 2000 and 2015.[4]

It is fitting that that the Nobel Prize went to researchers whose discoveries addressed parasitic diseases, because these have devastating consequences for the world's most vulnerable and poor inhabitants, an especially poignant issue in the twenty-first century, when many of the innovations, inventions, and discoveries in medicine benefit only the few who can afford exorbitant expenses for high-tech bionic replacement parts and procedures. The 2015 Nobel Prize discoveries weave together the companion themes of our book: folk medicine and science. We have seen the folk remedies of moldy bread for infected wounds (Chapter 35), the recipes of the Shropshire wife who used foxglove for dropsy (Chapter 13), the filtering of water with folded saris in South Asia to prevent cholera (Chapter 9), and now the use of wormwood for malaria.

There are many challenges for implementation. Youyou Tu's discovery could not have produced useful drugs for humanity without the help of the world's leading pharmaceutical companies. This was true also for Fleming (Chapter 35), Brotzu (Chapter 39), and Ehrlich (Chapter 33). In the twentieth and twenty-first centuries, huge financial commitments have become necessary to bring new discoveries to fruition, resources beyond the capacity of any one individual or institution.[5] In the case of Artemesia, it took the Mao-led Chinese government, the WHO, the United Nations Children's Fund, the United Nations Development Programme, the World Bank, Novartis, and many other intermediaries to implement the discovery.[6] The resultant combination therapy eradicates malaria completely.

Bridging the divide between traditional healing and bioscience is a major global challenge at this point. The WHO's endorsement of ACT[7] has caused conflict with traditional healers in Africa and elsewhere.

Herbalists, traditional birth attendants, bone setters, diviners, faith healers, traditional surgeons, spiritualists, and many others provide 80 percent of the healthcare in the countries where malaria is endemic, and 85 percent of treatments are based on herbal medicine.[8] The two major objections to ACT have been answered. High costs have been satisfactorily addressed by demonstration projects like the Affordable Medicines for Malaria (AMFM)[9] program, which has brought the prices down to levels comparable to less effective monotherapies, and the issue of adherence to the medication schedule has been addressed by new ACTS that are administered only twice daily.[10]

Nevertheless, less-effective folk remedies are more likely to be used in the very countries where malaria is endemic. Modern medicine has not yet satisfactorily addressed the disruptive effects of local commercialized growing of Artemesia, ingrown distrust of Western biomedicine by local cultures, fears of economic exploitation and medical coercion, and pride in traditional heritage.[11] It will take more than a Nobel Prize or two to overcome such issues.

Glossary

Aboriginal: Native or indigenous; referring to the original inhabitants of a land.

Alchemy: A scientific pursuit, not distinguished from chemistry until after the late seventeenth century; later associated with magic, fraud, and pseudoscience.

Allele: One of two or more alternative forms of a gene, found at the same place on a chromosome.

Amulet: A piece of jewelry or an ornament carried as a protection against evil or source of supernatural power.

Animalcules: Leeuwenhoek's name for microbes; literally, "little animals."

Antibody: A protein produced and used by the immune system to identify and attack bacteria, viruses, and other pathogens.

Antigen: A toxin or other substance that triggers an immune response in the body.

Aorta: The main artery of the body.

Artery: A vessel carrying blood from the heart to other parts of the body.

Asclepieion (plural, Asclepieia): A temple dedicated to Asklepios (the Greek god of healing), in which priestly physicians and a spa-like therapeutic environment contributed to patient cures.

Ayurveda: An ancient system of medicine with roots in the Indus River Valley civilization.

Bacillus: A genus of bacteria.

Black bile: In humoral theory, black bile (dry and cold) was the humor associated with earth and a melancholy disposition.

Black Death: An epidemic of bubonic plague that struck Europe in 1347 and killed as much as one third of the population.

Blood: In humoral theory, blood (wet and hot) was the humor associated with air and an optimistic (sanguine) disposition.

Cadaver: Corpse; dead body.

Caliph: A Muslim ruler, regarded as the successor to Muhammad.

Canopic jars: Containers for organs removed from Egyptian mummies.

Cataract: Clouding of the eye, usually age-related.

Cathartic: A purgative, meant to cause defecation.

Cautery (or cauterization): The act of burning a body part to remove it or close it off; this was once a routine way to prevent excessive bleeding during amputations or other surgeries.

Emetic: A medicine intended to cause vomiting.

Empirical: Based on experience or observation, as opposed to theory; hands-on.

Encephalitis: An inflammation of the brain.

Gangrene: Death of body tissues because of lost blood supply.

Hieroglyphic: Of a system of writing (such as that of ancient Egypt) in which pictographic and phonetic symbols may be combined.

Hippocratic Corpus: A collection of about 60 ancient Greek medical works attributed to or associated with Hippocrates; probably written between the fifth and the third centuries BC.

Humoral: Having to do with bodily fluids, or humors. Can refer to ancient humoral theory which claimed health depended on the balance among four basic humors—blood, black bile, phlegm, and yellow bile.

Hypothesis (plural, hypotheses): An explanation based on available evidence, proposed as a starting point for further investigation.

Incantation: Words spoken or chanted as part of a magical spell or charm.

Indigenous: Native to a place; (of a people) having lived there since before colonists arrived.

Inoculation: Vaccination; especially the introduction of a pathogen, possibly in weakened form, to stimulate the body's own immune system.

Leper: A person who has leprosy (Hansen's disease), or, in Biblical times, a person suffering from some chronic contagious disease affecting the skin.

Lesion: An area where disease or injury has damaged an organ or tissue; a wound, ulcer, tumor, or other reaction to disease or trauma.

Miasma theory: The belief that diseases (especially epidemic diseases) were spread by unwholesome air.

Microbes: Organisms too small to see without a microscope, such as the bacteria that cause disease or fermentation.

Mortality: Death, usually considered on a population-wide rather than individual basis, as in calculations of mortality rate: for every 1,000 individuals in a population, how many die each year of a given cause?

Mutation: Harmful change in a gene.

Neolithic: Relating to the later part of the Stone Age (the New Stone Age).

Neurosyphilis: Late stage syphilis that attacks the central nervous system, sometimes causing blindness, dementia, psychosis, and other symptoms. In the early twentieth century, these syphilis victims crowded mental hospitals.

Nestorian: A follower of Nestorius (AD 386 – 450), whose doctrine (considered heretical in the West) emphasized disunion between the divine and human natures of Jesus. Nestorian Christians, driven from Byzantium, established themselves in Sassanid Persia.

Obstetrics: Branch of medicine concerned with childbirth.

Pandemic: A severe, widespread epidemic; in 1918, a flu pandemic swept from the U.S. and Europe around the world, killing tens of millions.

Parasite: An organism that lives at the expense of another. Examples in medicine include viruses, bacteria, and parasitic worms.

Pathogen: A germ; an agent causing disease.

Pharaoh: Ruler of ancient Egypt.

Phlegm: In humoral theory, phlegm (cold and wet) was the humor associated with water and a stoic or unemotional disposition.

Plague: 1) A deadly pandemic, decimating large populations; or 2) bubonic plague, a disease caused by *Yersinia pestis*.

Polymorphisms: Genetic variations within a population.

Poultice: A moist soft mass that can be applied to a wounded or painful part of the body and held in place, typically with soft cloth. It may be heated and/or medicated.

Prosthesis (plural, prostheses): An artificial replacement for a missing limb, nose, or other body part.

Puerperal: Related to childbirth.

Ritual: A solemn ceremony in which actions must be performed and words spoken in a set order; often a religious observance.

Serum (plural, sera): Liquid that separates out when blood coagulates. Serum retains antibodies and can be used as the basis for vaccines and diagnostic tests.

Shaman: A person who can speak with and influence powers in the spirit world; in many prehistoric and contemporary indigenous cultures, shamans have served as healers.

Smallpox: A contagious disease, now extinct in the wild; historically, smallpox killed about 30% of its victims and left many others blind or disfigured.

Spontaneous generation, theory of: The old folk belief that living creatures (such as fleas) may arise from inanimate matter (such as dust); discredited by the experiments of Louis Pasteur.

Sushruta Samhita: Compendium of Sushruta; a collection of medical texts probably composed over time (c. 600 BC – AD 500) by a number of people and associated with the legendary physician Sushruta.

Suturing: Stitching up a wound so the flesh will heal.

Toxin: A poisonous substance, such as snake or spider venom.

Trepanation [sometimes spelled trephination]: Drilling, incising, or scraping a hole in the skull; a surgical intervention often practiced in prehistoric times.

Vector: An organism that transmits a disease or parasite from one host to another. Fleas are vectors of plague, deer ticks of Lyme disease, and mosquitoes of malaria, yellow fever, Zika, and other illnesses.

Vortex (plural, vortices): A swirl of fluid around an axis; seen in smoke rings, stirred coffee mugs, flushed toilets, etc.

Yellow bile, or choler: In humoral theory, yellow bile (hot and dry) was the humor associated with fire and an angry disposition.

Sources

Introduction: What Is Discovery?

Sources
Azizi, M. H., *et al.* "A Brief History of the Discovery of the Circulation of Blood in the Human Body." *Archive of Iranian Medicine* 11, 3 (May 2008): 345–50.
Krystal, John H., and Matthew W. State. "Psychiatric Disorders: Diagnosis to Therapy." *Cell* 157, 1 (March 2014): 201–14.

1. Ca. 3200 BC. The Iceman: Forensic Analysis of a Neolithic Killing

Sources
Bhanoo, Sindya N. "Lactose Intolerant, Before Milk Was on the Menu." *New York Times* (5 March 2006): www.nytimes.com/2012/03/06/science/iceman-had-brown-eyes-and-hair-and-was-lactose-intolerant.html.
Dickson, J. H., *et al.* "The Omnivorous Tyrolean Iceman: Colon Contents (Meat, Cereals, Pollen, Moss and Whipworm) and Stable Isotope Analyses." *Philosophical Transactions of the Royal Society of London B: Biological Sciences* 355, 1404 (2000): 1843–49.
Dorfer, L., *et al.* "A Medical Report from the Stone Age?" *The Lancet* 354 (18 September 1999): 1023–25.
Gostner, Paul, *et al.* "New Radiological Insights into the Life and Death of the Tyrolean Iceman." *Journal of Archaeological Science* 38, 12 (2011): 3425–31.
Hardy, Karen, Stephen Buckley, Matthew J. Collins, Almudena Estalrrich, Don Brothwell, *et al.* "Neanderthal Medics? Evidence for Food, Cooking, and Medicinal Plants Entrapped in Dental Calculus. *Naturwissenschaften* 99, 8 (2012): 617–26.
Knox, Richard. "Oetzi the Iceman May Be the Last in His Family." NPR (30 October 2008): www.npr.org/templates/story/story.php?storyId=96328080.
Magner, Lois N. *A History of Medicine*, 2d ed. New York: Taylor & Francis, 2005.
Ooi, Vincent E. C. and Fang Liu, "Immunomodulation and Anti-cancer Activity of Polysaccharide-protein Complexes," *Current Medical Chemistry* 7, 7 (2000): 715–29.
Peintner, U., *et al.*, "The Iceman's Fungi," *Mycological Research* 102, 10 (1998): 1153–62.
Saey, Tina Hesman. "Genome Paints a Better Portrait of the Iceman." *Science News* 181, 6 (24 March 2012): 5–6.
Samadelli, Marco, *et al.* "Complete Mapping of the Tattoos of the 5300-year-old Tyrolean Iceman." *Journal of Cultural Heritage* 16, 5 (2015): 753–58.
Wikipedia. "Ötzi." https://en.wikipedia.org/wiki/%C3%96tzi.
Wilford, John Noble. "Lessons in Iceman's Prehistoric Medicine Kit." *New York Times* (December 8, 1998). nytimes.com/1998/12/08/science/lessons-in-iceman-s-prehistoric-medicine-kit.html.

Additional Resources
Barbu, George. *Death of the Iceman*. BBC Horizon (2002): www.dailymotion.com/video/x225zgq_bbc-horizon-2002-death-of-the-iceman_shortfilms.
Eurac Research. "Iceman Photoscan." www.icemanphotoscan.eu/.
McQuilton, Michael. *Bushcraft Foraging: Piptoporus Betulinus*. YouTube (23 October 2015): https://www.youtube.com/watch?v=oXXyXaxP72Y.
Morelle, Rebecca. "Oetzi the Iceman Had a Stomach Bug, Researchers Say." BBC News, Science & Environment (8 January 2016): www.bbc.com/news/science-environment-35251892.
South Tyrol Museum of Archaeology. www.iceman.it/en/oetzi-the-iceman.
Spinosa, Ron. "Chaga: Chaga in the News." www.chagamushroom.com/chaga_in_the_news.htm.
Wade, Nicholas. "Ötzi the Iceman's Stomach Bacteria Offers Clues on Human Migration." *New York Times* (8 January 2016): www.nytimes.com/2016/01/08/science/otzi-the-iceman-stomach-bacteria-europe-migration.html.

2. A Parade of Ants: Magic and Folk Healing

Sources:
Aboriginal Art. *Traditional Aboriginal Bush Medicine*. Reen at Big River Internet (2000): www.aboriginalartonline.com/culture/medicine.php.
Cumes, David. "South African Indigenous Healing: How It Works." *Explore* 9, 1 (2013): 58–65.
Horrigan, Bonnie J. "Lyall Watson, Ph.D.: Healers, Healing, and the Nature of Reality." [interview]. *Explore* 2, 1 (2006): 47–54.
Lee, Hwa-Jin, *et al.* "Convergence of Dance and Korean Medicine: Focusing on the Therapeutic Function." *Oriental Pharmacy and Experimental Medicine* 15 (2015): 217–26.
Magner, Lois N. *A History of Medicine*, 2d ed. New York: Taylor & Francis, 2005.

Press, Irwin. "Urban Folk Medicine." *American Anthropologist* 80, 1 (1978): 71–84.
Sexton, Randall, and Ellen Anne Buljo Stabbursvik, "Healing in the Sámi North," *Culture, Medicine, and Psychiatry* 34 (2010): 571–89.
United Nations. "World Conference on Indigenous Peoples." (22–23 September 2014): www. un.org/en/ga/69/meetings/indigenous/background.shtml.
University of Ottawa. "Aboriginal Medicine and Healing Practices." Society, the Individual, and Medicine. (July 8, 2009): www.med.uottawa.ca/sim/data/Aboriginal_Medicine_e.htm.

Additional Resources:
American Museum of Natural History. "Journeys to Other Worlds: Rites of the Shamans." www. amnh.org/exhibitions/vietnam/journeys-to-other-worlds.
Burns, Corinne, and Randolph Arroo. "How to Cure the Stiffening of the Serpent: Herbal Medicine, Aztec Style." *Herbs* 30, 3 (2005): www.mexicolore.co.uk/aztecs/health/ herbal-medicine-aztec-style.
National Libraries of Medicine. "Native Voices: Native Peoples' Concepts of Health and Illness." www.nlm.nih.gov/nativevoices/.
Solomon, Andrew. "Naked, Covered in Ram's Blood, Drinking a Coke, and Feeling Pretty Good." *Esquire* (28 February 2014): www.esquire.com/news-politics/news/a27628/ notes-on-an-exorcism/.
Solomon, Andrew. "Notes on an Exorcism." *The Moth* (5 August 2014): http://themoth.org/posts/ episodes/1005.
Traditional Healers of South Africa. Revolvy. www.revolvy.com/main/index.php?s=Traditional%20 healers%20of%20South%20Africa.
van der Lee, Ton. *Zulu Sangoma and Spirit Healing.* Spirits of Africa. www.youtube.com/ watch?v=c4UQbozNFtM.

3. Massage: Rubbing Out Demons and Kinks

Sources:
Böck, Barbara. "When You Perform the Ritual of 'Rubbing': On Medicine and Magic in Ancient Mesopotamia." *Journal of Near Eastern Studies* 62 (2003): 1–16.
Celsus, A. Cornelius. *De Medicina (On Medicine)*, trans. by W. G. Spencer. v. 1, Book II. Loeb Classical Library, 1935. http://penelope.uchicago.edu/Thayer/E/Roman/Texts/Celsus/2*.html.
Crane, Justin D., *et al.* "Massage Therapy Attenuates Inflammatory Signaling after Exercise-Induced Muscle Damage." *Science Translational Medicine* 4, 119 (1 February 2012): http://stm.sciencemag.org/ content/4/119/119ra13.
Field, Tiffany. "Massage Therapy Research Review." *Complementary Therapies in Clinical Practice* 20 (2014): 224–29.
Mayo Clinic Staff. "Massage Therapy: Overview." www.mayoclinic.org/tests-procedures/ massage-therapy/home/ovc-20170282.
National Center for Complementary and Integrative Health. "Massage Therapy for Health Purposes." U.S. Department of Health and Human Services (2006–2015): https://nccih.nih.gov/ health/massage/massageintroduction.htm.
Petersen, Andrea. "Don't Call It Pampering: Massage Wants to Be Medicine." *Wall Street Journal* (Mar. 13, 2012): www.wsj.com/articles/SB10001424052702304537904577277303049173934.
Seppa, Nathan. "Massage May Accelerate Healing." *Science News* 181, 5 (10 March 2012): 17.

Additional Resources
Bakalar, Nicholas. "How Massage Heals Sore Muscles." *New York Times* (6 February 2012): http://well. blogs.nytimes.com/2012/02/06/how-massage-heals-sore-muscles/?_r=0.
Mark, Joshua J. "Health Care in Ancient Mesopotamia." *Encyclopedia of Ancient History* (21 May 2014): www.ancient.eu/article/687/.
Silicon Valley Massage Therapy. "A Short History of Massage." svmassagetherapy.com/ blog/2015/06/06/a-short-history-of-massage/.
Wikipedia. "Social Grooming." https://en.wikipedia.org/wiki/Social_grooming.

4. 1500 BC: Ancient Egyptian Mummifiers and Surgeons: Secrets of the Dead

Sources
Bishop, William John. *The Early History of Surgery.* New York: Barnes and Noble, 1960.
Blomstedt, Patric. "Cataract Surgery in Ancient Egypt." *Journal of Cataract and Refractive Surgery* 40, 3 (2014): 485–89.
Blomstedt, Patric. "Orthopedic Surgery in Ancient Egypt." *Acta Orthopaedica* 85, 6 (2014): 670–676.
Brandt-Rauf, P.W., and S.I. Brandt-Rauf. "History of Occupational Medicine: Relevance of Imhotep and the Edwin Smith Papyrus." *British Journal of Industrial Medicine* 44, 1 (1987): 68–70.
Čavka, Mislav, *et al.* "CT-Guided Endoscopic Recovery of a Foreign Object from the Cranial Cavity of an Ancient Egyptian Mummy." *Radiographics* 32 (2012): 2151–57.
Finlayson, James. "Ancient Egyptian Medicine." *The British Medical Journal* 1 1684, (1893): 748–52.
Magner, Lois N. *A History of Medicine.* New York: Marcel Dekker, 1992.

Muffly, Tyler M., *et al.* "The History and Evolution of Sutures in Pelvic Surgery." *Journal of the Royal Society of Medicine* 104, 3 (2011): 107–12.

Ritner, Robert K. "Innovations and Adaptations in Ancient Egyptian Medicine." *Journal of Near Eastern Studies* 59, 2 (2000): 107–17.

Thompson, Ethel E. "Doctors, Doctrines, and Drugs in Ancient Times." *Bulletin of the Medical Library Association* 50, 2 (1962): 236–42.

von Staden, H. "The Discovery of the Body: Human Dissection and Its Cultural Contexts in Ancient Greece." *Yale Journal of Biology and Medicine* 65, 3 (1992): 223–41.

Wade, Andrew D., *et al.* "A Synthetic Radiological Study of Brain Treatment in Ancient Egyptian Mummies." *HOMO Journal of Comparative Human Biology* 62 (2011): 248–69.

Zysk, Kenneth G. "The Evolution of Anatomical Knowledge in Ancient India, with Special Reference to Cross-Cultural Influences." *Journal of the American Oriental Society* 106, 4 (1986): 687–705.

Additional Resources

Behind the Scenes: Ant Stitches Aftermath." *Dual Survival.* www.discovery.com/tv-shows/dual-survival/videos/behind-the-scenes-ant-stitches-aftermath/.

Encyclopedia Smithsonian. "Egyptian Mummies." (2012). www.si.edu/Encyclopedia_SI/nmnh/mummies.htm.

Mystery Universe. "Prosthetic Screw in 3000-Year-Old Egypt Mummy Discovered." YouTube (16 July 2015): www.youtube.com/watch?v=y0mnni55l80.

National Museum of Natural History. "Eternal Life in Ancient Egypt." 2016. http://naturalhistory.si.edu/exhibits/eternal-life/.

Raupp, Michael J. "Jungle Raiders: Army Ants, *Eciton SP.*" Bug of the Week (7 February 2011): http://bugoftheweek.com/blog/2013/1/11/jungle-raiders-army-ants-ieciton-spi.

Rothschild, Anna. "Ancient Cataract Surgery." Gross Science. NOVA (24 September 2015): www.pbs.org/wgbh/nova/ancient/ancient-cataract.html.

5. 170 BC: Sleep Therapy at the Temples of Asklepios

Sources:

Askitopoulou, Helen, *et al.* "Surgical Cures under Sleep Induction in the Asklepieion of Epidauros." *International Congress Series* 1242 (2002): 11–17.

Beecher, H. K. "The Powerful Placebo." *Journal of the American Medical Association* 159, 17 (1955): 1602–06.

Blackwell, Barry, Saul S. Bloomfield, and C. Ralph Buncher. "Demonstration to Medical Students of Placebo Responses and Non-drug Factors." *The Lancet* 299 (7763): 1279–82.

Compton, Michael T. "The Union of Religion and Health in Ancient Asklepieia." *Journal of Religion and Health* 37, 4 (1998): 301–12.

Di Blasi, Zelda, and Jos Kleijnen. "Context Effects, Powerful Therapies, or Methodological Bias," *Evaluation & the Health Professions* 26, 2 (2003): 166–79.

Dillon, M.P.J. "The Didactic Nature of the Epidaurian Iamata." *Zeitschrift für Papyrologie und Epigraphik* 101 (1994): 239–60.

Edelstein, Emma Jeannette Levy, and Ludwig Edelstein. *Asclepius: Collection and interpretation of the Testimonies.* Baltimore: Johns Hopkins University Press, 1998.

Faraut, Brice, *et al.* "Immune, inflammatory and cardiovascular consequences of sleep restriction and recovery." *Sleep Medicine Reviews* 16 (2012): 137–49.

Homer. *The Iliad of Homer*, trans. Richmond Lattimore. Chicago: University of Chicago Press, 1951.

Louhiala, P., and R. Puustinen. "Rethinking the Placebo Effect." *Medical Humanities* 34, 2 (2008): 107–09.

National Heart, Lung, and Blood Institute. "Why Is Sleep Important?" www.nhlbi.nih.gov/health/health-topics/topics/sdd/why.

Pindar. "Pythian 3: For Hieron of Syracuse Horse Race ?474 B. C." Ed. Svarlien, Diane Arnson. *Perseus Digital Library.* Tufts University: 1990. www.perseus.tufts.edu/hopper/text?doc=Perseus%3Atext%3A1999.01.0162%3Abook%3DP.%3Apoem%3D3.

Traut, Eugene F., and Edwin W. Passarelli. "Placebos in the Treatment of Rheumatoid Arthritis and Other Rheumatic Conditions." *Annals of the Rheumatic Diseases* 16, 1 (1957): 18–22.

Waber, Rebecca L., *et al.* "Commercial Features of Placebo and Therapeutic Efficacy." *JAMA* 299, 9 (2008): 1016–17.

Walach, Harald. 2011. "Placebo Controls: Historical, Methodological and General Aspects." *Philosophical Transactions: Biological Sciences* 366, 1572 (2011): 1870–78.

Additional Sources

Antiqua Medicina from Homer to Vesalius. "Healing Cults and Sanctuaries: Asclepius and Votive Offerings." University of Virginia Historical Collections at the Claude Moore Health Sciences Library. http://exhibits.hsl.virginia.edu/antiqua/healercults/.

Atsma, Aaron J. "Asklepios." *Theoi Project* (2000–2015): theoi.com/Ouranios/Asklepios.html.

Bryce, Emma. *The Power of the Placebo effect.* TED-Ed. www.youtube.com/watch?v=z03FQGlGgoo.

Science Museum: Brought to Life. "Visit the Asklepion."
    www.sciencemuseum.org.uk/broughttolife/themes/belief/asklepion_temple.
University of Warwick, Faculty of the Art. "Sanctuary of Asklepios, Epidaurus." www2.warwick.
    ac.uk/fac/arts/classics/students/modules/greekreligion/database/clumcc/.
Wikipedia. "Asclepeion." https://en.wikipedia.org/wiki/Asclepeion.

6. AD 200: Galen Discovers Nerves and Humors

Sources

Gross, Charles G. "Galen and the Squealing Pig." *Neuroscientist* 4 (1998): 216–21.
Nutton, Vivian. "The Fatal Embrace: Galen and the History of Ancient Medicine." *Science in Context*
    18, 1 (March 2005): 111–21.
Nutton, Vivian. "Galen and Roman Medicine: Or Can a Greek Become a Latin?" *European Review* 20,
    4 (October 2012): 534–42.
Nutton, Vivian. "Logic, Learning, and Experimental Medicine." *Science, New Series* 295, 5556 (1 Febru-
    ary 2002): 800–01.
"Origins & History of Chinese Medicine." Sacred Lotus (2001–2015): www.sacredlotus.com/go/
    foundations-chinese-medicine/get/origins-history-chinese-medicine.
Pachuta, Donald M. "Chinese Medicine: The Law of Five Elements," *India International Centre Quarterly*
    18, 2/3 (1991): 41–68.
Scarborough, John. "The Galenic Question." *Sudhoffs Archiv* 65, 1 (1981): 1–31.
Varma, Daya R. "From Witchcraft to Allopathy: Uninterrupted Journey of Medical Science." *Eco-
    nomic and Political Weekly* 41, 33 (2006): 3605–11.
Wikipedia. "Huangdi Neijing." https://en.wikipedia.org/wiki/Huangdi_Neijing.

Additional Resources

Antiqua Medicina from Homer to Vesalius: "Galen: Greek Physician, Surgeon, and Philosopher in
    the Roman Empire." University of Virginia Historical Collections at the Claude Moore Health
    Sciences Library.
    http://exhibits.hsl.virginia.edu/antiqua/galen/.
India: Ayurveda. Full Episodes on Discovery. www.discovery.com/tv-shows/other-shows/videos/
    discovery-atlas-india-ayurveda/.
Mootz, Denis. *Ancient Discoveries.* www.historychannel.com.au/teachers-guide/ancient-discoveries/.
Nordqvist, Christian. *What is ancient Roman Medicine.* Medical News Today. www.medicalnewstoday.
    com/info/medicine/ancient-roman-medicine.php.
Ogden, Aimee. *How Galen's Mistake Misled Medicine for Centuries.* Mental_Floss. mentalfloss.com/
    article/66738/how-galens-mistake-misled-medicine-centuries.
Origins and History of Chinese Medicine. Sacred Lotus: Chinese Medicine. www.sacredlotus.com/go/
    foundations-chinese-medicine/get/origins-history-chinese-medicine.
Science Museum: Brought to Life. "Humours."
    www.sciencemuseum.org.uk/broughttolife/techniques/humours.

7. 900: Al-Razi and Evidence-Based Medicine in the Middle Ages

Al-Ghazal, Sharif Khaf. "The Origin of Bismaristans (Hospitals) in Islamic Medical History." Man-
    chester, UK: Foundation for Science, Technology, and Civilization, April 2007. www.muslim-
    heritage.com/uploads/The_Origin_of_Bimaristans_in_Islamic_Medical_History.pdf.
Cochrane, Steve. "Asian Centres of Learning and Witness before 1000 C.E.: Insights for Today."
    Transformation 26, 1 (2009): 30–39.
Hajar, Rachel. "The Air of History (Part IV): Great Muslim Physicians Al Rhazes." *Heart Views* 14
    (2013): 93–95. www.heartviews.org/text.asp?2013/14/2/93/115499.
Hourani, Albert. *A History of the Arab Peoples.* Cambridge, MA: The Belknap Press, 1991, 2002.
Houston, G. W. "An Overview of Nestorians in Inner Asia," *Central Asiatic Journal* 24, 1/2 (1980):
    60–68.
Mackensen, Ruth Stellhorn. "Background of the History of Moslem Libraries (Continued)." *The
    American Journal of Semitic Languages and Literatures* 52, 1 (1935): 22–33.
Magner, Lois N. *A History of Medicine.* New York: Marcel Dekker, 1992.
Miller, A. C. "Jundi-Shapur, Bimaristans, and the Rise of Academic Medical Centres." *Journal of the
    Royal Society of Medicine* 99, 12 (2006): 615–17.
Pormann, Peter E. "Qualifying and Quantifying Medical Uncertainty in
    10th Century Baghdad: Abu Bakr al-Razi." *JLL Bulletin: Commentar-
    ies on the History of Treatment Evaluation* (2013): www.jameslindlibrary.org/articles/
    qualifying-and-quantifying-medical-uncertainty-in-10th-century-baghdad-abu-bakr-al-razi/.
Tibi, Selma. "Al-Razi and Islamic Medicine in the 9th Century." *JLL Bulletin: Commen-
    taries on the History of Treatment Evaluation* (2005): www.jameslindlibrary.org/articles/
    al-razi-and-islamic-medicine-in-the-9th-century/.
Whipple, Allen O. "Role of the Nestorians as the Connecting Link between Greek and Arabic Medi-
    cine." *Bulletin of the New York Academy of Medicine* 12, 7 (1936): 446–62.
Zarrintan, Sina, *et al.* "Early Contributions of Abu Bakr Muhammad ibn Zakariya Razi (865–925) to
    Evidence-Based Medicine." *International Journal of Cardiology* 168, 1 (20 September 2013): 604–05.

Additional Resources

Ali, Sara. "Medical Education in Medieval Islam." *Hektoen International* 8, 1 (Winter 2016): www.hektoeninternational.org/index.php?option=com_content&view=article&id=164:medical-education-in-medieval-islam&catid=18&Itemid=435.

Savage-Smith, Emilie. "The Art as a Profession." *Islamic Culture and the Medical Arts.* Bethesda, MD: National Library of Medicine, 1994. https://www.nlm.nih.gov/exhibition/islamic_medical/islamic_13.html.

8. 1508: DaVinci's Heart

Sources

Bissell, M.M., E. Dall'Armellina, and R.P. Choudhury. "Flow Vortices in the Aortic Root: In vivo 4D-MRI Confirms Predictions of Leonardo da Vinci." *European Heart Journal* 35, 20 (2014): 1344.

Boon, B. "Leonardo da Vinci on Atherosclerosis and the Function of the Sinuses of Valsalva." *Netherlands Heart Journal* 17, 12 (2009): 496–99.

Chiarelli, Leonard C. "Muslim Sicily and the Beginnings of Medical Licensing in Europe." *Journal of the Islamic Medical Association of North America* 31, 2 (1999). http://jima.imana.org/article/view/5551/31_2-8.

Ghosh, Sanjib Kumar. "Human Cadaveric Dissection: A Historical Account from Ancient Greece to the Modern Era." *Anatomy & Cell Biology* 48, 3 (2015): 153–69.

Keele, Kenneth D. "Leonardo da Vinci's Influence on Renaissance Anatomy." *Medical History* 8, 4 (1964): 360–70.

Khan, Ijaz A., Samantapudi K. Daya, and Ramesh M. Gowda. "Evolution of the Theory of Circulation." *International Journal of Cardiology* 98, 3 (2005): 519–21.

Martins e Silva, Joao. "Leonardo da Vinci and the First Hemodynamic Observations." *Revista portuguesa de cardiología* 27, 2 (2008): 243–72. www.ncbi.nlm.nih.gov/pubmed/18488922.

Mesquita, E.T., C.V. de Souza Junior, and T.R. Ferreira. "Andreas Vesalius 500 Years - A Renaissance That Revolutionized Cardiovascular Knowledge." *Revista Brasileira de Cirurgía Cardiovascular* 30, 2 (2015): 260–65.

Wells, Francis C. *The Heart of Leonardo.* Heidelberg: Springer, 2013.

West, John B. "Ibn al-Nafis, the Pulmonary Circulation, and the Islamic Golden Age." *Journal of Applied Physiology* (1985) 105, 6 (2008): 1877–80. www.ncbi.nlm.nih.gov/pmc/articles/PMC2612469/?report=classic.

Additional Sources

Roxby, Phillippa. "What Leonardo Taught Us about the Heart." BBC News (28 June 2014): www.bbc.comnews/health-28054468.

Royal Collection Trust. "Leonardo da Vinci: The Mechanics of Man." Edinburgh: The Queen's Gallery, Palace of Holyroodhouse, 2013. www.royalcollection.org.uk/exhibitions/leonardo-da-vinci-the-mechanics-of-man.

Sellmer, Rory. "Anatomy and Art in the Renaissance." *The Proceedings of the 10th Annual History of Medicine Days*, 80–82. Calgary, Alberta: Faculty of Medicine, University of Calgary, March 23 – 24, 2001. www.ucalgary.ca/uofc/Others/HOM/Dayspapers2001.pdf.

Sooke, Alastair. "Leonardo da Vinci: Anatomy of an Artist." *Daily Telegraph* (July 28, 2013): www.telegraph.co.uk/culture/art/leonardo-da-vinci/10202124/Leonardo-da-Vinci-Anatomy-of-an-artist.html.

Van Doren, Charles. "The Renaissance Man." From *A History of Knowledge: Past, Present, and Future* (New York: Ballantine Books, 1991). http://alexpetrov.com.memes/hum/renaissance-man.html.

Vesalius. "de Humani Corporis Fabrica." https://ceb.nlm.nih.gov/proj/ttp/flash/vesalius/vesalius.html.

Wells, Francis. *Leonardo da Vinci.* The Prince's Teaching Institute, 2013. https://vimeo.com/56980795.

9. 1660: The Chamberlen Family Secret

Sources

Dunn, Peter M. "The Chamberlen Family (1560–1728) and Obstetric Forceps." *Archives of Disease in Childhood - Fetal and Neonatal Edition* 81, 3 (November 1, 1999): F232–34. http://fn.bmj.com/content/81/3/F232.

Girl Museum. "STEM Girls: Agnodice." (4 March 2015): www.girlmuseum.org/stem-girls-agnodice/.

Hibbard, Bryan M. *The Obstetrician's Armamentarium: Historical Obstetrical Instruments and Their Inventors.* San Anselmo, California: Norman Publishing, 2000.

Hyginus, Caius Julius. "274. Inventors and Their Inventions." *Fabulae.* Tr. Mary Grant. Classical E-Text: Hyginus, Fabulae 200 – 277. www.theoi.com/Text/HyginusFabulae5.html.

Lingo, Alison Klairmont. "Obstetrics and Midwifery." *Encyclopedia of Children and Childhood in History and Society.* www.faqs.org/childhood/Me-Pa/Obstetrics-and-Midwifery.html.

Lurie, Samuel. "Caesarean Section in Ancient Greek Mythology." *Acta med-hist Adriat* 13, no. 1 (2015): 209–16.

Massey, Lyle. "Pregnancy and Pathology: Picturing Childbirth in Eighteenth-Century Obstetric Atlases." *The Art Bulletin* 87, 1 (2005): 73–91.

Radosh, Polly F. "Midwives in the United States: Past and Present." *Population Research and Policy Review* 5, 2 (1986): 129–146.

Raju, Tonse N.K. "The Birth of Caesar and the Cesarean Misnomer." *American Journal of Perinatology* 24, 10 (2007): 567–68.

Sheikh, Sukhera, Inithan Ganesaratnam, and Haider Jan. "The Birth of Forceps." *Journal of the Royal Society of Medicine Short Reports* 4 (2013): 1–4.

Soranus, of Ephesus. *Soranus' Gynecology*. Tr. Owsei Temkin. Baltimore, MD: Johns Hopkins Press, 1956.

Additional Resources

Helmuth, Laura. "The Disturbing, Shameful History of Childbirth Deaths." *Slate* (10 September 2013): www.slate.com/articles/health_and_science/science_of_longevity/2013/09/death_in_childbirth_doctors_increased_maternal_mortality_in_the_20th_century.html.

McRobbie, Linda Rodriguez. *Four Historical Royal Birthing Traditions*. Mental_Floss. http://mentalfloss.com/article/51781/4-historical-royal-birthing-traditions.

Sewell, Jane Eliot. *Cesarian Section – A Brief History*. History of Medicine. Washington, DC: U. S. National Library of Medicine, 1993–2013. www.nlm.nih.gov/exhibition/cesarean/part1.html.

10. 1670: Looking Through Van Leeuwenhoek's Tiny Microscopes

Sources

Anderson, Douglas. "Still Going Strong: Leeuwenhoek at Eighty." *Antonie van Leeuwenhoek Journal of Microbiology* 105, 4 (2014): http://lensonleeuwenhoek.net/sites/default/files/avl_at_80.pdf.

Baker, Henry. "An Account of Mr. Leeuwenhoek's Microscopes." *Philosophical Transactions* 41 (1 January 1739): 503–19.

Ford, Brian J. "The Royal Society and the Microscope." *Notes and Records of the Royal Society of London* 55, 1 (January 2001): 29–49.

Gest, Howard. "The Discovery of Microorganisms by Robert Hooke and Antoni van Leeuwenhoek, Fellows of the Royal Society." *Notes and Records of the Royal Society of London* 58, 2 (May 2004): 187–201.

Palm, Lodewijk C. "The Edition of Leeuwenhoek's Letters: Changing Demands, Changing Policies." *Text* 17 (2005): 265–76.

Royal Society. "History." royalsociety.org/about-us/history/.

Ruestow, Edward G. "Leeuwenhoek and the Campaign against Spontaneous Generation." *Journal of the History of Biology* 17, 2 (Summer 1984): 225–48.

Wikipedia, "Gresham College and the Formation of the Royal Society," en.wikipedia.org/wiki/Gresham_College_and_the_formation_of_the_Royal_Society.

Additional Resources

British Library. "Fleas, Mould, and Plant Cells: Under a 17th Century Microscope with Robert Hooke." (27 July 2014): http://britishlibrary.typepad.co.uk/collectioncare/2014/07/roberthooke.html.

Famous Scientists. "Robert Hooke." www.famousscientists.org/robert-hooke/.

Hooke, Robert. "Micropraphia." https://ceb.nlm.nih.gov/proj/ttp/flash/hooke/hooke.html.

Lane, Nick. "The Unseen World: Reflections on Leeuwenhoek (1677) 'Concerning Little Animals'." *Philosophical Transactions B* 370, 1666 (2015): http://rstb.royalsocietypublishing.org/content/370/1666/20140344.

Loncke, Hans. "Making an Antonie van Leeuwenhoek Microscope Replica." www.microscopy-uk.org.uk/mag/indexmag.html?http://www.microscopy-uk.org.uk/mag/artjul07/hl-loncke2.html.

Philipszoon, Thonis. "Antonj van Leeuwenhoek, 1632–1723 A.D. Peter W. Pedrotti, Jr., AntonieVanLeeuwenhoek.com (2010): www.vanleeuwenhoek.com/.

11. 1721: Fighting Smallpox and Public Opinion in Colonial Boston

Sources:

Coss, Stephen. *The Fever of 1721: The Epidemic That Revolutionized Medicine and American Politics*. New York: Simon & Schuster, 2016.

Fenner, Frank. "Smallpox: Emergence, Global Spread, and Eradication." *History and Philosophy of the Life Sciences* 15, 3 (1993): 397–420.

Gross, Cary P., and Kent A. Sepkowitz. "The Myth of the Medical Breakthrough: Smallpox, Vaccination, and Jenner Reconsidered." *International Journal of Infectious Diseases* 3, 1 (1998): 54–60.

Jones, David S. *Rationalizing Epidemics: Meanings and Uses of American Indian Mortality since 1600*. Cambridge, MA: Harvard University Press, 2004.

Leung, Angela Ki Che. "'Variolation' and Vaccination in Late Imperial China, Ca 1570–1911." Chapter 2 in *History of Vaccine Development*, edited by Stanley A. Plotkin, 5–12. New York: Springer, 2011.

Mann, Charles O. *1491: New Revelations of the Americas Before Columbus*. New York: Vintage, 2011.

Mayor, Adrienne. "The Nessus Shirt in the New World: Smallpox Blankets in History and Legend." *The Journal of American Folklore* 108, 427 (1995): 54–77.

Riedel, Stefan. "Edward Jenner and the History of Smallpox and Vaccination." Proceedings (Baylor University. Medical Center) 18, 1 (2005): 21–25.

Small, Parker A. and S. Small Natalie. "Mankind's Magnificent Milestone: Smallpox Eradication." *The American Biology Teacher* 58, 5 (1996): 264–71.

Wikipedia. "Smallpox." https://en.wikipedia.org/wiki/Smallpox.

Wikipedia. "Variolation." https://en.wikipedia.org/wiki/Variolation.

World Health Organization. "Smallpox: Eradicating an Ancient Scourge." Chapter 1 in *Bugs, Drugs, and Smoke: Stories from Public Health*, 3–11. World Health Organization, 2011. www.who.int/about/history/publications/public_health_stories/en/.

Additional Resources

Contagion: Historical Views of Diseases and Epidemics. "The Boston Smallpox Epidemic, 1721." Harvard University Library Open Collection Program. http://ocp.hul.harvard.edu/contagion/smallpox.html.

The College of Physicians of Philadelphia. "Smallpox Lesions 2." The History of Vaccines, Gallery. www.historyofvaccines.org/content/smallpox-lesions-2.

Flight, Colette. "Smallpox: Eradicating the Scourge." BBC (Feb 17, 2011): www.bbc.co.uk/history/british/empire_seapower/smallpox_01.shtml.

McEleney, Brenda. "Smallpox: A Primer." The Counterproliferation Papers, Future Warfare Series No. 9. Maxwell Air Force Base, AL: Air University, [2000]. www.au.af.mil/au/awc/awcgate/cpc-pubs/biostorm/mceleney.pdf.

National Geographic. "Smallpox Mystery." http://video.nationalgeographic.com/video/smallpox-sci.

Science Museum: Brought to Life. "Smallpox: Innoculation and vaccination." www.sciencemuseum.org.uk/broughttolife/themes/diseases/smallpox.

12. 1747: Limeys and the Conquest of Scurvy

Sources

Baron, Jeremy Hugh. "Sailors' Scurvy before and after James Lind—A Reassessment." *Nutrition Reviews* 67, 6 (2009): 315–32.

Centers for Disease Control and Prevention. "Executive Summary," *Second National Report on Biochemical Indicators of Diet and Nutrition in the U.S. Population.* Atlanta, GA: National Center for Environmental Health, 2012. cdc.gov/nutritionreport/index.html.

Eijkman, Christiaan. "Nobel Lecture." nobelprize.org/nobel_prizes/medicine/laureates/1929/eijkman-lecture.html.

Gordon, Eleanora C. "Scurvy and Anson's Voyage Round the World 1740–1744: An Analysis of the Royal Navy's Worst Outbreak." *American Neptune* 44 (1984): 155–65. www.mv.helsinki.fi/home/hemila/history/Gordon_1984.pdf.

Harrison, M. "Scurvy on Sea and Land: Political Economy and Natural History, 1780–1850." *Journal for Maritime Research* 15, 1 (2013): 7–25.

Hoenig, Leonard J., and Walter H. C. Burgdorf. "Scurvy Aboard Ferdinand Magellan's Voyage of Circumnavigation." *JAMA Dermatology* 150, 7 (2014): 742.

Kodicek, Egon H., and Frank G. Young. "Captain Cook and Scurvy." *Notes and Records of the Royal Society of London* 24, 1 (1969): 43–63.

Kumar, Saravana. "Closing the Evidence-Practice Gaps: The Challenges and Opportunities." *AQ: Australian Quarterly* 83, 4 (2012): 22–25, 32.

Lloyd, C. C. "The Conquest of Scurvy." The British Journal for the History of Science 1, no. 4 (1963): 357–63.

MedlinePlus. "Vitamin C." National Library of Medicine. nlm.nih.gov/medlineplus/ency/article/002404.htm.

Milne, Iain. "Who Was James Lind, and What Exactly Did He Achieve?" *JLL Bulletin: Commentaries on the History of Treatment Evaluation* (2012): www.jameslindlibrary.org/articles/who-was-james-lind-and-what-exactly-did-he-achieve/.

Norton, Louis Arthur. "Maritime Occupational Disease: 'The Scurvy.'" *The Northern Mariner/le marin du nord* XX, 1 (2010): 57–70.

Pimentel, Laura. "Scurvy: Historical Review and Current Diagnostic Approach." *American Journal of Emergency Medicine* 21, 4 (July 2003): 328–32.

Zuckerman, Arnold. "Scurvy and the Ventilation of Ships in the Royal Navy: Samuel Sutton's Contribution." *Eighteenth-Century Studies* 10, 2 (1976): 222–34.

Additional Sources

Black, Annetta. "Scurvy: By the End, Death Is a Mercy." Atlas Obscura (1 May 2012): www.atlasobscura.com/articles/scurvy.

Brown, Karen. "The Pulse: Scurvy Cropping up in New England." Rhode Island Public Radio (4 August 2016): http://ripr.org/post/pulse-scurvy-cropping-new-england.

Ceglowski, Maciej. "Scott and Scurvy." (7 March 2010): http://idlewords.com/2010/03/scott_and_scurvy.htm.

The Mariner's' Museum. "Life at Sea in the Age of Captain Cook." http://ageofex.marinersmuseum.org/?type=webpage&id=55.

National Institutes of Health, Office of Dietary Supplements. "Vitamin C." https://ods.od.nih.gov/factsheets/VitaminC-HealthProfessional/.
O'Sullivan, Nancy. *Vitamins and Minerals.* www.youtube.com/watch?v=ORmO23Ui5E4&feature=youtu.be.
Trinh Nguyen, Ginnie. *How do vitamins work?* TEDEd. www.youtube.com/watch?v=ISZLTJH5lYg.
University of Maryland Medical Center. "Vitamin B1 (Thiamine)." http://umm.edu/health/medical/altmed/supplement/vitamin-b1-thiamine.

13. 1776: A Folk Remedy for Congestive Heart Failure

Sources

Biggs, R.D. "Medicine, Surgery, and Public Health in Ancient Mesopotamia." *Journal of Assyrian Academic Studies* 19, 1 (2005): 1.
Estes, J. Worth, and Paul Dudley White. "William Withering and the Purple Foxglove." *Scientific American* 212 (June 1965): 111–19.
Krikler, Dennis M. "The Foxglove, 'The Old Woman from Shropshire,' and William Withering." *Journal of the American College of Cardiology* 5, 5 (May 1985), 3A – 9A.
Rahimtoola, S. H. "Digitalis and William Withering, the Clinical Investigator." *Circulation* 52 (1975): 969–71.
Teall, Emily K. "Medicine and Doctoring in Ancient Mesopotamia." *Grand Valley Journal of History* 3, 1 (2014).
True, Rodney H. "Folk Materia Medica." *Journal of American Folklore* 14, 53 (1901): 105–14.
Withering, William. *An Account of the Foxglove and Some of Its Medical Uses: With Practical Remarks on Dropsy and Other Diseases.* Birmingham: GGJ and J Robinson, 1785. https://archive.org/details/mobot31753000722048.
"William Withering." *Nature* 3724 (15 March 1941): 325.

Additional Resources

Behrens, Julia. *A History of Herbal Medicine.* Heritage Lottery Fund. www.youtube.com/watch?v=S8SHvgM1bMc.
Blackwell, Elizabeth. *A Curious Herbal.* https://ceb.nlm.nih.gov/proj/ttp/flash/blackwell/blackwell.html.
Medline Plus. *Herbal Medicine.* https://medlineplus.gov/herbalmedicine.html?session=LZOOor1MnPkiXKgYdG43aYtwDa.
Norman, Jeremy N. "William Withering and the Purple Foxglove: A Bicentennial Tribute." *Historyof Science.com* (1985): www.historyofscience.com/articles/jmnorman-william-withering.php.
Science Museum: Brought to Life. "Exploring the History of Medicine: British Herbalism." www.sciencemuseum.org.uk/broughttolife/themes/traditions/herbalism.
University of Maryland Medical Center. *Herbal medicine.* http://umm.edu/health/medical/altmed/treatment/herbal-medicine.

14. 1799: Heroic Bloodletting, Leech Mania, and What Doesn't Work

Sources

Christopoulou-Aletra, Helen and Papavramidou, Niki. "Cupping: An Alternative Surgical Procedure Used by Hippocratic Physicians." *The Journal of Alternative and Complementary Medicine* 14, 8 (2008): 899–902. http://online.liebertpub.com/doi/abs/10.1089/acm.2008.0238?journalCode=acm.
Deppisch, Ludwig M. "Andrew Jackson and American Medical Practice: Old Hickory and His Physicians." *Tennessee Historical Quarterly* 62, 2 (2003): 130–51.
Dixon, Mim, and Scott Kirchner. " 'Poking,' an Eskimo Medical Practice in Northwest Alaska." *Études/Inuit/Studies* 6, 2 (1982): 109–25.
Hussain, Altaf. "Kashmir Hospitals Using Leeches." *BBC News* (4 April 2008): http://news.bbc.co.uk/2/hi/south_asia/7328369.stm.
Kahn, Linda, and Alfredo Morabia. "Using the Numerical Method in 1836, James Jackson Bridged French Therapeutic Epistemology and American Medical Pragmatism." *Journal of Clinical Epidemiology* 68, 4 (2014): www.researchgate.net/publication/270008477_Using_the_numerical_method_in_1836_James_Jackson_bridged_French_therapeutic_epistemology_and_American_medical_pragmatism.
Kirk, Robert G. W., and Neil Pemberton. "Re-imagining Bleeders: The Medical Leech in the Nineteenth Century Bloodletting Encounter." *Medical History* 55, 3 (July 2011): 355–60. www.ncbi.nlm.nih.gov/pmc/articles/PMC3143864/.
Magner, Lois N. *A History of Medicine,* 2d ed. New York: Taylor & Francis, 2005.
Morabia, Alfredo. "Pierre-Charles-Alexandre Louis and the Evaluation of Bloodletting." *Journal of the Royal Society of Medicine* 99 (2006): 158–60.
Morens, David. "Death of a President." *New England Journal of Medicine* 341, 24 (1999): 1845–49.
Papavramidou, N., V. Thomaidis, and A. Fiska. "The Ancient Surgical Bloodletting Method of Arteriotomy." *Journal of Vascular Surgery* 54, 6 (2011): 1842–44.
Parapia, Liakat Ali. "History of Bloodletting by Phlebotomy." *British Journal of Haematology* 143 (2008): 490–95. http://onlinelibrary.wiley.com/doi/10.1111/j.1365-2141.2008.07361.x/full.

Tandeter, Howard, Mirta Grynbaum, and Jeffrey Borkan. "A Qualitative Study on Cultural Blood-letting among Ethiopian Immigrants." *Israel Medical Association Journal* 3, 12 (2001): 937–39. www.researchgate.net/publication/11563702_A_qualitative_study_on_cultural_bloodletting_among_Ethiopian_immigrants.

Whitaker, I.S., *et al.* "Hirudo Medicinalis: Ancient Origins of, and Trends in the Use of Medicinal Leeches throughout History." *British Journal of Oral & Maxillofacial Surgery* 42, 2 (2004): 133–37.

Wikipedia. "George Washington." https://en.wikipedia.org/wiki/George_Washington.

Additional Resources

Bloodletting (Phlebotomy). The Old Operating Theatre Museum and Herb Garret. www.thegarret.org.uk/collectionbloodletting.htm.

Davis, Audrey, and Tony Appel. *Bloodletting Instruments in the National Museum of History and Technology.* Washington, DC: Smithsonian Institutions, 1979. www.gutenberg.org/files/33102/33102-h/33102-h.htm.

"English Caricature: Heroic Medicine—Bloodletting, Emetics, and Laxatives." *Very Ill! The Many Faces of Medical Caricature.* University of Virginia. Historical Collections at the Claude Moore Health Sciences Library. http://exhibits.hsl.virginia.edu/caricatures/en2-heroic.

Hanna, Brad. From Bloodletting to Evidence-Based Medicine. http://skeptvet.com/Blog/wp-content/uploads/2011/06/2011-Equine-Guelph-Bloodletting-to-EBM-May19.pdf.

"Medicinal Leech." Wildscreen Arkive. www.arkive.org/medicinal-leech/hirudo-medicinalis/.

Mitgang, Herbert. "Death of a President: A 200-Year-Old Malpractice Debate." *New York Times* (14 December 1999): www.nytimes.com/1999/12/14/health/death-of-a-president-a-200-year-old-malpractice-debate.html.

Reynolds, Gretchen, and Karen Crouse. "What Are the Purple Dots on Michael Phelps? Cupping Has an Olympic Moment." *New York Times* (8 August 2016): http://well.blogs.nytimes.com/2016/08/08/what-are-the-purple-dots-on-michael-phelps-cupping-has-an-olympic-moment/?_r=0.

Science Museum: Brought to Life. "Cupping." www.sciencemuseum.org.uk/broughttolife/techniques/cupping.

Vadakan, Vibul V. "A Physician Looks at the Death of Washington." *The Early American Review* 6, 1 (2005): www.earlyamerica.com/early-america-review/volume-9/washingtons-death/.

15. 1816: René Laennec Invents the Stethoscope

Sources

Cheng, Tsung O. "How Laënnec Invented the Stethoscope." *International Journal of Cardiology* 118 (2007): 281–285.

Duffin, Jacalyn M. "The Medical Philosophy of R.T.H. Laennec (1781–1826)." *History and Philosophy of the Life Sciences* 8, 2 (1986): 195–219.

Finlayson, James. "Galen [a Biblographical Demonstration in the Library of the Faculty of Physicians and Surgeons of Glasgow, December 9th, 1891] (Concluded)." *The British Medical Journal* 1, 1632 (1892): 771–74.

Furst, Lilian R. "Introduction: From Speculation to Science," 1–21. In *Medical Progress and Social Reality: A Reader in Nineteenth-Century Medicine and Literature.* Albany: State University of New York, 2000.

Ghasemzadeh, Nima, and A. Maziar Zafari. "A Brief Journey into the History of the Arterial Pulse." *Cardiology Research and Practice* 2011, Article ID 164832 (2011).

Hajar, Rachel. "The Air of History: Early Medicine to Galen (Part I)." *Heart Views* 13, 3 (Jul 2012): 120–08.

Hajar, Rachel. "The Air of History (Part V): Ibn Sina (Avicenna)." *Heart Views* 14, 4 (2013): 196–201.

O'Neal, John C. "Auenbrugger, Corvisart, and the Perception of Disease." *Eighteenth-Century Studies* 31, 4 (Summer, 1998): 473–89.

Scherer, John R. "Before Cardiac MRI: Rene Laennec (1781–1826) and the Invention of the Stetho-scope." *Cardiology Journal* 14, 5 (2007): 518–19.

Thadepalli, Haragopal. "Women Gave Birth to the Stethoscope: Laennec's Introduction of the Art of Auscultation of the Lung." *Clinical Infectious Diseases* 35, 5 (Sep. 1, 2002): 587–88.

Additional Resources

How Stuff Works. *The Story of the Stethoscope: Stuff of Genius.* YouTube (2 April 2013): www.youtube.com/watch?v=F3bqVNXQCXE.

Peacock, Pamela. "World Health Day 2013: A Short History of Sphygmomanometers and Blood Pressure Measurement." https://museumofhealthcare.wordpress.com/2013/04/07/world-health-day-2013-a-short-history-of-sphygmomanometers-and-blood-pressure-measurement/.

Salber, Patricia. *Eko's Digital Stethoscope Lets You See Heart Sounds.* https://thedoctorweighsin.com/ekos-digital-stethoscope-lets-you-see-heart-sounds/.

Science Museum: Brought to Life. "Pulse-measurement, Sphygmometers and Sphygmographs." www.sciencemuseum.org.uk/broughttolife/techniques/pulsemeasure.

Virtual EMS Museum. "1816: The Stethoscope." www.emsmuseum.org/virtual-museum/by_era/articles/398118-1816-The-Stethoscope.

16. 1828: Cutting for Stone

Sources
Chakravorty, R.C. "Urinary Stones, Their Cause and Treatment, as Described in the Sushrutas-amhita." *Hist Sci Med* 17, Spec 2 (1982): 328–32. . www.biusante.parisdescartes.fr/sfhm/hsm/HSMx1982x017xspec2/HSMx1982x017xspec2x0328.pdf.
Duhaime, Lloyd. "1828: The First Recorded Medical Malpractice Litigation." Law Museum. 26 September 2011. duhaime.org/LawMuseum/LawArticle-1324/1828-The-First-Recorded-Medical-Malpractice-Litigation.aspx.
Herr, H. W. "'I Will Not Cut . . .' : The Oath That Defined Urology." *BJU International* 102, 7 (September 2008): 769–71.
Jones, Roger. "Thomas Wakley, Plagiarism, Libel, and the Founding of *The Lancet*." *The Lancet* 371 (April 26, 2008): 1410–11.
Mayo Clinic. "Kidney Stones." mayoclinic.org/diseases-conditions/kidney-stones/basics/definition/con-20024829.
Osman, Mahmoud M., *et al*. "5-year-follow-up of Patients with Clinically Insignificant Residual Fragments after Extracorporeal Shockwave Lithotripsy." *European Urology* 47 (2005): 860–64.
Pearle, Margaret S. "Shock-Wave Lithotripsy for Renal Calculi." *New England Journal of Medicine* 367 (2012): 50–57.
Shah, J., and H.N. Whitfield. "Urolithiasis through the Ages." *British Journal of Urology International* 89, 8 (2002): 801–10.
[Wakley, Thomas.] "The Operation of Lithotomy, by Mr. Bransby Cooper, Which Lasted Nearly One Hour!!" *The Lancet* 1827 – 28, v. 1 (March 29, 1828): 959–60.
Zhong, Wen, *et al*. "Percutaneous Nephrolithotomy for Renal Stones Following Failed Extracorporeal Shockwave Lithotripsy: Different Performances and Morbidities." *Urolithiasis* 41 (2013): 165–168.

Additional Resources
"The Diary of Samuel Pepys: Monday 26 March 1660." www.pepysdiary.com/diary/1660/03/26/.
Fitzharris, Lindsey. "Cutting for the Stone: The Case of Stephen Pollard." *The Chirurgeon's Apprentice* (4 October 2011): http://thechirurgeonsapprentice.com/2011/10/04/cutting-for-the-stone-the-case-of-stephen-pollard/.
"Kidney Stones In-Depth Report." *New York Times*. www.nytimes.com/health/guides/disease/kidney-stones/print.html.
Macfarlane, Ross. "Samuel Pepys and His 'Old Pain.'" *Early Medicine* (1 January 2010). blog.wellcome-library.org/2010/01/samuel-pepys-and-his-old-pain/.

17. 1846: Laughing Gas

Sources
Abdel-Azeem, Ahmed M. "The History, Fungal Biodiversity, Conservation, and Future Perspectives for Mycology in Egypt." *IMA Fungus* 1, 2 (December 2010): 123–42.
Aptowicz, Cristin O›Keefe. *Dr. Mütter's Marvels: A True Tale of Intrigue and Innovation at the Dawn of Modern Medicine*. New York: Avery, 2015.
Guzman, Gaston. "Hallucinogenic Mushrooms in Mexico: An Overview." *Economic Botany* 62, 3 (2008): 404–12.
Hobbs, Christopher. Medicinal Mushrooms, A Clinician's Overview. www.christopherhobbs.com/webdocs/presentations/Medicinal-Mushrooms-2014.pdf.
Leake, Chauncey D. "The Historical Development of Surgical Anesthesia." *Scientific Monthly* 20, 3 (1925): 304–28.
López-Valverde, A., *et al*. "The Discovery of Surgical Anesthesia: Discrepancies Regarding Its Authorship." *Journal of Dental Research* 90, 1 (2011): 31–34.
Poovey, Mary. "'Scenes of an Indelicate Character': The Medical 'Treatment' of Victorian Women." *Representations* 14 (Spring, 1986): 137–68.
Stallings, Shirley and Michael Montagne. "A Chronicle of Anesthesia Discovery in New England." *Pharmacy in History* 35, 2 (1993): 77–80.
Underwood, E. Ashworth. "Before and after Morton: A Historical Survey of Anaesthesia." *The British Medical Journal* 2, 4475 (1946): 525–31.

Additional Resources
History of Anaesthesia Society. "Timeline." www.histansoc.org.uk/timeline.html.
Jay, Mike. "'O, Excellent Air Bag': Humphrey Davis and Nitrous Oxide." *The Public Domain Review*: http://publicdomainreview.org/2014/08/06/o-excellent-air-bag-humphry-davy-and-nitrous-oxide/.
McHigh, Anna. *Mushrooms in History – The Greeks and Egyptians*. Crazy about Mushrooms. http://blog.crazyaboutmushrooms.com/mushrooms-history-greeks-egyptians/#more-1448.
The Wood Library-Museum of Anesthesiology. "History of Anesthesia." www.woodlibrarymuseum.org/history-of-anesthesia/.

18. 1847: Wash Your Hands

Sources

Aptowicz, Cristin O'Keefe. *Dr. Mütter's Marvels: A True Tale of Intrigue and Innovation at the Dawn of Modern Medicine*. New York: Avery, 2015.

Dolman, C. E. "The Sanitarian's Place in Public Health." *Canadian Journal of Public Health / Revue Canadienne de Santé Publique* 39, no. 2 (1948): 41–51.

Fee, Elizabeth, and Theodore M. Brown. "The Public Health Act of 1848." *Bulletin of the World Health Organization* 83, 11 (2005): 866–67. www.who.int/bulletin/volumes/83/11/866.pdf.

Gill, Christopher J. and Gillian C. Gill. "Nightingale in Scutari: Her Legacy Reexamined." *Clinical Infectious Diseases* 40, 12 (2005): 1799–805.

Gillies, Donald. "Hempelian and Kuhnian Approaches in the Philosophy of Medicine: The Semmelweis Case." *Studies in History and Philosophy of Biological and Biomedical Sciences* 36 (2005): 159–81.

Johnson, Steven. *The Ghost Map*. New York: Riverhead Books, 2006.

Magnello, M. Eileen. "Victorian Statistical Graphics and the Iconography of Florence Nightingale's Polar Area Graph." *BSHM Bulletin* 27 (2012): 13–37.

Miller, Patti J. "Semmelweis." *Infection Control* 3, 5 (1982): 405–09.

Persson, Johannes. "Semmelweis's Methodology from the Modern Stand-point: Intervention Studies and Causal Ontology." *Studies in History and Philosophy of Biological and Biomedical Sciences* 40 (2009): 204–09.

Ringen, Knut. "Edwin Chadwick, the Market Ideology, and Sanitary Reform: On the Nature of the 19th-Century Public Health Movement." *International Journal of Health Services* 9, 1 (1979): 107–20.

Additional Resources

Biographies of Women Mathematicians. "Polar Area Graph." www.agnesscott.edu/lriddle/women/nightpiechart.htm.

Centers for Disease Control. "Put Your Hands Together." www.youtube.com/watch?v=SyRtMl4a1FE.

Lane, Hilary, Nava Blum, and Elizabeth Fee. "Oliver Wendell Holmes (1809 – 1894) and Ignatz Philipp Semmelweis (1818–1865): Preventing the Transmission of Puerperal Fever." *American Journal of Public Health* 100, 6 (2010): 1008–09. www.ncbi.nlm.nih.gov/pmc/articles/PMC2866610/.

Markel, Howard. "In 1850 Ignaz Semmelweis Saved Lives with Three Words: Wash Your Hands." PBS Newshour (May 15, 2015): www.pbs.org/newshour/updates/ignaz-semmelweis-doctor-prescribed-hand-washing/.

O'Connor, Anahad. "Getting Doctors to Wash their Hands." *New York Times* (September 1, 2011): http://well.blogs.nytimes.com/2011/09/01/getting-doctors-to-wash-their-hands/?_r=1.

Semmelweis Society International. "Dr. Semmelweis' Biography." http://semmelweis.org/about/dr-semmelweis-biography/.

19. 1848: Monster Soup

Sources

Dolman, C. E. "The Sanitarian's Place in Public Health." *Canadian Journal of Public Health / Revue Canadienne de Santé Publique* 39, 2 (1948): 41–51.

Fee, Elizabeth, and Theodore M. Brown. "The Public Health Act of 1848." *Bulletin of the World Health Organization* 83, 11 (2005): 866–67.

Gray, Harold Farnsworth. "Sewerage in Ancient and Mediaeval Times." *Sewage Works Journal* 12, 5 (1940): 939–46.

Jansen, M. "Water Supply and Sewage Disposal at Mohenjo-Daro." *World Archaeology* 21, 2 (1991): 177–92.

Johnson, Steven. *The Ghost Map*. New York: Riverhead Books, 2006.

Subramanian, T.S. "The Rise and Fall of a Harappan City." *Frontline: India's National Magazine* 27, 12 (June 5-18, 2010): www.frontline.in/static/html/fl2712/stories/20100618271206200.htm.

Wikipedia. "Edwin Chadwick." https://en.wikipedia.org/wiki/Edwin_Chadwick.

Additional Resources

Carr, T. J. The Harappan Civilization. Archeology Online. http://archaeologyonline.net/artifacts/harappa-mohenjodaro.

Chadwick, Edwin. Report on the Sanitary Condition of the Labouring Population and on the Means of its Improvement. London. May 1842. www.deltaomega.org/documents/ChadwickClassic.pdf.

JeetoBharat. *Indus Valley Civilization*. Compete India. www.youtube.com/watch?v=juc3msgLMoc.

"Mencken's History of the Bathtub." hoaxes.org/archive/permalink/the_history_of_the_bathtub.

Wald, Chelsea. "The Secret History of Ancient Toilets." *Nature News* 533, 7604 (2016): www.nature.com/news/the-secret-history-of-ancient-toilets-1.19960.

WikiLeaks. *History of Potable Water Supply and Sanitation*. YouTube. www.youtube.com/watch?v=DUON8qpcyZg.

20. 1854: Cholera and Epidemiology

Sources
Ball, Laura. "Cholera and the Pump on Broad Street: The Life and Legacy of John Snow." *The History Teacher* 43, 1 (2009): 105–19.
Bingham, P., *et al.* "John Snow, William Farr and the 1849 Outbreak of Cholera That Affected London: A Reworking of the Data Highlights the Importance of the Water Supply." *Public Health* 118 (2004): 387–94.
Centers for Disease Control. "Cholera: General Information." cdc.gov/cholera/general/index.html.
Colwell, Rita R., *et al.* "Reduction of Cholera in Bangladeshi Villages by Simple Filtration." *Proceedings of the National Academy of Sciences* 100, 3 (2003): 1051–55. pnas.org/content/100/3/1051.full.pd.
Evans, Richard J. "Epidemics and Revolutions: Cholera in Nineteenth-Century Europe." *Past & Present* 120 (August 1988): 123–146.
Johnson, Steven. *The Ghost Map.* New York: Riverhead Books, 2006.
Lacey, Stephen W. "Cholera: Calamitous Past, Ominous Future." *Clinical Infectious Diseases* 20, 5 (May 1995): 1409–19.
Levy, Sharon. "Cholera's Life Aquatic." *BioScience* 55, no. 9 (2005): 728–32.
Tuite, Ashleigh R., Christina H. Chan and David N. Fisman. "Cholera, Canals, and Contagion: Rediscovering Dr. Beck's Report." *Journal of Public Health Policy* 32, 3 (2011): 320–33.

Additional Resources
Contagion: Historical Views of Diseases and Epidemics. "Cholera Epidemics in the 19th Century." http://ocp.hul.harvard.edu/contagion/cholera.html.
City of Westminster Archives. "Cholera and the Thames." www.choleraandthethames.co.uk/.
Ewald, Paul. "Can We Domesticate Germs?" TED (2007): www.ted.com/talks/paul_ewald_asks_can_we_domesticate_germs.
"Mapping the 1854 London Cholera Outbreak." www.udel.edu/johnmack/frec682/cholera/.
Medical London. "John Snow and the Cholera Outbreak of 1854 with Mike Jay." Wellcome Collection. YouTube (2008): www.youtube.com/watch?v=Pq32LB8j2K8.
The Story of Cholera. Global Health Media Project. www.youtube.com/watch?v=jG1VNSCsP5Q.
Tuthill, Kathleen. "John Snow and the Broad Street Pump: On the Trail of an Epidemic." *Cricket* 31, 3 (2003): 23–31. www.ph.ucla.edu/epi/snow/snowcricketarticle.html.
UCLA Department of Epidemiology. www.ph.ucla.edu/epi/snow.html.

21. 1865: Gregor Mendel's Observations about Inherited Traits

Sources
Bizzo, Nelio, and Charbel N. El-Hani. "Darwin and Mendel: Evolution and Genetics." *Journal of Biological Education* 43, 3 (2009): 108–14.
de Beer, Gavin. "Mendel, Darwin, and Fisher (1865–1965)." *Notes and Records of the Royal Society of London* 19, 2 (1964): 192–226.
De Castro, Mauricio. "Johann Gregor Mendel: Paragon of Experimental Science." *Molecular Genetics & Genomic Medicine* 4, 1 (2016): 3–8.
Dunn, P. M. "Gregor Mendel, OSA (1822–1884), Founder of Scientific Genetics." *Archives of Disease in Childhood: Fetal and Neonatal Edition* 88, 6 (November 2003): F537–39.
Hackett, Shannon, Kevin Feldheim and Mark Alvey. "Genes and Genius: The Inheritance of Gregor Mendel." *DNA and Cell Biology* 25, 12 (2006): 655–58.
Harbou, D. J. "Gregor Johann Mendel: A Biographical Sketch." *The Scientific Monthly* 40, 4 (1935): 313–22.
Luzzatto, Lucio. "Sickle Cell Anaemia and Malaria." *Mediterranean Journal of Hematology and Infectious Diseases* 4, 1 (2012): http://dx.doi.org/10.4084/mjhid.2012.065.
Offner, Susan. "Mendel's Peas & the Nature of the Gene: Genes Code for Proteins & Proteins Determine Phenotype." *The American Biology Teacher* 73, 7 (2011): 382–87. http://dx.doi.org/10.1525/abt.2011.73.7.3.
World Health Organization. "New Report Signals Country Progress in the Path to Malaria Elimination." News Release (December 9, 2015): www.who.int/mediacentre/news/releases/2015/report-malaria-elimination/en/.
World Health Organization. "Sickle-cell Disease and Other Haemoglobin Disorders." Fact Sheet 308 (2011): www.who.int/mediacentre/factsheets/fs308/en/.

Additional Resources
McNeil, Donald G., Jr. "Biochemistry: Scientists Decode the Protective Element Sickle Cell Offers Against Malaria." *New York Times* (November 14, 2011): www.nytimes.com/2011/11/15/health/biochemistry-scientists-decode-the-protective-element-sickle-cell-anemia-offers-against-malaria.html?_r=0.
"Mendel's Genetics." http://anthro.palomar.edu/mendel/mendel_1.htm.
Py-Lieberman, Beth. "Evolution World Tour: Mendel's Garden, Czech Republic." *Smithsonian Magazine* (January 2012): www.smithsonianmag.com/evotourism/evolution-world-tour-mendels-garden-czech-republic-6088291/?no-ist.

Roach, Margaret. "Planting Peas, with Mendel in Mind." A Way to Garden.com (2013): http://away-togarden.com/planting-peas-with-mendel-in-mind/.
Sant, Joseph. "Mendel, Darwin and Evolution." (2016): www.scientus.org/Mendel-Darwin.html.
Understanding Evolution. "The 'Bad' Gene." http://evolution.berkeley.edu/evolibrary/article/misconcep_04.
Wikipedia. "Gregor Mendel." https://en.wikipedia.org/wiki/Gregor_Mendel.

22. 1870: Discovering Ancient Skull Surgeries

Sources

Clower, William T., and Stanley Finger. "Discovering Trepanation: The Contribution of Paul Broca." *Neurosurgery* 49, 6 (2001): 1417–25.
Finger, Stanley, and Hiran R. Fernando. "E. George Squier and the Discovery of Cranial Trepanation: A Landmark in the History of Surgery and Ancient Medicine." *Journal of the History of Medicine* 56 (2001): 353–81.
Lee, K. S. "History of Chronic Subdural Hematoma." *Korean Journal of Neurotrauma* 11, 2 (2015): 27–34.
Lv, X., Z. Li, and Y. Li. "Prehistoric Skull Trepanation in China." *World Neurosurgery* 80, 6 (2013): 897–99.
May, Brian, Takako Tomoda, and Michael Wang. "The Life and Medical Practice of Hua Tuo." *Pacific Journal of Oriental Medicine* 14 (2000): 40–54. www.academia.edu/8266309/The_Life_and_Medical_Practice_of_Hua_Tuo.
Papagrigorakas, Manolis J., *et al.* "Neurosurgery During the Bronze Age: A Skull Trepanation in 1900 BC Greece." *World Neurosurgery* 81, 2 (2014): 431–35.
Tsermoulas, G., A. Aidonis, and G. Flint. "The Skull of Chios: Trepanation in Hippocratic Medicine." *Journal of Neurosurgery* 121, 2 (2014): 328–32.

Additional Resources

Chan, Eugene. "Hua Tuo, the Father of Chinese Surgery." *Hist. Ophthalm. Int.* 3 (1985): 307–12. http://histoph.com/wp-content/uploads/2015/03/Chan-Chinese-Surgery.pdf.
Chang, Rhonda. "Making Theoretical Principles for New Chinese Medicine." *Health and History* 16, 1 (2014): 66–86.
Costandi, Mo. "An Illustrated History of Trepanation." *Neurophilosophy* (13 June 2007): https://neurophilosophy.wordpress.com/2007/06/13/an-illustrated-history-of-trepanation/.
Funami, Shaw. "Hu Tuo and a Jail Guard." Ezine @rticles (11 March 2011): http://ezinearticles.com/?Dr-Hua-Tuo-and-a-Jail-Guard&id=6066146.
Garofalo, Michael. Frolics of the Five Animals (2013). www.egreenway.com/qigong/animalfrolics.htm.
Irving, Jenni. "Trephination." Ancient History Encyclopedia (May 1, 2013): www.ancient.eu/Trephination/.
Konnikova, Maria. "The Man Who Couldn't Speak and How He Revolutionized Psychology." *Scientific American* (8 February 8): http://blogs.scientificamerican.com/literally-psyched/the-man-who-couldnt-speakand-how-he-revolutionized-psychology/.

23. 1881: Spontaneous Generation and the Germ Theory of Disease

Sources

Cameron, Hector C. "Lord Lister and the Evolution of Modern Surgery." *British Medical Journal* 2, 2189 (1902): 1844–48.
Cope, Zachary. "Joseph Lister, 1827–1912." *British Medical Journal* 2, 5543 (1967): 7–8.
Egerton, Frank N. "A History of the Ecological Sciences, Part 12: Invertebrate Zoology and Parasitology During the 1500s." *Bulletin of the Ecological Society of America* 85, 1 (2004): 27–31.
Francoeur, Jason R. "Joseph Lister: Surgeon Scientist (1827–1912)." *Journal of Investigative Surgery* 13 (2000): 129–32.
Furst, Lilian R. *Medical Progress and Social Reality: A Reader in Nineteenth-century Medicine and Literature.* Albany: State University of New York Press, 2000.
Keen, W. W. "Before and after Lister." *Science* 41, 1067 (1915): 845–53.
Lathan, S. Robert. "Caroline Hampton Halsted: The First to Use Rubber Gloves in the Operating Room." *Proceedings* (Baylor University Medical Center) 23, 4 (2010): 389–92.
Lawson, Anton E. "Human Traits Vs. Crucial Experiments." *The American Biology Teacher* 36, 6 (1974): 334–48.
Pasteur, Prof. [Louis]. "On the Germ Theory." *Science* 2, 62 (1881): 420–22.
Porter, Stephen. *The Great Plague.* Stroud, Gloucestershire: Sutton Publishing, 1999.
Ruestow, Edward G. "Leeuwenhoek and the Campaign against Spontaneous Generation." *Journal of the History of Biology* 17, 2 (Summer, 1984): 225–48.
Smith, Kendall. "Louis Pasteur, the Father of Immunology?" *Frontiers in Immunology* 3, Article 68 (10 April 2012): www.ncbi.nlm.nih.gov/pmc/articles/PMC3342039/.
Weiss, Harry B. "Francesco Redi, the Father of Experimental Entomology." *The Scientific Monthly* 23, 3 (1926): 220–24.
Wikipedia. "Spontaneous Generation." https://en.wikipedia.org/wiki/Spontaneous_generation.

Additional Resources

Dapple, Dap. "Bacteriology: Louis Pasteur & Robert Koch." www.youtube.com/
  watch?v=rR4sC9RDaKY.
Gawande, Atul. "Slow Ideas." *The New Yorker* (July 23, 2013): www.newyorker.com/
  magazine/2013/07/29/slow-ideas.
Lidwell, O. M. "Joseph Lister and Infection from the Air." *Epidemiology and Infection* 99, 3 (1987): 568–
  78. www.ncbi.nlm.nih.gov/pmc/articles/PMC2249236/.
Markel, Howard. "How 'Going Under the Knife' Became Much Less Deadly."
  PBS Newshour (26 July 2013): www.pbs.org/newshour/rundown/
  how-going-under-the-knife-became-much-less-deadly/.
Science Museum: Brought to Life. "Gloves, Gowns, and Clothing." www.sciencemuseum.org.uk/
  broughttolife/techniques/clothing.
Worboys, Michael. "Joseph Lister and the Performance of Antiseptic Surgery." *Notes and Records of the
  Royal Society of London* 67, 3 (2013): 199–209.

24. 1882: Tuberculosis Emerges from the Miasma

Sources

Abrams, Jeanne E. "'Spitting Is Dangerous, Indecent, and against the Law!' Legislating Health
  Behavior during the American Tuberculosis Crusade." *Journal of the History of Medicine and Allied Sci-
  ences* 68, 3 (2013): 416–50.
Barnes, David S. "Historical Perspectives on the Etiology of Tuberculosis." *Microbes and Infection* 2
  (2000): 431–40.
Bell, Michael. "Vampires and Death in New England, 1784 to 1892." *Anthropology and Humanism* 31, 2
  (2006): 124–40.
Daniel, Thomas M. "The History of Tuberculosis." *Respiratory Medicine* 100 (2006): 1862–70.
Flynn, JoAnne L., and John Chan. "Tuberculosis: Latency and Reactivation." Ed. D. A. Portnoy.
  Infection and Immunity 69,7 (2001): 4195–4201. PMC. www.ncbi.nlm.nih.gov/pmc/articles/
  PMC98451/.
Frith, John. "History of Tuberculosis. Part 2 - the Sanatoria and the Discoveries of the Tubercle
  Bacillus." *Journal of Military and Veterans' Health* 22, 2 (2016).
Garetier, Marc, and Jean Rousset. "Thoracic Balls." *CMAJ/JAMC* 183, 14 (2011): e1091. www.ncbi.
  nlm.nih.gov/pmc/articles/PMC3185102/.
Grzybowski, Stefan, and Edward A. Allen. "History and Importance of Scrofula." *The Lancet* 346, 8988
  (1995): 1472–74.
Johnson, Steven. *The Ghost Map.* New York: Riverhead Books, 2006.
Pease, Arthur Stanley. "Some Remarks on the Diagnosis and Treatment of Tuberculosis in Antiq-
  uity." *Isis* 31, 2 (1940): 380–93.
Sabbatani, S. "[Historical Insights into Tuberculosis. Girolamo Fracastoro's Intuition on the Transmission of Tuberculosis and His Opponents.]" *Le Infezioni in Medicina* 12, 4 (2004): 284–91. www.
  ncbi.nlm.nih.gov/pubmed/15729021.
Warren, Peter. "The Evolution of the Sanatorium: The First Half-Century, 1854–1904." *Canadian Bulletin of Medical History* 23, 2 (2006): 457–70. www.cbmh.ca/index.php/cbmh/article/
  viewFile/1239/1230.
Wikipedia. "Royal Touch." https://en.wikipedia.org/wiki/Royal_touch.
World Health Organization. "Tuberculosis: Fact Sheet 104." www.who.int/mediacentre/factsheets/
  fs104/en/.

Additional Resources

Atlas Obscura. "The Mummies of Vác, Hungary." www.atlasobscura.com/places/
  mummies-v-c-hungary.
Centers for Disease Control Fact Sheets. "Tuberculosis: General Information." www.cdc.gov/tb/
  publications/factsheets/general/tb.htm.
Contagion: Historical Views of Diseases and Epidemics. "Tuberculosis in Europe and North America." http://ocp.hul.harvard.edu/contagion/tuberculosis.html.
How to Survive a Tuberculosis Infection. They will Kill You. www.youtube.com/
  watch?v=ld7As7Vy2Oo.
McNeil, Donald G., Jr. "Vietnam's Battle with Tuberculosis." *New York Times* (3/28/2016): www.
  nytimes.com/2016/03/29/health/vietnam-tuberculosis.html?_r=0.
Science Museum: Brought to Life. "King's Evil and the Royal Touch." www.sciencemuseum.org.uk/
  broughttolife/techniques/kingsevil.

25. 1894: A Barrel of Snakes and an Antitoxin

Sources

Bochner, Rosany. "Paths to the Discovery of Antivenom Serotherapy in France." *Journal of Venomous
  Animals and Toxins including Tropical Diseases* 22, 1 (2016): 1–7.
Centers for Disease Control. "Your Immune System." www.cdc.gov/bam/diseases/immune/immune-
  sys.html.

Ditmars, Raymond L. "Deadly Snakes Now Conquered by Science." *The Science News-Letter* 11, 321 (Jun. 4, 1927): 349–50 + 355–56.

Ehrlich, Paul. "Partial Cell Functions." Nobel Lecture (December 11, 1908). www.nobelprize.org/ nobel_prizes/medicine/laureates/1908/ehrlich-lecture.html.

Guénel, Annick. "The Creation of the First Overseas Pasteur Institute, or the Beginning of Albert Calmette's Pastorian Career." *Medical History* 43 (1999): 1–25.

"The Immune System: In Defense of Our Lives." *Nobel Prize.org.* Nobel Media AB (September 6, 2010). nobelprize.org/educational/medicine/immuneresponses/overview/.

Kaufmann, Stefan H.E. "Élie Metchnikoff's and Paul Ehrlich's Impact on Infection Biology." *Microbes and Infection* 10 (2008): 1417–19.

Luttenberger, Franz. "Arrhenius vs. Ehrlich on Immunochemistry: Decisions about Scientific Progress in the Context of the Nobel Prize." *Theoretical Medicine* 13, 2 (1992): 137–73.

The Nobel Prize in Physiology or Medicine 1908." NobelPrize.org. Nobel Media AB 2014. www. nobelprize.org/nobel_prizes/medicine/laureates/1908/.

Wikipedia. "Albert Calmette." https://en.wikipedia.org/wiki/Albert_Calmette.

Wikipedia. "Mithridates VI of Pontus." https://en.wikipedia.org/wiki/Mithridates_VI_of_Pontus.

Additional Resources

SciShow. *How to Make Anti-Venom* (May 13, 2013): www.youtube.com/watch?v=0yqVow4J4oA.

"The Immune System: In Defense of Our Lives." Nobel Prize.org (September 6, 2010): www.nobel-prize.org/educational/medicine/immuneresponses/overview/.

"The Immune System—Pioneers." NobelPrize.org. www.nobelprize.org/educational/medicine/ immunity/immune-pioneers.html.

"The Immune System Game." Nobel Prize.org. www.nobelprize.org/educational/medicine/ immunity/.

Wikipedia. "Side-chain Theory." https://en.wikipedia.org/wiki/Side-chain_theory.

26. 1896: The Discovery of X-rays

Sources

Frankel, Richard I. "Centennial of Röntgen's Discovery of X-Rays." *Western Journal of Medicine* 164, 6 (1996): 497–501. www.ncbi.nlm.nih.gov/pmc/articles/PMC1303625/.

Glasser, Otto. "W. C. Roentgen and the Discovery of the Roentgen Rays." *American Journal of Roentgenology* 165 (1995): 1033–40.

Langevin-Joliot, H. "Radium, Marie Curie and Modern Science." Radiation Research 150, no. 5 (1998): S3–S8.

Riesz, Peter B. "The Life of Wilhelm Conrad Roentgen." *American Journal of Roentgenology* 165 (1995): 1533–37.

Wikipedia. "Crookes Tube." https://en.wikipedia.org/wiki/Crookes_tube.

Additional Resources

American Institute of Physics. "The Top 5 Ways Medical Physics Has Changed Health Care." *EurekAlert! AAAS* (28 February 2008): www.eurekalert.org/pub_releases/2008-02/aiop-ttf022808.php.

Donya, Mohamed, *et al.* "Radiation in Medicine: Origins, Risks, and Aspirations." *Global Cardiology Science & Practice* (February 2015): www.qscience.com/doi/abs/10.5339/gcsp.2014.57.

NDT Resource Center. "X-Rays and Gamma Rays." www.nde-ed.org/EducationResources/High-School/Radiography/hs_rad_index.htm.

Schwartz, Rob. "Watch This Lenard Tube Demonstration Go Horribly Right." *Stranger Dimensions* (20 August 2014): www.strangerdimensions.com/2014/08/20/ watch-lenard-tube-demonstration-go-horribly-right/.

Shields, Brenton. "The History of the X-Ray Machine." eHow. www.ehow.com/about_5368638_history-ray-machine.html.

Waters, Hannah. "The First X-Ray, 1895." *The Scientist* (July 1, 2011): www.the-scientist.com/?articles. view/articleNo/30693/title/The-First-X-ray--1895/.

Wikipedia. "Shoe-fitting Fluoroscope." https://en.wikipedia.org/wiki/Shoe-fitting_fluoroscope.

27. 1898: A Small Game Hunter Fights Bubonic Plague

Sources

Bibel, David J. and T.H. Chen. "Diagnosis of Plague: An Analysis of the Yersin-Kitasato Controversy." *Bacteriological Reviews* 40, 3 (September 1976): 633–51.

Centers for Disease Control. "Plague." www.cdc.gov/plague/index.html.

Cohn, Samuel K., Jr. "The Black Death: End of a Paradigm." *The American Historical Review* 107, 3 (2002): 703–38.

Crawford, Edward A., Jr. "Paul-Louis Simond and His Work on Plague." *Perspectives in Biology and Medicine* 39, 3 (1996): 446–58.

Gross, Ludwik. "How the Plague Bacillus and Its Transmission Through Fleas Were Discovered: Reminiscences from My Years at the Pasteur Institute in Paris." *Proceedings of the National Academy of Sciences of the United States of America* 92, 17 (August 1995): 7609–11.

Haensch, Stephanie, *et al.* "Distinct Clones of *Yersinia pestis* Caused the Black Death." *PLoS Pathogens* 6, 10 (2010): http://journals.plos.org/plospathogens/article?id=10.1371/journal.ppat.1001134.

Little, Lester K., ed. *Plague and the End of Antiquity: The Pandemic of 541–750.* New York: Cambridge University Press: 2007.

McCormick, Michael. "Rats, Communications, and Plague: Toward an Ecological History." *The Journal of Interdisciplinary History* 34, 1 (2003): 1–25.

National Institute of Allergies and Infectious Diseases. "Types of Plague." 2015. https://www.niaid.nih.gov/topics/plague/Pages/forms.aspx.

Tran, T. N. *et al.* "Brief Communication: Co-detection of *Bartonella quintana* and *Yersinia pestis*." *American Journal of Physical Anthropology* 145, 3 (2011): 489–94.

Twigg, Graham. *The Black Death: A Biological Reappraisal.* London: Batsford, 1984.

Wagner, D.M., *et al.* "*Yersinia pestis* and the Plague of Justinian 541–543 AD: A Genomic Analysis." *The Lancet. Infectious diseases* 14, 4 (2014): 319–26.

Wikipedia. "Waldemar Haffkine." en.wikipedia.org/wiki/Waldemar_Haffkine.

Additional Resources:

BBC Timewatch. "Plague Rat Experiment." (6 September 2010): www.youtube.com/watch?v=lDwiLdEKyuo.

The Black Death. archive.org/web/20080625094232/http://www.channel4.com/history/microsites/H/history/a-b/blackdeath.html.

Fitzharris, Lindsey. "The Plague Doctor." Under the Knife. www.youtube.com/watch?v=Per1onjC1ug.

PBS Science Odyssey. "Bubonic Plague Hits San Francisco: 1900–1909." www.pbs.org/wgbh/aso/databank/entries/dm00bu.html.

World Health Organization. "Plague." www.who.int/topics/plague/en/.

28. 1898: Viruses Borrow Life Support from Tobacco Leaves and Humans

Sources

Bauer, J. H. "Yellow Fever." *Public Health Reports (1896–1970)* 55, 9 (1940): 362–71.

Bos, L. "Beijerinck's Work on Tobacco Mosaic Virus: Historical Context and Legacy." *Philosophical Transactions: Biological Sciences* 354, 1383 (29 March 1999): 675–85.

Fredericks, David N., and David A. Relman. "Sequence-Based Identification of Microbial Pathogens: A Reconsideration of Koch's Postulates." *Clinical Microbiology Reviews* 9, 1 (1996): 18–33.

Frierson, J. Gordon. "The Yellow Fever Vaccine: A History." *The Yale Journal of Biology and Medicine* 83, 2 (2010): 77–85. www.ncbi.nlm.nih.gov/pmc/articles/PMC2892770/.

Lipkin, W. Ian. "Microbe Hunting in the 21st Century." *Proceedings of the National Academy of Sciences* 106, 1 (2009): 6–7.

"Nobel Prize 1951." *British Medical Journal* 2, 4738 (1951): 1020.

Porterfield, J. S. "Yellow Fever in West Africa: A Retrospective Glance." *British Medical Journal* 299, 6715 (1989): 1555–57.

Rivers, Thomas M. "Viruses and Koch's Postulates." *Journal of Bacteriology* 33, 1 (1937): 1–12.

Stanley, W. M. "Progress in the Conquest of Virus Diseases." *Science* 101, 2617 (1945): 185–88.

Woolhouse, Mark et al. "Human Viruses: Discovery and Emergence." *Philosophical Transactions of the Royal Society B: Biological Sciences* 367, 1604 (2012): 2864–71. www.ncbi.nlm.nih.gov/pmc/articles/PMC3427559/.

World Health Organization. "Yellow Fever." www.who.int/mediacentre/factsheets/fs100/en/.

Additional Resources

"Are Viruses Alive?" DNews (6 March 6): www.youtube.com/watch?v=VvTfkMhEw3g.

History of Vaccines. "Timeline: Yellow Fever." www.historyofvaccines.org/content/timelines/yellow-fever.

MacDonald, Fiona. "Viruses ARE Alive, and They're Older than Modern Cells, New Study Suggests." *Science Alert* (28 September 2015): www.sciencealert.com/viruses-are-alive-and-they-re-older-than-modern-cells-new-study-suggests.

Rockefeller Foundation. "Yellow Fever." http://rockefeller100.org/exhibits/show/health/yellow-fever.

Villarreal, Luis P. "Are Viruses Alive?" *Scientific American* (8 August 2008): www.scientificamerican.com/article/are-viruses-alive-2004/.

29. 1900: Marie Curie's Lab Glows in the Dark

Sources

Curie, Marie. "The Discovery of Radium." Excerpted from *Pierre Curie*, 1923. Lateral Science (8 July 2012): http://lateralscience.blogspot.com/2012/07/the-discovery-of-radium-by-marie-curie.html.

Dutreix, Jean, *et al.* "The Hazy Dawn of Brachytherapy." *Radiotherapy and Oncology* 49 (1998): 223–32.

Fox, B. W. "The History of Radium in Medicine in Manchester." *Clinical Oncology* 10 (1998): 115–24.

Fröman, Nancy. "Marie and Pierre Curie and the Discovery of Polonium and Radium." Nobelprize. org (December 1996): www.nobelprize.org/nobel_prizes/themes/physics/curie/.

Ham, Denise. "Marie Sklodowska Curie: The Woman Who Opened the Nuclear Age." *21st Century* (Winter 2002–2003): 30–68. www.21stcenturysciencetech.com/articles/wint02-03/Marie_Curie.pdf.

Harvie, David I. "The Radium Century." *Endeavour* 23, 3 (1999): 100–05.

Mazeron, Jean-Jacques, and Alain Gerbaulet. "The Centenary of Discovery of Radium." *Radiotherapy and Oncology* 49 (1998): 205–16.

Rockwell, Sara. "The Life and Legacy of Marie Curie." *Yale Journal of Biology and Medicine* 76 (2003): 167–80.

U.S. Department of Commerce. *Measures for Progress: A History of the National Bureau of Standards.* "Chapter VI: The Time of the Great Depression." Washington, DC: U.S. Department of Commerce, 1966. www.nist.gov/nvl/upload/MP275_11_Chapter_VI-__THE_TIME_OF_THE_GREAT_DEPRESSION.pdf.

Wikipedia. "Marie Curie." https://en.wikipedia.org/wiki/Marie_Curie.

Additional Resources

Damelin, Dan. "Henri Becquerel and Marie Curie." Chemistry 101, Chemsite. http://chemsite.lsrhs.net/AtomicTheory/Radioactivity.html.

Nobelprize.org. Henri Becquerel: Biographical. www.nobelprize.org/nobel_prizes/physics/laureates/1903/becquerel-bio.html.

Science of E. *The Genius of Marie Curie.* YouTube (10 April 2015): www.youtube.com/watch?v=do41AJwIjZE.

30. 1901: Making Blood Transfusions Safe

Sources

Baskett, Thomas F. "The Resuscitation Greats: James Blundell: The First Transfusion of Human Blood." *Resuscitation* 52 (2002): 229–33.

DeKleine, William. "The Blood Plasma Reservoir." The American Journal of Nursing 41, 5 (1941): 572–73.

"History of Blood Transfusion." *The British Medical Journal* 1, 4280 (Jan. 16, 1943): 74.

Landsteiner, Karl. "Individual Differences in Human Blood." *Science, New Series* 73, 1894 (Apr. 17, 1931): 403–09.

Pelis, Kim. "Blood Clots: The Nineteenth-Century Debate over the Substance and Means of Transfusion in Britain." *Annals of Science* 54 (1997): 331–60.

Pinkerton, Peter H. "Norman Bethune, Eccentric, Man of Principle, Man of Action, Surgeon, and His Contribution to Blood Transfusion in War." *Transfusion Medicine Reviews* 21, 3 (2007): 255–64.

Sturgis, Cyrus C. "The History of Blood Transfusion." *Bulletin of the Medical Library Association* 30, 2 (1942): 105–12. www.ncbi.nlm.nih.gov/pmc/articles/PMC193993/.

Wikipedia. "ABO Blood Group System." en.wikipedia.org/wiki/ABO_blood_group_system.

Wikipedia. "Charles R. Drew." en.wikipedia.org/wiki/Charles_R._Drew.

Additional Resources

"A Brief History of Blood Transfusion." *The Biomedical Scientist* (2005). www.ibms.org/go/nm/history-blood-transfusion.

March of Dimes. "Rh Disease." marchofdimes.org/complications/rh-disease.aspx.

NIH. National Heart, Lung, and Blood Institute. "What Is a Blood Transfusion?" www.nhlbi.nih.gov/health/health-topics/topics/bt.

Nobelprize.org. "Karl Landsteiner – Biographical." www.nobelprize.org/nobel_prizes/medicine/laureates/1930/landsteiner-bio.html.

Nobelprize.org. "The Blood Typing Game." www.nobelprize.org/educational/medicine/bloodtypinggame/.

Seeker Network. *The Bizarre History of Blood Transfusions.* YouTube (21 April 2015): www.youtube.com/watch?v=nU9Rah_cP5E.

Wikipedia. "ABO Blood Group System." https://en.wikipedia.org/wiki/ABO_blood_group_system.

31. 1905: Hormones and Endocrinology

Sources

Associated Press. "Tanya Angus, Woman Who Couldn't Stop Growing, Dies at 34." CBS News (17 January 2013): www.cbsnews.com/news/tanya-angus-woman-who-couldnt-stop-growing-dies-at-34/.

Genel, Myron. "The Olympic Games and Athletic Sex Assignment." *JAMA* 316, 13 (October 4, 2016): 1359–60.

Henriksen, J. H., and O. B. Schaffalitzky de Muckadell. "Secretin, Its Discovery, and the Introduction of the Hormone Concept." *Scandinavian Journal of Clinical and Laboratory Investigation* 60 (2000): 463–72.

López-Muñoz, F., *et al.* "An Historical View of the Pineal Gland and Mental Disorders." *Journal of Clinical Neuroscience* 18 (2011): 1028–37.

Macchi, M. Mila, and Jeffrey N. Bruce. "Human Pineal Physiology and Functional Significance of Melatonin." *Frontiers in Neuroendocrinology* 25, 3 (2004): 175–95.

MedlinePlus. "Endocrine Diseases." https://medlineplus.gov/endocrinediseases.html.

Ralph, Charles L. "Evolution of Pineal Control of Endocrine Function in Lower Vertebrates." *American Zoologist* 23, 3 (1983): 597–605.

Tata, Jamshed R. "100 Years of Hormones." *EMBO Reports* 6, 6 (2005): 490–96.

Tunbridge, W. Michael G. "La Mujer Barbuda by Ribera, 1631: A Gender Bender." *QJM* 104, 8 (2011): 733–36.

Young, Simon N. "How to Increase Serotonin in the Human Brain without Drugs." *Journal of Psychiatry & Neuroscience* 32, 6 (2007): 394–99.

Additional Resources

Crash Course. "Endocrine System, Part 1: Glands & Hormones." (June 22, 2015): www.youtube.com/watch?v=eWHH9je2zG4.

Mayo Clinic. "100th Anniversary of Thyroid Hormone Discovery." December 19, 2014): www.youtube.com/watch?v=sXorW2r3YGk.

Spiegel, Alix. "When It Comes to Depression, Serotonin Isn't the Whole Story." Morning Edition, NPR (January 23, 2012): www.npr.org/sections/health-shots/2012/01/23/145525853/when-it-comes-to-depression-serotonin-isnt-the-whole-story.

Wikipedia. "Endocrine System." https://en.wikipedia.org/wiki/Endocrine_system.

32. 1907: Typhoid Mary Becomes the World's Most Notorious Cook

Sources

Brightman, Christopher. "Typhoid Fever: Yesterday, Today and Unfortunately Still Tomorrow." *Trends in Urology & Men's Health* 6, 6 (2015): http://onlinelibrary.wiley.com/doi/10.1002/tre.491/abstract.

Moorhead, Robert. "William Budd and Typhoid Fever." *Journal of the Royal Society of Medicine* 95, 11 (2002): 561–564. www.ncbi.nlm.nih.gov/pmc/articles/PMC1279260/.

Mortimer, Philip P. "Mr N the Milker, and Dr Koch's Concept of the Healthy Carrier." *The Lancet* 353, 9161 (1999): 1354–56.

Prescott, Heather Munro. "Sending Their Sons into Danger: Cornell University and the Ithaca Typhoid Epidemic of 1903." *New York History* 78, 3 (July 1997: 273–308.

Soper, George A. "The Curious Career of Typhoid Mary." *Bulletin of the New York Academy of Medicine* 15, 10 (1939): 698–712. www.ncbi.nlm.nih.gov/pmc/articles/PMC1911442/.

World Health Organization. "Typhoid Fever." www.who.int/topics/typhoid_fever/en/.

Additional Resources

Centers for Disease Control. "Typhoid Fever." 2013. www.cdc.gov/nczved/divisions/dfbmd/diseases/typhoid_fever/.

Leavitt, Judith Walzer. "Typhoid Mary: Villain or Victim?" NOVA (October 12, 2004): www.pbs.org/wgbh/nova/body/typhoid-mary-villain-or-victim.html.

McGrath Jane. "Who Was Typhoid Mary?" *How Stuff Works: Culture.* http://history.howstuffworks.com/historical-figures/typhoid-mary.htm.

Marineli, Filio, Gregory Tsoucalas, Marianna Karamanou, and George Androutsos. "Mary Mallon (1869–1938) and the History of Typhoid Fever." *Annals of Gastroenterology* 26, 2 (2013): 132–134. www.ncbi.nlm.nih.gov/pmc/articles/PMC3959940/.

Plackett, Benjamin. "The Real Cause of Typhoid Fever Accidentally Discovered." *Inside Science News Service* (19 July, 2013): www.insidescience.org/content/real-cause-typhoid-fever-accidentally-discovered/1212).

Science Channel. Dark Matters. *True Story Behind Typhoid Mary.* YouTube (2013): www.youtube.com/watch?v=XE8HwwNqHG4.

33. 1909: Ehrlich's Magic Bullet and the Beginnings of Chemotherapy

Sources

Bosch, Fèlix, and Laia Rosich. "The Contributions of Paul Ehrlich to Pharmacology: A Tribute on the Occasion of the Centenary of His Nobel Prize." *Pharmacology* 82 (2008): 171–79.

Buchwalow, Igor, Werner Boecker and Markus Tiemann. "The Contribution of Paul Ehrlich to Histochemistry: A Tribute on the Occasion of the Centenary of His Death." *Virchows Archiv* 466 (2015): 111–16.

Hofmann, Heinz. "Columbus and Epic Recusatio: Fracastoro's Syphilis." In *The Classical Tradition and the Americas*, edited by Wolfgang Haase and Meyer Reinhold, vol I. Berlin, New York: Walter De Gruyter, 1994.

Parascandola, John. "From Mercury to Miracle Drugs: Syphilis Therapy over the Centuries." *Pharm Hist* 51, 1 (2009): 14–23.
Principe, Lawrence M. *The Secrets of Alchemy.* Chicago: University of Chicago Press, 2013.
Rothschild, Bruce M. "History of Syphilis." *Clinical Infectious Diseases* 40, 10 (2005): 1454–63.
Travis, Anthony S. "Science as Receptor of Technology: Paul Ehrlich and the Synthetic Dyestuffs Industry." *Science in Context* 3 (1989): 383–408.
Webster, Charles. "Paracelsus, and 500 Years of Encouraging Scientific Inquiry." *British Medical Journal* 306, 6878 (1993): 597–98.
Wikipedia. "William Henry Perkin." https://en.wikipedia.org/wiki/William_Henry_Perkin.
Williams, K. J. "The Introduction of 'Chemotherapy' Using Arsphenamine—the First Magic Bullet." *Journal of the Royal Society of Medicine* 102, 8 (August 2009): 343–48.
Winau, Florian, Otto Westphal, and Rolf Winau. "Paul Ehrlich—In Search of the Magic Bullet." *Microbes and Infection* 6 (2004): 786–89.

Additional Resources
Dapple, Dap. "The Immune System – Paul Erlich and Elie Metchnikoff." www.youtube.com/watch?v=HGEuopke-Ck.

34. 1921: Controlling Diabetes

Sources
Bliss, M. "The Eclipse and Rehabilitation of JRR Macleod, Scotland's Insulin Laureate." *Journal of the Royal College of Physicians of Edinburgh* 43 (2013): 366–73.
Bliss, Michael. "Dr. Frederick Banting: Getting out of Town." *Canadian Medical Association Journal* (May 1, 1984): 1215–21.
Collip, J. B. "Frederick Grant Banting, Discoverer of Insulin." *The Scientific Monthly* 52, 5 (May 1941): 472–74.
Columbia Doctors. "The Pancreas and Its Functions." http://columbiasurgery.org/pancreas/pancreas-and-its-functions.
"The Discovery of Insulin." Nobelprize.org. www.nobelprize.org/educational/medicine/insulin/discovery-insulin.html.
Helmstädter, A. "Antidiabetic Drugs Used in Europe Prior to the Discovery of Insulin." *Pharmazie* 62, 9 (2007): 717–20.
Karamitsos, Dimitrios T. "The Story of Insulin Discovery." *Diabetes Research and Clinical Practice* 93S (2011): S2–S8.
Science Museum: Brought to Life. "Leonard Thompson (1908–35)." www.sciencemuseum.org.uk/broughttolife/people/frederickbanting.
Sawyer, Warren A. "Frederick Banting's Misinterpretations of the Work of Ernest L. Scott as Found in Secondary Sources." *Perspectives in Biology and Medicine* 29, 4 (1986): 611–18.
Sjöquist, J. "Physiology or Medicine 1923: Presentation Speech." Nobelprize.org. www.nobelprize.org/nobel_prizes/medicine/laureates/1923/press.html.
Wikipedia. "History of Diabetes." https://en.wikipedia.org/wiki/History_of_diabetes.

Additional Resources
Markel, Howard. "How a Boy Became the First to Beat Back Diabetes." PBS News Hour (2013): www.pbs.org/newshour/rundown/how-a-dying-boy-became-the-first-to-beat-diabetes/.

35. 1929: Fleming's Dirty Dishes Give Us Penicillin

Sources
Abraham, Edward. "Penicillin and Its Successors: A Personal View." *Bulletin of the American Academy of Arts and Sciences* 39, 1 (1985): 8–27.
Chain, Ernst. "Thirty Years of Penicillin Therapy." *Proceedings of the Royal Society of London. Series B, Biological Sciences* 179, 1057 (1971): 293–319.
Fleming, Alexander. "Penicillin." *British Medical Journal* 2, 4210 (1941): 386.
Florey, H. W. "Penicillin: A Survey." *British Medical Journal* 2, 4361 (1944): 160–71.
Hofmann, Heinz. "Columbus and Epic Recusatio: Fracastoro's Syphilis." In *The Classical Tradition and the Americas,* edited by Wolfgang Haase and Meyer Reinhold, vol I. Berlin, New York: Walter De Gruyter, 1994.
Houbraken, Jos, Jens C. Frisvad, and Robert A. Samson. "Fleming's Penicillin Producing Strain Is Not *Penicillium Chrysogenum* but *P. Rubens.*" *IMA Fungus: The Global Mycological Journal* 2, 1 (2011): 87–95.
Ligon, B. Lee. "Penicillin: Its Discovery and Early Development." *Seminars in Pediatric Infectious Diseases* 15, 1 (2004): 52–57.
Ligon, B. Lee. "Sir Alexander Fleming: Scottish Researcher Who Discovered Penicillin." *Seminars in Pediatric Infectious Diseases* 15, 1 (2004): 58–64.
Parascandola, John. "From Mercury to Miracle Drugs: Syphilis Therapy over the Centuries." *Pharm Hist* 51, 1 (2009): 14–23.

Persson, Sheryl. *Smallpox, Syphilis and Salvation: Medical Breakthroughs That Changed the World*. Wollombi, NSW: Exisle Publishing, 2009.Principe, Lawrence M. *The Secrets of Alchemy*. Chicago: University of Chicago Press, 2013.

Rothschild, Bruce M. "History of Syphilis." *Clinical Infectious Diseases* 40, 10 (2005): 1454–63.

Travis, Anthony S. "Science as Receptor of Technology: Paul Ehrlich and the Synthetic Dyestuffs Industry." *Science in Context* 3 (1989): 383–408.

Wainwright, Milton. "Moulds in Ancient and More Recent Medicine." *The Mycologist* (1989): www.fungi4schools.org/Reprints/Mycologist_articles/Post-16/Medical/V03pp021-023folk_medicine.pdf.

Wainwright, Milton. "Moulds in Folk Medicine." *Folklore* 100, 2 (1989): 162 –66.

Webster, Charles. "Paracelsus, and 500 Years of Encouraging Scientific Inquiry: Stood for Sensitivity to the Environmental, Social, Spiritual, and Moral Dimensions of Health." *British Medical Journal* 306, 6878 (1993): 597–98.

Williams, K. J. "The Introduction of 'Chemotherapy' Using Arsphenamine—the First Magic Bullet." *J R Soc Med* 102, 8 (August 2009): 343–48.

Winau, Florian, Otto Westphal, and Rolf Winau. "Paul Ehrlich—In Search of the Magic Bullet." *Microbes and Infection* 6 (2004): 786–89.

Additional Resources

Brienne, Pierre. *The Discovery of Penicillin*. Encore. Wellcome. www.youtube.com/watch?v=VGC5JOLQoGo.

Encyclopedia.com. "Antibiotics: Fleming Discovers Penicillin." www.encyclopedia.com/utility/print-topic.aspx?id=54051.

Hermann, Thomas. "Lecture 2: History of Antibiotics." *Chemistry 259: Medicinal History of Modern Antibiotics*. San Diego: University of California (2012). http://tch.ucsd.edu/chem259/259_lecture_02_2012.pdf.

Markel, Howard. "The Real Story behind Penicillin." PBS Newshour (27 September 2013): www.pbs.org/newshour/rundown/the-real-story-behind-the-worlds-first-antibiotic/.

Peoria Historical Society. "Exhibit Penicillin—Accidental Discovery." www.peoriahistoricalsociety.org/!/Exhibits-PenicillinDiscovery.

Science Museum: Brought to Life. "Petri Dish Showing the Effect of Penicillin on Bacteria, United Kingdom, 1944." www.sciencemuseum.org.uk/broughttolife/objects/display?id=5762.

36. 1935: Psychosurgery

Sources

Charles Barber, "The Brain: A Mindless Obsession," *The Wilson Quarterly* 32, 1 (2008): 32–44.

Collins, Brianne M., and Hendrikus J. Stam. "Freeman's Transorbital Lobotomy as an Anomaly: A Material Culture Examination of Surgical Instruments and Operative Spaces." *History of Psychology* 18, 2 (20154): 119–31.

Collins, Brianne M., and Hendrikus J. Stam. "A Transnational Perspective on Psychosurgery: Beyond Portugal and the United States." *Journal of the History of the Neurosciences* 23, 4 (2014): 335–54.

"Egas Moniz—Facts." *Nobelprize.org*. nobelprize.org/nobel_prizes/medicine/laureates/1949/moniz-facts.html.

Miller, A. "The Lobotomy Patient a Decade Later: A Follow-up Study of a Research Project Started in 1948." *Canadian Medical Association Journal* 96 (April 15, 1967): 1095–1103.

NPR. "'My Lobotomy': Howard Dully's Journey." (Nov 16, 2005): npr.org/2005/11/16/5014080/my-lobotomy-howard-dullys-journey.

Raz, Mical. "Psychosurgery, Industry and Personal Responsibility, 1940–1965." *Social History of Medicine* 23, 1 (2010): 116–33.

Robinson, R. Aaron, *et al.* "Surgery of the Mind, Mood, and Conscious State: An Idea in Evolution." *World Neurosurgery* 80, 3/4 (2013): S2–S26.

Tan, Siang Yan, and Angela Yip. "António Egas Moniz (1874–1955): Lobotomy Pioneer and Nobel Laureate." *Singapore* 55, 4 (2014): 175–76.

Tsay, Cynthia J. "Julius Wagner-Jauregg and the Legacy of Malarial Therapy for the Treatment of General Paresis of the Insane." *Yale Journal of Biology and Medicine* 86, 2 (2013): 245–54.

Wikipedia. "Rosemary Kennedy." en.wikipedia.org/wiki/Rosemary_Kennedy.

Additional Sources

BBC News. "Howard Dully on Recovery from 'Ice-Pick' Lobotomy." (October 16, 2013): bbc.com/news/world-us-canada-24551691.

Day, Elizabeth. "He Was Bad, So They Put an Ice Pick in His Brain." *The Guardian* (January 13, 2008): www.theguardian.com/science/2008/jan/13/neuroscience.medicalscience.

Nobelprize.org. "Julius Wagner-Jauregg—Facts." www.nobelprize.org/nobel_prizes/medicine/laureates/1927/wagner-jauregg-facts.html.

Nuland, Sherwin. "How Electricoshock Therapy Changed Me." TED Talks (February 2001): ted.com/talks/sherwin_nuland_on_electroshock_therapy?language=en.

Raz, Mical. "Looking Back: Interpreting Lobotomy—The Patients' Stories." *The Psychologist* 27 (January, 2014): 56–59.

United States Department of Health and Human Services. "Information on Protection of Human Subjects in Research Funded or Regulated by U.S. Government." www.hhs.gov/1946inoculationstudy/protection.html.

United States Holocaust Memorial. "Nuremberg Code." www.ushmm.org/information/exhibitions/online-features/special-focus/doctors-trial/nuremberg-code.

Wikipedia. "Frontal Lobe." https://en.wikipedia.org/wiki/Frontal_lobe

37. 1939: Rat Poison for a U.S. President

Sources

"In Science Fields." *The Science News-Letter* 40, 3 (1941): 40–41.

Kingsbury, John M. "Commentary: One Man's Poison." *BioScience* 30, 3 (1980): 171–76.

Lichtenstein, A. "Award Ceremony Speech." The Nobel Prize in Physiology or Medicine 1943. www.nobelprize.org/nobel_prizes/medicine/laureates/1943/press.html.

Link, Karl Paul. "The Discovery of Dicumarol and Its Sequels." *Circulation* 19 (1959): 534–38.

Mueller, Richard L., and Stephen Scheidt. "History of Drugs for Thrombotic Disease: Discovery, Development, and Directions for the Future." *Circulation* 89, 1 (1994): 432–49.

Scully, Mike. "Warfarin Therapy: Rat Poison and the Prevention of Thrombosis." *The Biochemist* (2002): 15–17. www.biochemist.org/bio/02401/0015/024010015.pdf.

Additional Resources

Alberta Agriculture and Forestry. "Sweet Clover Poisoning: Frequently Asked Questions." www1.agric.gov.ab.ca/$department/deptdocs.nsf/all/faq8154?opendocument.

Meek, Thomas. "This Month in 1939: How Dead Cattle Led to the Discovery of Warfarin." PM Live (27 June 2013): www.pmlive.com/pharma_news/how_dead_cattle_led_to_the_discovery_of_warfarin_485464.

Snowbeck, Christopher. "Farmer, Sick Herd, and Persistent UW Scientist Results in Warfarin." *Twin Cities Pioneer Press* (7 October 2011): www.twincities.com/2011/10/07/farmer-sick-herd-and-persistent-uw-scientist-results-in-warfarin/.

38. 1944: Discovering DNA

Sources

Amsterdamska, Olga. "From Pneumonia to DNA: The Research Career of Oswald T. Avery." *Historical Studies in the Physical and Biological Sciences* 24, 1 (1993): 1–40.

Collins, Francis S., *et al.* "The Human Genome Project: Lessons from Large-Scale Biology." *Science* 300, 5617 (2003): 286–90.

Dahm, Ralf. "Friedrich Miescher and the Discovery of DNA." *Developmental Biology* 278 (2005): 274–88.

de Sojo, Áurea Anguera, Juan Ares, María Aurora Martínez, *et al.* "Serendipity and the Discovery of DNA." *Foundations of Science* 19 (2014): 387–401.

Dubos, R. J. "Oswald Theodore Avery, 1877–1955." *Biographical Memoirs of Fellows of the Royal Society* 2 (November 1956): 35–48.

Maderspacher, Florian. "Rags before the Riches: Friedrich Miescher and the Discovery of DNA." *Current Biology* 14, 15 (2004): R608.

Magner, Lois N. *A History of Medicine*, 2d ed. New York: Taylor & Francis, 2005.

National Cancer Institute. "BRCA1 and BRCA2: Cancer Risk and Genetic Testing." www.cancer.gov/about-cancer/causes-prevention/genetics/brca-fact-sheet.

National Institutes of Health. "Bacterial Pneumonia Caused Most Deaths in 1918 Influenza Pandemic." News Release (19 August 2008): www.nih.gov/news-events/news-releases/bacterial-pneumonia-caused-most-deaths-1918-influenza-pandemic.

Ponder, Bruce. "Genetic Testing for Cancer Risk." *Science* 278, 5340 (1997): 1050–54.

Portin, Petter. "The Birth and Development of the DNA Theory of Inheritance: Sixty Years since the Discovery of the Structure of DNA." *Journal of Genetics* 93, 1 (2014): 293–302.

Portugal, Frank. "Oswald T. Avery: Nobel Laureate or Noble Luminary?" *Perspectives in Biology and Medicine* 53, 4 (2010): 558–70.

U. S. Army Medical Department. *The Medical Department of the United States Army in the World War*, Chapter XXV. http://history.amedd.army.mil/booksdocs/wwi/adminamerexp/chapter25.html.

Watson, James D., and Francis H.C. Crick. "Molecular Structure of Nucleic Acids: A Structure for Deoxyribose Nucleic Acid." *Nature* 171 (1953): 737–38.

Wikipedia. "Griffith's Experiment." https://en.wikipedia.org/wiki/Griffith%27s_experiment.

Additional Resources

Crow, Ernest W. and James F. Crow. "100 Years Ago: Walter Sutton and the Chromosome Theory of Heredity." *Genetics* 160, 1 (2002): 1–4. www.genetics.org/content/160/1/1.

Guerra, Claudio. Rosalind. Franklin. DNA's unsung Hero. TED-Ed. www.youtube.com/watch?v=BIPolYrdirI.

National Institutes of Health. National Human Genome Institute. Deoxyribonucleic Acid (DNA). www.genome.gov/25520880.

Understanding Science. "The Structure of DNA: Cooperation and Competition." http://undsci. berkeley.edu/article/dna_01.

U.S. National Library of Medicine. "What Is DNA?" *Genetics Home Reference: Your Guide to Understanding Genetic Conditions* (3/28/2016): https://ghr.nlm.nih.gov/handbook/basics/dna.

Watson, James D. *The Double Helix: A Personal Account of the Discovery of the Structure of DNA.* New York: Atheneum, 1968.

Wikipedia. "DNA." https://en.wikipedia.org/wiki/DNA.

39. 1945: A Miracle Drug in the Sewage

Sources

Abraham, Edward. "Penicillin and Its Successors: A Personal View." *Bulletin of the American Academy of Arts and Sciences* 39, 1 (1985): 8–27.

Bo, G. "Giuseppe Brotzu and the Discovery of Cephalosporins." *Clinical Microbiology and Infection* 6, S3 (2000): 6–8.

Brotzu, Giuseppe. "Research on a New Antibiotic." Translated by R. Pompei and G. Cornaglia. *Publications of the Cagliari Institute of Hygiene* (1948): 6–19. pacs.unica.it/brotzu/brotzuen.pdf.

Orrù, Beniamino, *et al.* "Giuseppe Brotzu and the Discovery of Cephalosporins." Cologne: 8th European Conference of Medical and Health Libraries (2002): researchgate.net/publication/33496496_Giuseppe_Brotzu_and_the_Discovery_of_Cephalosporins.

Scarpa, B. "Homage from One Sardinian to Another." *Clinical Microbiology and Infection* 6, S3 (2000): 3–5.

Wainwright, Milton. "Moulds in Folk Medicine." Folklore 100, 2 (1989): 162–66.

Additional Resources

Bailey, Dan. "The Making of a Miracle Drug." Smells Like Science. http://smellslikescience.com/the-making-of-a-miracle-drug/.

Science Clarified. "Antibiotics." www.scienceclarified.com/Al-As/Antibiotics.html.

40. 1945: Saving Lives with Sausage Casings, Washing Machines, and Juice Cans

Sources

Dunphy, Lynne M. "Iron Lungs." *American Journal of Nursing* 103, 5 (2003): 641.

Kolff, Willem. "An Artificial Heart Inside the Body." *Scientific American* 213, 5 (November 1965): 38–46. www.nature.com.uri.idm.oclc.org/scientificamerican/journal/v213/n5/pdf/scientificamerican1165-38.pdf.

Kolff, Willem J. "The Artificial Kidney and Its Effect on the Development of Other Artificial Organs." *Nature Magazine* 8, 10 (October 2002): 1063–65.

Mayo Clinic Staff. "Acute Kidney Failure." mayoclinic.org/diseases-conditions/kidney-failure/basics/definition/con-20024029.

Schwid, Stephen A., and Willem J. Kolff. "Closed Sleeve Bandage to Protect Dialysis Shunts." *JAMA* 202, 2 (1967): 156.

Shinaberger, James H. "Quantitation of Dialysis: Historical Perspective." *Seminars in Dialysis* 14, 4 (2001): 238–45.

Stanley, Theodore H. "A Tribute to Dr Willem J. Kolff: Innovative Inventor, Physician, Scientist, Bioengineer, Mentor, and Significant Contributor to Modern Cardiovascular Surgical and Anesthetic Practice." *Journal of Cardiothoracic and Vascular Anesthesia* 27, 3 (June 2013): 600–13.

Wikipedia. "Dialysis." https://en.wikipedia.org/wiki/Dialysis.

Wikipedia. "Iron Lung." https://en.wikipedia.org/wiki/Iron_lung.

Additional Resources

Academy of Achievement. "Willem Kolff Biography." Academy of Achievement (2013). www.achievement.org/autodoc/page/kol0bio-1.

Blakeslee, Sandra. "Willem Kolff, Doctor Who Invented Kidney and Heart Machines, Dies at 97." *New York Times* (12 February 2009): www.nytimes.com/2009/02/13/health/13kolff.html?_r=0.

History of Vaccines. "History of Polio." www.historyofvaccines.org/content/timelines/polio.

J. Willard Marriott Library. "Willem J. Kolff, 1911 – 2009." University of Utah. www.lib.utah.edu/collections/photo-exhibits/willem_kolf.php.

41. 1951: Frankenstein and the Heart Machines

Sources

Aquilina, Oscar. "A Brief History of Cardiac Pacing." *Images in Paediatric Cardiology* 8, 2 (2006): 17–81.

Friedman, Lester D. "It's *Still Alive: Victor Frankenstein*." *The Pharos* (Spring 2016): 49–52. http://alphaomegaalpha.org/pharos/PDFs/2016-2-Movies.pdf.

Rosenbaum, Jean B., and Darwood Hansen. "Simple Cardiac Pacemaker and Defibrillator." *JAMA* 155, 13 (1954): 1151.

"Jean Rosenbaum: Health Association Executive, Fitness Physician." Prabook: prabook.org/web/person-view.html?profileId=596729.

Smithsonian. National Museum of American History. "Yorick, the Bionic Skeleton." http://americanhistory.si.edu/ collections/search/object/nmah_1203675.

Ward, Catherine, Susannah Henderson, and Neil H. Metcalfe. "A Short History on Pacemakers." *International Journal of Cardiology* 169 (2013): 244–48.

Wikipedia. "Artificial Cardiac Pacemaker." https://en.wikipedia.org/wiki/Artificial_cardiac_pacemaker.

Wolfson, Susan J. "'*This* Is My Lightning' or; Sparks in the Air." *Studies in English Literature 1500 – 1900* 55, 4 (2015): 751–86.

Additional Resources

Brown, Alan S. "The Science That Made Frankenstein." Inside Science (October 27, 2010): www.insidescience.org/content/science-made-frankenstein/1116.

Mandrola, John. "What's Electrophysiology?" www.drjohnm.org/about-electrophysiology/.

Whale, James, director. *Frankenstein: The Man Who Made a Monster.* Clip showing monster animated by electricity: www.youtube.com/watch?v=1qNeGSJaQ9Q.

42. 1967: Baruch Blumberg Discovers a Cancer-Causing Virus

Sources

Blumberg, B. S., *et al.* "The Relation of Infection with the Hepatitis B Agent to Primary Hepatic Carcinoma." *American Journal of Pathology* 81, 3 (1975): 669–82.

Blumberg, Baruch S. "Baruch S. Blumberg – Biographical." Nobelprize.org (1976; addendum 2006): www.nobelprize.org/nobel_prizes/medicine/laureates/1976/blumberg-bio.html.

Blumberg, Baruch S. "The Hepatitis B Virus." *Public Health Reports* 95, 5 (1980): 427–35.

Blumberg, Baruch S. "Hepatitis B Virus, the Vaccine, and the Control of Primary Cancer of the Liver." *Proceedings of the National Academy of Science* 94, 14 (1997): 7121–25.

McPherson, Mary Patterson, *et al.* "Baruch S. Blumberg: 28 July 1925 5 April 2011." *Proceedings of the American Philosophical Society* 155, 3 (2011): 301–11.

National Cancer Institute. "Cancer Vaccines." www.cancer.gov/about-cancer/causes-prevention/vaccines-fact-sheet#q8.

Segelken, H. Roger. "Baruch S. Blumberg," *New York Times* (6 April 2011): nytimes.com/2011/04/07/health/07blumberg.html?_r=0.

Senior, John R., W. Thomas London, and Alton I. Sutnick. "The Australia Antigen and Role of the Late Philadelphia General Hospital in Reducing Post-Transfusion Hepatitis and Sequelae." *Hepatology* 54, 3 (2011): 753–56.

World Health Organization. "World Health Report: Infectious Diseases and Cancer," 1996: who.int/whr/1996/media_centre/press_release/en/index7.html.

Additional Resources

Hepatitis B Foundation. "Hepatitis B and Primary Liver Cancer." (Last modified 3/6/2014). www.hepb.org/liver-cancer/hepb_and_liver_cancer.htm.

NASA Astrobiology Institute. http://nai.nasa.gov/.

Segelken, H. Roger. "Baruch S. Blumberg, Who Discovered and Tackled Hepatitis B, Dies at 85." *New York Times* (April 6, 2011): www.nytimes.com/2011/04/07/health/07blumberg.html?_r=0.

Smith, Adam. "Interview with Baruch S. Blumberg." (March 2009): www.nobelprize.org/mediaplayer/index.php?id=1245.

43. 1967: The First Heart Transplant

Sources

Altman, Lawrence K. "Christiaan Barnard, Surgeon for First Heart Transplant, Dies." *New York Times* (September 3, 2001). nytimes.com/2001/09/03/world/christiaan-barnard-78-surgeon-for-first-heart-transplant-dies.html.

Ankney, R. N. "Miracle in South Africa: A Historical Review of US Magazines' Coverage of the First Heart Transplant." *Ecquid Novi: African Journalism Studies* 19, 2 (1998): 26–38.

"Balancing the Drug Dosage." *Science News* 93, 1 (1968): 7–8.

Barnard, Christiaan N. "Heart Transplants Fell into Disrepute." *New York Times* Arts and Leisure, D1 (November 26, 1972). query.nytimes.com/gst/abstract.html?res=9A02EFDF1F3DE533A25755C2A9679D946390D6CF.

"First Human Hearts Transplanted." *Science News* 92, 25 (1967): 581.

Holloway, Marguerite. "Graft and Host, Together Forever." *Scientific American* 296, 2 (2007): 32–33.

"Peter Medawar - Biographical." *Nobelprize.org.* www.nobelprize.org/nobel_prizes/medicine/laureates/1960/medawar-bio.html.

"Ss. Cosmas and Damian, the Patron Saints of Medicine." *British Medical Journal* 2, 2180 (1902): 1176–77.

Starzl, Thomas E. "The Landmark Identical Twin Case." *JAMA* 251, 19 (1984): 2572–73.

Starzl, Thomas E. "History of Clinical Transplantation." *World Journal of Surgery* 24, 7 (2000): 759–82.

Starzl, Thomas E. "The Birth of Clinical Organ Transplantation." *Journal of the American College of Surgeons* 192, 4 (2001): 431–46.

Starzl, Thomas E. "Peter Brian Medawar: Father of Transplantation." *Journal of the American College of Surgeons* 180, 3 (1995): 332–36.

Starzl, Thomas E., and Clyde Barker. "The Origin of Clinical Organ Transplantation Revisited." *JAMA* 301, 19 (May 20, 2009): 2041–43.

Watson, C. J. E. and J. H. Dark. "Organ Transplantation: Historical Perspective and Current Practice." *British Journal of Anaesthesia* 108, suppl 1 (January 1, 2012): i29–42.

Wikipedia. "Brain Death." https://en.wikipedia.org/wiki/Brain_death.

Wright, Irving S. "A New Challenge to Ethical Codes: Heart Transplants." *Journal of Religion and Health* 8, 3 (1969): 226–41.

Additional Resources

Lieberman, Dan. "The Waiting Game: 9 Organ Transplant Patients Fight to Survive." ABC News (May 1, 2012): http://abcnews.go.com/Health/waiting-game-organ-transplant-patients-fight-survive/story?id=16245341.

National Institutes of Health. "Human Leukocyte Antigens." U.S. National Library of Medicine. https://ghr.nlm.nih.gov/primer/genefamily/hla.

U.S. Department of Health and Human Services. "Organ Matching Process." www.organdonor.gov/about/organmatching.html.

44. 1972: A Magic Bullet from Ancient Chinese Medicine

Sources

Chang, Rhonda. "Making Theoretical Principles for New Chinese Medicine." *Health and History* 16, 1 (2014): 66–86.

Dunning, Brian. "Mao's Barefoot Doctors: The Secret History of Chinese Medicine." *Skeptoid* Podcast #259 (May 24, 2011): https://skeptoid.com/episodes/4259.

"From Branch to Bedside: Youyou Tu Is Awarded the 2011 Lasker-DeBakey Clinical Medical Research Award for Discovering Artemesinin as a Treatment for Malaria." *Journal of Clinical Investigation* 121, 10 (2011): 3768–73.

Levinovitz, Alan. "Chairman Mao Invented Traditional Chinese Medicine." Slate.com (22 October 2013): www.slate.com/articles/health_and_science/medical_examiner/2013/10/traditional_chinese_medicine_origins_mao_invented_it_but_didn_t_believe.single.html.

McKenna, Phil. "Malaria's Nemesis." *New Scientist* 212, 2838 (12 November 2011).

Miller, Louis H., and Xinzhuan Su. "Artemisinin: Discovery from the Chinese Herbal Garden." *Cell* 146, 6 (2011): 855–88.

Stone, Richard. "Lifting the Veil on Traditional Chinese Medicine." *Science* 319, 5864 (February 8, 2008): 709–10.

Tu Youyou. "The Discovery of Artemisinin (Qinghausu) and Gifts from Chinese Medicine." *Nature Medicine* 17, 10 (2011): 1217–20.

World Health Organization. "WHO/UNICEF Report: Malaria MDG Target Achieved amid Sharp Drop in Cases and Mortality, But 3 Billion People Remain at Risk." www.who.int/mediacentre/news/releases/2015/malaria-mdg-target/en/.

Additional Resources

Dambeck, Susanne. "The Modest Nobel Laureate: Youyou Tu." Lindau Nobel Laureate Meetings (12 October 2015): www.lindau-nobel.org/the-modest-nobel-laureate-youyou-tu/.

Hatton, Celia. "Nobel Prize Winner Tu Youyou Helped by Ancient Chinese Remedy." BBC News (October 6, 2015): www.bbc.com/news/blogs-china-blog-34451386.

National Center for Complementary and Integrative Health. "Traditional Chinese Medicine: In Depth." https://nccih.nih.gov/health/whatiscam/chinesemed.htm.

45. 1978: The First Test Tube Baby

Sources

Biggers, John D. "IVF and Embryo Transfer: Historical Origin and Development." *Reproductive Biomedicine Online* 25 (2012): 118–27.

Brooks, Carol Flora. "The Early History of the Anti-Contraceptive Laws in Massachusetts and Connecticut." *American Quarterly* 18, 1 (1966): 3–23.

Connell, Elizabeth B. "Contraception in the Prepill Era." *Contraception* 59 (1999): 7S–10S.

Dyer, Clare. "White Couple Can Keep Mixed Race Twins after IVF Blunder." *BMJ* 325, 7372 (2002): 1055.

Grady, Denise. "Lesley Brown, Mother of the World's First 'Test-Tube Baby,' Dies at 64." *New York Times* (24 June 2012) www.nytimes.com/2012/06/24/health/lesley-brown-mother-of-first-test-tube-baby-dies-at-64.html.

Greenhouse, Linda and Reva B. Siegel. "Before (and after) Roe V. Wade: New Questions About Backlash." *Yale Law Journal* 120, 8 (2011): 2028–87.

Henig, Robin Marantz. "Lesley Brown, b. 1964." *New York Times* (December 30, 2012): www.nytimes. com/interactive/2012/12/30/magazine/the-lives-they-lived-2012.html?view=Lesley_Brown.

Hoffman, Jessica R. "You Say Adoption, I Say Objection: Why the Word War over Embryo Disposition Is More Than Just Semantics." *Family Law Quarterly* 46, 3 (2012): 397–417.

Human Fertilisation & Embryo Authority, "About Infertility," (1 June 2012): www.hfea.gov.uk/ infertility.html.

Joffe, Carole. "Portraits of Three 'Physicians of Conscience': Abortion before Legalization in the United States." *Journal of the History of Sexuality* 2, 1 (1991): 46–67.

Johnson, Martin H. "Robert Edwards: Nobel Laureate in Physiology or Medicine." Nobel Lecture, 2010. www.nobelprize.org/nobel_prizes/medicine/laureates/2010/edwards-lecture.html.

Mroz, Jacqueline. "One Sperm Donor, 150 Offspring." New York Times (6 September 2011): www. nytimes.com/2011/09/06/health/06donor.html.

Powderly, Kathleen E. "Contraceptive Policy and Ethics Illustrations from American History." *The Hastings Center Report* 25, 1 (1995): S9–S11.

Rowland, Robyn. "Donor Insemination to in Vitro Fertilization: The Confusion Grows." *Politics and the Life Sciences* 12, 2 (1993): 192–93.

Simpson, Bob. "Making 'Bad' Deaths 'Good': The Kinship Consequences of Posthumous Conception." *Journal of the Royal Anthropological Institute* 7, 1 (2001): 1–18.

Simpson, Bob. "Managing Potential in Assisted Reproductive Technologies: Reflections on Gifts, Kinship, and the Process of Vernacularization." *Current Anthropology* 54, S7 (2013): S87–S96.

Stein, Marc. "The Supreme Court's Sexual Counter-Revolution." *OAH Magazine of History* 20, 2 (2006): 21–25.

Ward, Victoria. "Louise Brown, the First IVF Baby, Reveals Family Was Bombarded with Hate Mail." *The Telegraph* (July 24, 2015): www.telegraph.co.uk/news/health/11760004/Louise-Brown-the-first-IVF-baby-reveals-family-was-bombarded-with-hate-mail.html.

Watts, Geoff. "IVF Pioneer Robert Edwards Wins Nobel Prize for Medicine." *BMJ: British Medical Journal* 341, 7776 (2010): 747.

Additional Resources

Enriquez, Juan. "We Can Reprogram Life—How to Do It Wisely." TED Talks (2015): www.ted. com/talks/juan_enriquez_we_can_reprogram_life_how_to_do_it_wisely#t-677446.

Stock, Gregory. "To Upgrade Is Human." TED Talks (2003): www.ted.com/talks/ gregory_stock_to_upgrade_is_human.

World Medical Assembly. "WMA Statement on In-Vitro Fertilization and Embryo Transplantation." *Adopted by the 39th World Medical Assembly Madrid, Spain, October 1987 and rescinded at the WMA General Assembly, Pilanesberg, South Africa, 2006.* www.wma.net/en/30publications/10policies/20archives/e5/.

46. 1983: Preventing Cancers

Sources

American Cancer Society. "The History of Cancer." cancer.org/cancer/cancerbasics/ thehistoryofcancer/the-history-of-cancer-what-is-cancer.

Annas, George J., and Edward R. Utley. *The Nazi Doctors and the Nuremberg Code: Human Rights in Human Experimentation.* New York: Oxford University Press, 1992.

Casper, Monica J., and Adele E. Clarke. "Making the Pap Smear into the 'Right Tool' for the Job: Cervical Cancer Screening in the USA, circa 1940–95." *Social Studies of Science* 28, 2 (1998): 255–90.

Dawar, Meenakshi, Shelley Deeks, and Simon Dobson. "Human Papillomavirus Vaccines Launch a New Era in Cervical Cancer Prevention." *Canadian Medical Association Journal* 177, 5 (2007): 456–61.

Denny, Lynette, et al. "Cervical Cancer." In *Cancer: Disease Control Priorities,* Third Edition (Volume 3), edited by H. Gelband et al. Washington (DC): The World Bank, 2015.

Higby, Gregory J. "Tuskegee Syphilis Study Revisited." *Pharmacy in History* 41, 4 (1999): 169–70.

Lederer, Susan. "Experimentation on Human Beings." *OAH Magazine of History* 19, 5 (2005): 20–22.

Mukherjee, Siddhartha. *The Emperor of All Maladies: A Biography of Cancer.* New York: Scribner, 2010: 287.

National Cancer Institute. "Causes and Prevention: Risk Factors for Cancer." cancer.gov/ about-cancer/causes-prevention/risk.

Sandlow, L.J. "Oaths, Codes, and Charters in Medicine over the Ages." *Hektoen International* (Fall 2011): hektoeninternational.org/index.php?option=com_content&view=article&id=399:oaths-codes-and-charters-in-medicine-over-the-ages&catid=71&Itemid=716.

Southam, Chester M., et al. "Homotransplantation of Human Cell Lines." *Science, New Series* 125, 3239 (25 January 1957): 158–60.

Vollmann, Jochen, and Rolf Winau. "Informed Consent in Human Experimentation before the Nuremberg Code." *BMJ: British Medical Journal* 313, 7070 (1996): 1445–47.

Wikipedia. "Nuremberg Code." en.wikipedia.org/wiki/Nuremberg_Code.

Wynder, Ernest L. "Environmental Factors in Cervical Cancer: An Approach to Its Prevention." *British Medical Journal* 1, 4916 (1955): 743–47.

Zur Hausen, Harald. "Biographical." Nobelprize.org. nobelprize.org/nobel_prizes/medicine/laureates/2008/hausen-bio.html.

Zur Hausen, Harald. "Papillomaviruses in the Causation of Human Cancers—A Brief Historical Account." *Virology* 384 (2009): 260–65.

Additional Resources
Krock, Lexi. "Accidental Discoveries." NOVA (27 February 2001): pbs.org/wgbh/nova/body/accidental-discoveries.html.
Murchison, Elizabeth. "Fighting a Contagious Cancer." TED Talks (July 2011): ted.com/talks/elizabeth_murchison?language=en#t-754618.
Yong, Ed. "The Curious Case of a Contagious Cancer." *The Atlantic* (January 7, 2016): theatlantic.com/science/archive/2016/01/second-contagious-cancer-in-tasmanian-devils-baffles-scientists/423012/.

47. 1998: MMR Vaccine, Autism, Discovery, and Fraud

Sources
Centers for Disease Control. "Autism Spectrum Disorder (ASD) Data & Statistics." www.cdc.gov/ncbddd/autism/data.html.
Flaherty, Dennis K. "The Vaccine-Autism Connection: A Public Health Crisis Caused by Fraudulent Science." *Annals of Pharmacotherapy* 45 (October 2011): 1302–04.
Hendriks, Jan, and Stuart Blume. "Measles Vaccination before the Measles-Mumps-Rubella Vaccine." *American Journal of Public Health* 103, 8 (2013): 1393–1401.
Jain, Anjali, *et al.* "Autism Occurrence by MMR Vaccine Status Among US Children With Older Siblings With and Without Autism." *Journal of the American Medical Association* 313, 15 (2015): 1534–40.
Meacham, William. "Postinfection Immunity to Measles Was Known to Common Folk Well Before Its Discovery by Science." *American Journal of the Medical Sciences* 347, 6 (June 2014): 502–03.
Poland, Gregory A. "MMR Vaccine and Autism: Vaccine Nihilism and Postmodern Science." *Mayo Clinic Proceedings* 86, 9 (September 2011): 869–71.
St. Louis Children's Hospital. "Case Study: July 'First Disease.'" www.stlouischildrens.org/health-care-professionals/publications/doctors-digest/september-october-2013/case-study-july-first-d.
Stark, Cynthia. "MMR Vaccine and Autism—A Mother's Journey to Heal Her Child." Vaccine Choice Canada (February 2013): http://vaccinechoicecanada.com/personal-stories/mmr-vaccine-and-autism-a-mothers-journey-to-heal-her-child/.
Wikipedia. "Leo Kanner." https://en.wikipedia.org/wiki/Leo_Kanner.
World Health Organization. Media Centre. "Measles Fact Sheet." Reviewed March 2016. www.who.int/mediacentre/factsheets/fs286/en/.

Additional Resources
CNN Wire. "Retracted Autism Study an 'Elaborate Fraud,' British Journal Finds." CNN (5 January 2011): www.cnn.com/2011/HEALTH/01/05/autism.vaccines/.
Donvan, John, and Caren Zucker. "Autism's First Child." *The Atlantic* (2010): www.theatlantic.com/magazine/archive/2010/10/autisms-first-child/308227/.
O'Callaghan, Martine. "MMR and Autism: Our Story." Voices for Vaccines: Parents Speaking Up for Immunization. www.voicesforvaccines.org/mmr-and-autism-our-story/.
Stallard, Brian. "Deadly Measles Is Back in the U.S., but Why?" Nature World News (5 February 2015): www.natureworldnews.com/articles/12575/20150206/deadly-measles-back-why.htm.
Szalavitz, Maria. "Autism—It's Different in Girls." *Scientific American* (1 March 2016): www.scientificamerican.com/article/autism-it-s-different-in-girls/#.

48. 2011: Bionic Parts

Sources:
"Advanced Delivery Devices - Implantable Drug-Eluting Devices: A Novel Approach to Patient Care." *Drug Development and Delivery* (2015): www.drug-dev.com/Main/Back-Issues/ADVANCED-DELIVERY-DEVICES-Implantable-DrugEluting-1006.aspx.
Chen, Stephen. "'This Is Just the Beginning': China Approves World's First 3D-Printed Hip Joint for General Use." *South China Morning Post* (1 September 2015): www.scmp.com/tech/science-research/article/1854369/just-beginning-china-approves-worlds-first-3d-printed-hip.
Dabizzi, E. and P. G. Arcidiaco. "Update on Enteral Stents." *Current Treatment Options in Gastroenterology* 14, 2 (2016): 178–84.
Gaviria, Laura, John Paul Salcido, Teja Guda, and Joo L. Ong. "Current Trends in Dental Implants." *Journal of the Korean Association of Oral and Maxillofacial Surgeons* 40, 2 (2014): 50–60.
Grose, Thomas K. "Human Spare Parts." *ASEE Prism* 24, 6 (2015): 24–29.
Hohenforst-Schmidt, Wolfgang, *et al.* "Drug Eluting Stents for Malignant Airway Obstruction: A Critical Review of the Literature." *J Cancer* 7, 4 (01/13/ 2016): 377–90.
Kohnen, Thomas, Martin Baumeister, Daniel Kook, Oliver K. Klaproth, and Christian Ohrloff. "Cataract Surgery with Implantation of an Artificial Lens." *Deutsches Ärzteblatt International* 106, 43 (10/23/ 2009): 695–702.

Moy, Brian T. and John W. Birk. "An Update to Hepatobiliary Stents." *Journal of Clinical and Translational Hepatology* 3, 1 (2015): 67-77.

Roehr, Bob. "Vaginal Ring Offers Hope in HIV Prevention." *Scientific American* (February 24, 2016): scientificamerican.com/article/vaginal-ring-offers-hope-in-hiv-prevention/.

Spangehl, Mark. "Hip Resurfacing: An Alternative to Conventional Hip Replacement?" Mayo Clinic (14 February 2014): http://www.mayoclinic.org/hip-resurfacing/expert-answers/faq-20057913.

"Sbu Systematic Review Summaries." In *Drug-Eluting Stents in Coronary Arteries.* Stockholm: Swedish Council on Health Technology Assessment, 2014.

Theobald, Stacy. "Custom Surgery Creates Normal Hips for 30-Year-Old." Mayo Clinic (27 October 2011): http://sharing.mayoclinic.org/discussion/custom-surgery-creates-normal-hips-for-30-year-old/.

Van Brabandt, Hans, Mattias Neyt, and Frank Hulstaert. "Transcatheter Aortic Valve Implantation (TAVI): Risky and Costly." *BMJ: British Medical Journal* 345, 7868 (2012): 24–27.

Ventola, C. Lee. "Medical Applications for 3D Printing: Current and Projected Uses." *Pharmacy and Therapeutics* 39, 10 (2014): 704–711.

Additional Resources

American Academy of Orthopedic Surgeons. "Questions and Answers about Metal on Metal Hip Implants." http://orthoinfo.aaos.org/topic.cfm?topic=a00625.

Boyd, Kierstan. "IOL Implants: Lens Replacement and Cataract Surgery." American Academy of Ophthalmologists (1 March 2016): www.aao.org/eye-health/diseases/cataracts-iol-implants.

Future of Things. "7 Major Advancements 3D Printing is Making in the Medical Field." http://thefutureofthings.com/8973-7-major-advancements-3d-printing-is-making-in-the-medical-field/.

Mayo Clinic. "3D Printer Helps Hip." www.mayoclinic.org/tests-procedures/hip-replacement-surgery/multimedia/vid-20078391.

Tillemann-Dick, Charity. "Singing after a Double Lung Transplant." TEDmed (2010): www.ted.com/talks/charity_tillemann_dick_singing_after_a_double_lung_transplant#t-363304.

49. 2013: Poop Therapy for the Human Microbiome

Sources

Cammarota, Giovanni, *et al.* "Gut Microbiota Modulation: Probiotics, Antibiotics or Fecal Microbiota Transplantation?" *Internal and Emergency Medicine* 9 (2014): 365–73.

CDC Press Room. "Nearly Half a Million Americans Suffered from *Clostridium difficile* Infections in a Single Year." (25 February 2015): www.cdc.gov/media/releases/2015/p0225-clostridium-difficile.html.

Hsiao, William W.L., and Claire M. Fraser-Liggett. "Human Microbiome Project—Paving the Way to a Better Understanding of Ourselves and Our Microbes." *Drug Discovery Today* 14, 7 (2009): 331–33.

Orenstein, Robert, *et al.* "Moving Fecal Microbiota Transplantation into the Mainstream." *Nutrition in Clinical Practice* 28, 5 (2013): 589–98.

van Nood, Els, *et al.* "Duodenal Infusion of Donor Feces for Recurrent *Clostridium difficile.*" *New England Journal of Medicine* 368, 5 (January 13, 2013): 407–15.

Van Schooneveld, Trevor C., *et al.* "Duodenal Infusion of Donor Feces for Recurrent *Clostridium difficile:* To the Editor." *New England Journal of Medicine* 368, 22 (May 30, 2013): 2143.

Vyas, Dinesh, *et al.* "Fecal Transplant Policy and Legislation." *World Journal of Gastroenterology* 21, 1 (2015): 6–11.

Zimmer, Carl. "Fecal Transplants Can Be Life-Saving, but How?" *New York Times* (15 July 2016): nytimes.com/2016/07/15/science/fecal-transplants-bacteria-viruses.html?_r=0.

Additional Resources

Berkeley Wellness. "Probiotics Pros and Cons." 3 March 2014. www.berkeleywellness.com/supplements/other-supplements/article/probiotics-pros-and-cons.

Centers for Disease Control. "*Clostridium difficile* Infection Information for Patients. 24 February 2015. www.cdc.gov/hai/organisms/cdiff/Cdiff-patient.html.

McKenna, Maryn. "Transplants Become Routine for Debilitating Diarrhea?" *Scientific American* (1 December 2011): www.scientificamerican.com/article/swapping-germs/.

National Center for Complementary and Integrative Health. "Probiotics: In Depth." May 4, 2016. https://nccih.nih.gov/health/probiotics/introduction.htm.

50. 2016: Researching the Zika Virus

Sources

Brazil. Ministry of Health. "Ministry of Health Confirmed 1,709 Cases of Microcephaly." (July 16, 2016): https://translate.google.com/translate?hl=en&sl=pt&u=http://portalsaude.saude.gov.br/&prev=search.

CDC. "Zika Virus." cdc.gov/zika/index.html.

McNeil, Donald G., Jr. *Zika: The Emerging Epidemic.* New York: W. W. Norton, 2016.

Paixão, Enny S., *et al.* "History, Epidemiology, and Clinical Manifestations of Zika: A Systematic Review." *American Journal of Public Health* 106, 4 (April 2016): 606–12.

Weaver, Scott C., *et al.* "Zika Virus: History, Emergence, Biology, and Prospects for Control." *Antiviral Research* 130 (2016): 69–80.

World Health Organization. "Zika Virus and Complications." who.int/emergencies/zika-virus/en/.

Additional Resources

Belluck, Pam. "Confronting a Lingering Question about Zika: How It Enters the Womb." *New York Times* (18 July 2016): nytimes.com/2016/07/19/health/zika-virus-placenta.html.

Saint Louis, Catherine. "Microcephaly, Spotlighted by Zika Virus, Has Long Afflicted and Mystified." *New York Times* (31 January 2016): nytimes.com/2016/02/01/health/microcephaly-spotlighted-by-zika-virus-has-long-afflicted-and-mystified.html.

Weintraub, Karen. "Scientists Link Zika Firmly to Paralysis, As Patients in Tahiti Know Too Well." STAT (29 February 2016): statnews.com/2016/02/29/zika-guillain-barre-tahiti/.

Wolfe, Nathan. "What's Left to Explore?" TED Talks (February 2012): ted.com/talks/nathan_wolfe_what_s_left_to_explore.

Conclusion

Sources

"Ancient Chinese Anti-fever Cure Becomes Panacea for Malaria: An Interview with Zhou Yiqing." *Bulletin of the World Health Organization* 87 (2009): 743–744. www.who.int/bulletin/volumes/87/10/09-051009.pdf.

Andersson, Jan, *et al.* "Avermectin and Artemisinin: Revolutionary Therapies against Parasitic Diseases." www.nobelprize.org/nobel_prizes/medicine/laureates/2015/advanced-medicine-prize2015.pdf.

Brooker, Simon. "Estimating the Global Distribution and Disease Burden of Intestinal Nematode Infections: Adding up the Numbers – a Review." *International Journal for Parasitology* 40, 10 (04/27/2010): 1137–44. http://scialert.net/fulltext/?doi=rjphyto.2010.154.161&org=10.

Falodun, A. "Herbal Medicine in Africa: Distribution, Standardization and Prospects." *Research Journal of Phytochemistry*, 4 (2010): 154–161.

Hsu, Elisabeth. "Reflections on the 'Discovery' of the Antimalarial Qinghao." *British Journal of Clinical Pharmacology* 61, 6 (2006): 666–70.

Meier zu Biesen, Caroline. "The Rise to Prominence of *Artemisia Annua* L.—The Transformation of a Chinese Plant to a Global Pharmaceutical." *African Sociological Review* 14, 2 (2010): 24–46.

Novartis Malaria Initiative. "First-in-Class Treatment." Novartis (2015): www.malaria.novartis.com/malaria-initiative/treatment/first-in-class-treatment/index.shtml.

Talisuna, Ambrose O., *et al.* "The Affordable Medicines Facility-malaria—A Success in Peril." *Malaria Journal* 11 (2012): 370. www.ncbi.nlm.nih.gov/pmc/articles/PMC3506461/.

World Health Organization. "Malaria Fact Sheet." (April 2016): www.who.int/mediacentre/factsheets/fs094/en/.

World Health Organization. "WHO Position Statement: Effectiveness of Non-Phamaceutical Forms of Artemesia Annua L. Against Malaria." June 2012. www.who.int/malaria/publications/atoz/position_statement_herbal_remedy_artemisia_annua_l/en/.

Additional Resources

Freeman, Colin. "Nobel Prize for Chinese Traditional Medicine Expert Who Developed Malaria Cure." *Telegraph* (5 October 2015): www.telegraph.co.uk/news/worldnews/asia/china/11912754/Nobel-Prize-for-Chinese-traditional-medicine-expert-who-developed-malaria-cure.html.

Guo, Jeff. "How a Secret Chinese Military Drug Based on an Ancient Herb Won the Nobel Prize." *Washington Post* (6 October 2015): washingtonpost.com/news/wonk/wp/2015/10/06/how-a-secret-chinese-military-drug-based-on-an-ancient-herb-won-the-nobel-prize/.

UnitAid. "Affordable Medicines for Malaria." www.unitaid.eu/en/amfm.

Endnotes

Introduction

1. Azizi, M. H. *et al.*, "A Brief History of the Discovery of the Circulation of Blood in the Human Body," *Archive of Iranian Medicine* 11, 3 (May 2008): 345–50.
2. John H. Krystal and Matthew W. State, "Psychiatric Disorders: Diagnosis to Therapy," *Cell* 157, 1 (March 2014): 201–14.

Chapter 1

1. Paul Gostner *et al.*, "New Radiological Insights into the Life and Death of the Tyrolean Iceman," *Journal of Archaeological Science* 38, 12 (2011): 3425–31.
2. James H. Dickson *et al.*, "The Omnivorous Tyrolean Iceman," *Philosophical Transactions of the Royal Society B: Biological Sciences* 355, 1404 (2000): 1843–1849.
3. Richard Knox, "Oetzi the Iceman May Be the Last in His Family," NPR (30 October 2008): www.npr.org/templates/story/story.php?storyId=96328080.
4. Tina Hesman Saey, "Genome Paints a Better Portrait of the Iceman," *Science News* 181, 6 (24 March 2012): 5–6.
5. Sindya N. Bhanoo, "Lactose Intolerant, Before Milk Was on the Menu," *New York Times* (5 March 2006): www.nytimes.com/2012/03/06/science/iceman-had-brown-eyes-and-hair-and-was-lactose-intolerant.html.
6. Gostner *et al.*, "New Radiological Insights."
7. Lois N. Magner, *A History of Medicine*, 2d ed. (New York: Taylor & Francis, 2005), 12.
8. Dickson *et al.*, "The Omnivorous."
9. Marco Samadelli, *et al.*, "Complete Mapping of the Tattoos of the 5300-year-old Tyrolean Iceman," *Journal of Cultural Heritage* 16, 5 (2015): 753–58.
10. L. Dorfer *et al.*, "A Medical Report from the Stone Age?" *The Lancet* 354 (September 18, 1999): 1023–25.
11. U. Peintner *et al.*, "The Iceman's Fungi," *Mycological Research* 102, 10 (1998): 1153–62.
12. John Noble Wilford, "Lessons in Iceman's Prehistoric Medicine Kit," *New York Times* (December 8, 1998). www.nytimes.com/1998/12/08/science/lessons-in-iceman-s-prehistoric-medicine-kit.html.
13. Wikipedia, "Ötzi," en.wikipedia.org/wiki/%C3%96tzi; Wikipedia, "*Fomes fomentarius*," en.wikipedia.org/wiki/Fomes_fomentarius.
14. Vincent E. C. Ooi and Fang Liu, "Immunomodulation and Anti-cancer Activity of Polysaccharide-protein Complexes," *Current Medical Chemistry* 7, 7 (2000): 715–29.
15. Karen Hardy *et al.*, "Neanderthal Medics?" *Naturwissenschaften* 99, 8 (2012): 617–26.
16. Hardy *et al.*, "Neanderthal Medics?"

Chapter 2

1. Bonnie J. Horrigan, "Lyall Watson, Ph.D.: Healers, Healing, and the Nature of Reality," *Explore* 2, 1 (2006): 47–54.
2. United Nations, "World Conference on Indigenous Peoples" (September 22–23, 2014), www.un.org/en/ga/69/meetings/indigenous/background.shtml.
3. Aboriginal Art, *Traditional Aboriginal Bush Medicine*, www.aboriginalartonline.com/culture/medicine.php; Randall Sexton and Ellen Anne Buljo Stabbursvik, "Healing in the Sámi North," *Culture, Medicine, and Psychiatry* 34 (2010): 571–89.
4. Irwin Press, "Urban Folk Medicine," *American Anthropologist* 80, 1 (1978): 71–84.
5. Press, "Urban Folk Medicine."
6. Aboriginal Art, *Traditional Aboriginal Bush Medicine*.
7. University of Ottawa, "Aboriginal Medicine and Healing Practices," *Society, the Individual, and Medicine* (July 8, 2009): www.med.uottawa.ca/sim/data/Aboriginal_Medicine_e.htm.
8. Hwa-Jin Lee *et al.*, "Convergence of Dance and Korean Medicine: Focusing on the Therapeutic Function," *Oriental Pharmacy and Experimental Medicine* 15 (2015): 217–26.
9. Lois N. Magner, *A History of Medicine*, 2d ed. (New York: Taylor & Francis, 2005), 17.
10. Cumes, David. "South African Indigenous Healing: How It Works." *Explore* 9, 1 (2013): 58–65.
11. Cumes, "South African Indigenous Healing."

Chapter 3

1. Barbara Böck, "When You Perform the Ritual of 'Rubbing,'" *Journal of Near Eastern Studies* 62 (2003): 1–16.
2. Celsus, *De Medicina (On Medicine)*, penelope.uchicago.edu/Thayer/E/Roman/Texts/Celsus/2*.html.
3. Mayo Clinic Staff, "Massage Therapy: Overview," www.mayoclinic.org/tests-procedures/massage-therapy/home/ovc-20170282.
4. Andrea Petersen, "Don't Call It Pampering," *Wall Street Journal* (13 March 2012): www.wsj.com/articles/SB10001424052702304537904577277303049173934.
5. Mayo Clinic, "Massage Therapy."
6. Justin D. Crane *et al.*, "Massage Therapy Attenuates Inflammatory Signaling," *Science Translational Medicine* 4, 119 (Feb. 1, 2012).
7. National Center for Complementary and Integrative Health, "Massage Therapy for Health Purposes," nccih.nih.gov/health/massage/massageintroduction.htm.
8. Celsus, *De Medicina*.
9. Tiffany Field, "Massage Therapy Research Review," *Complementary Therapies in Clinical Practice* 20 (2014): 224–29.

10. Field, "Massage Therapy."
11. Nathan Seppa, "Massage May Accelerate Healing," *Science News* 181, 5 (3/10/2012).
12. National Center, "Massage Therapy."

Chapter 4
1. Lois N. Magner, *A History of Medicine* (New York: Marcel Dekker, 1992).
2. Mislav Čavka *et al.*, "CT-Guided Endoscopic Recovery of a Foreign Object from the Cranial Cavity of an Ancient Egyptian Mummy," *Radiographics* 32 (2012): 2151–57.
3. Andrew D. Wade *et al.*, "A Synthetic Radiological Study of Brain Treatment in Ancient Egyptian Mummies," *HOMO Journal of Comparative Human Biology* 62 (2011): 248–69.
4. Wade *et al.*, "Synthetic Radiological Study."
5. Čavka *et al.*, "CT-Guided Endoscopic Recovery."
6. Robert K. Ritner, "Innovations and Adaptations in Ancient Egyptian Medicine," *Journal of Near Eastern Studies* 59, 2 (2000): 107-17.
7. P.W. Brandt-Rauf and S.I. Brandt-Rauf, "History of Occupational Medicine: Relevance of Imhotep and the Edwin Smith Papyrus," *British Journal of Industrial Medicine* 44, 1 (1987): 68–70.
8. Brandt-Rauf and Brandt-Rauf, "History of Occupational Medicine."
9. James Finlayson, "Ancient Egyptian Medicine," *The British Medical Journal* 1, 1684 (1893): 748–52.
10. Patric Blomstedt, "Cataract Surgery in Ancient Egypt," *Journal of Cataract and Refractive Surgery* 40, 3 (2014): 485–89.
11. Patric Blomstedt, "Orthopedic Surgery in Ancient Egypt," *Acta Orthopaedica* 85, 6 (2014): 670–676.
12. William John Bishop, *The Early History of Surgery* (New York: Barnes and Noble, 1960).
13. H. von Staden, "The Discovery of the Body: Human Dissection and Its Cultural Contexts in Ancient Greece," *The Yale Journal of Biology and Medicine* 65, 3 (1992): 223–41.
14. Kenneth G. Zysk, "The Evolution of Anatomical Knowledge in Ancient India, with Special Reference to Cross-Cultural Influences," *Journal of the American Oriental Society* 106, 4 (1986): 687–705.
15. Zysk, "The Evolution of Anatomical Knowledge."
16. Ethel E. Thompson, "Doctors, Doctrines, and Drugs in Ancient Times," *Bulletin of the Medical Library Association* 50, 2 (1962): 236–42.
17. Tyler M. Muffly *et al.*, "History and Evolution of Sutures," *Journal of the Royal Society of Medicine* 104, 3 (2011): 107–12.
18. Muffly *et al.*, "History and Evolution of Sutures."

Chapter 5
1. Michael T. Compton, "The Union of Religion and Health in Ancient Asklepieia," *Journal of Religion and Health* 37, 4 (1998): 301–12.
2. Askitopoulou, Helen *et al.*, "Surgical Cures under Sleep Induction in the Asklepieion of Epidauros." *International Congress Series* 1242 (2002): 11– 17.
3. Askitopoulou *et al.*, "Surgical Cures."
4. Compton, "Union of Religion and Health."
5. Compton, "Union of Religion and Health."
6. Emma and Ludwig Edelstein, *Asclepius* (Baltimore: Johns Hopkins University Press, 1998).
7. M.P.J. Dillon, "The Didactic Nature of the Epidaurian Iamata," *Zeitschrift für Papyrologie und Epigraphik* 101 (1994): 239–60.
8. Askitopoulou *et al.*, "Surgical Cures."
9. Compton, "Union of Religion and Health."
10. Askitopoulou *et al.*, "Surgical Cures."
11. National Heart, Lung, and Blood Institute, "Why Is Sleep Important?" www.nhlbi.nih.gov/health/health-topics/topics/sdd/why.
12. Brice Faraut *et al.*, "Immune, inflammatory and cardiovascular consequences of sleep restriction and recovery," *Sleep Medicine Reviews* 16 (2012): 137–49.
13. Pindar, "Pythian 3," perseus.tufts.edu/hopper/text?doc=Perseus%3Atext%3A1999.01.0162%3Abook%3DP.%3Apoem%3D3.
14. Homer, *The Iliad of Homer*, trans. Richmond Lattimore (Chicago: University of Chicago Press, 1951), 95.
15. H. K. Beecher, "The Powerful Placebo," *Journal of the American Medical Association* 159, 17 (1953): 1602–06.
16. Eugene F. Traut and Edwin W. Passarelli, "Placebos in the Treatment of Rheumatoid Arthritis and Other Rheumatic Conditions," *Annals of the Rheumatic Diseases* 16, 1 (1957): 18–22.
17. Rebecca L. Waber *et al.*, "Commercial Features of Placebo and Therapeutic Efficacy," *JAMA* 299, 9 (2008): 1016–17.
18. Barry Blackwell *et al.*, "Demonstration to Medical Students of Placebo Responses and Non-drug Factors," *The Lancet* 299 (7763): 1279–82.
19. Beecher, "The Powerful Placebo," *Journal of the American Medical Association* 159, 17 (1955): 1602–06.
20. Harald Walach, "Placebo Controls," *Philosophical Transactions: Biological Sciences* 366, 1572 (2011): 1870–78.
21. Zelda Di Blasi and Jos Kleijnen, "Context Effects, Powerful Therapies, or Methodological Bias," *Evaluation & the Health Professions* 26, 2 (2003): 166–79.
22. P. Louhiala and R. Puustinen, "Rethinking the Placebo Effect," *Medical Humanities* 34, 2 (2008): 107–09.

Chapter 6
1. Vivian Nutton, "Galen and Roman Medicine," *European Review* 20, 4 (2012): 534–42.
2. Charles G. Gross, "Galen and the Squealing Pig," *Neuroscientist* 4 (1998): 216–21.

3. Vivian Nutton, "Logic, Learning, and Experimental Medicine," *Science, New Series* 295, 5556 (2002): 800–01.
4. John Scarborough, "The Galenic Question," *Sudhoffs Archiv* 65, 1 (1981): 1–31.
5. Vivian Nutton, "The Fatal Embrace: Galen and the History of Ancient Medicine," *Science in Context* 18, 1 (2005): 111–21.
6. Scarborough, "Galenic Question."
7. Nutton, "Logic, Learning, and Experimental Medicine."
8. Daya R. Varma, "From Witchcraft to Allopathy: Uninterrupted Journey of Medical Science," *Economic and Political Weekly* 41, 33 (2006): 3605–11.
9. "Origins & History of Chinese Medicine," Sacred Lotus (2001–2015), www.sacredlotus.com/go/foundations-chinese-medicine/get/origins-history-chinese-medicine.
10. "Origins & History of Chinese Medicine"; Wikipedia, "Huangdi Neijing," en.wikipedia.org/wiki/Huangdi_Neijing.
11. Donald M. Pachuta, "Chinese Medicine: The Law of Five Elements," *India International Centre Quarterly* 18, 2/3 (1991): 41–68.

Chapter 7

1. Sharif Khaf Al-Ghazal, "The Origin of Bismaristans (Hospitals) in Islamic Medical History" (Manchester, UK: Foundation for Science, Technology, and Civilization, April 2007): www.muslimheritage.com/uploads/The_Origin_of_Bimaristans_in_Islamic_Medical_History.pdf.
2. Albert Hourani, *A History of the Arab Peoples* (Cambridge, MA: The Belknap Press, 2002), 76.
3. G. W. Houston, "An Overview of Nestorians in Inner Asia," *Central Asiatic Journal* 24, 1/2 (1980): 60–68; Steve Cochrane, "Asian Centres of Learning and Witness before 1000 C.E.: Insights for Today," *Transformation* 26, 1 (2009): 30–39. 2009."
4. Al-Ghazal, "The Origin of Bismaristans."
5. Magner, *A History of Medicine.*

6. Ruth Stellhorn Mackensen, "Background of the History of Moslem Libraries (Continued)," *The American Journal of Semitic Languages and Literatures* 52, 1 (1935): 22–33.
7. Al-Ghazal, "The Origin of Bismaristans."
8. Al-Ghazal, "The Origin of Bismaristans."
9. Selma Tibi, "Al-Razi and Islamic Medicine in the 9th Century," *JLL Bulletin: Commentaries on the History of Treatment Evaluation* (2005): www.jameslindlibrary.org/articles/al-razi-and-islamic-medicine-in-the-9th-century/.
10. Peter E. Pormann, "Qualifying and Quantifying Medical Uncertainty in 10th Century Baghdad: Abu Bakr al-Razi," *JLL Bulletin* (2013): www.jameslindlibrary.org/articles/qualifying-and-quantifying-medical-uncertainty-in-10th-century-baghdad-abu-bakr-al-razi/.
11. Sina Zarrintan *et al.*, "Early Contributions of Abu Bakr Muhammad ibn Zakariya Razi (865–925) to Evidence-Based Medicine," *International Journal of Cardiology* 168, 1 (September 20, 2013): 604–05.
12. Tibi, "Al-Razi."
13. Zarrintan *et al.*, "Early Contributions."
14. Tibi, "Al-Razi."
15. Pormann, "Qualifying and Quantifying."
16. Tibi, "Al-Razi."
17. A. C. Miller, "Jundi-Shapur, Bimaristans, and the Rise of Academic Medical Centres," *Journal of the Royal Society of Medicine* 99, 12 (2006): 615–17.
18. G. W. Houston, "An Overview of Nestorians in Inner Asia," *Central Asiatic Journal* 24, 1/2 (1980): 60–68; Steve Cochrane, "Asian Centres of Learning and Witness before 1000 C.E.: Insights for Today," *Transformation* 26, 1 (2009): 30–39.
19. Allen O. Whipple, "Role of the Nestorians as the Connecting Link between Greek and Arabic Medicine," *Bulletin of the New York Academy of Medicine* 12, 7 (1936): 446–62.
20. Houston, "Overview of Nestorians."

Chapter 8

1. B. Boon, "Leonardo da Vinci on Atherosclerosis and the Function of the Sinuses of Valsalva," *Netherlands Heart Journal* 17, 12 (2009): 496–99.
2. Joao Martins e Silva, "Leonardo da Vinci and the First Hemodynamic Observations," *Revista portuguesa de cardiologia* 27, 2 (2008): 243–72.
3. Boon, "Leonardo da Vinci,"
4. Sanjib Kumar Ghosh, "Human Cadaveric Dissection: A Historical Account from Ancient Greece to the Modern Era," *Anatomy & Cell Biology* 48, 3 (2015): 153–69.
5. Martins e Silva, "Leonardo and the First Hemodynamic Observations."
6. Martins e Silva, "Leonardo and the First Hemodynamic Observations."
7. Francis C. Wells, *The Heart of Leonardo* (Heidelberg: Springer, 2013).
8. Boon, "Leonardo da Vinci."
9. Boon, "Leonardo da Vinci."
10. M. M. Bissell *et al.*, "Flow Vortices in the Aortic Root: *In vivo* 4D-MRI Confirms Predictions of Leonardo da Vinci," *European Heart Journal* 35, 20 (2014): 1344.
11. Boon, "Leonardo da Vinci."
13. John B. West, "Ibn al-Nafis, the Pulmonary Circulation, and the Islamic Golden Age," *Journal of Applied Physiology* (1985) 105, 6 (2008): 1877–80.
14. Ijaz A. Khan, Samantapudi K. Daya, and Ramesh M. Gowda, "Evolution of the Theory of Circulation," *International Journal of Cardiology* 98, 3 (2005): 519–21.
15. Wells, *The Heart of Leonardo.*

16. Kenneth D. Keele, "Leonardo da Vinci's Influence on Renaissance Anatomy," *Medical History* 8, 4 (1964): 360–70.
17. Leonard C. Chiarelli, "Muslim Sicily and the Beginnings of Medical Licensing in Europe," *Journal of the Islamic Medical Association of North America* 31, 2 (1999).
18. Ghosh, "Human Cadaveric Dissection," *Anatomy & Cell Biology* 48, 3 (2015): 153–69.
19. E. T. Mesquita *et al.*, "Andreas Vesalius 500 Years: A Renaissance That Revolutionized Cardiovascular Knowledge," *Revista Brasileira de Cirurgia Cardiovascular* 30, 2 (2015): 260–65.

Chapter 9

1. Peter M. Dunn, "The Chamberlen Family (1560–1728) and Obstetric Forceps," *Archives of Disease in Childhood - Fetal and Neonatal Edition* 81, 3 (November 1, 1999): F232–34.
2. Alison Klairmont Lingo, "Obstetrics and Midwifery," *Encyclopedia of Children and Childhood in History and Society*. www.faqs.org/childhood/Me-Pa/Obstetrics-and-Midwifery.html.
3. Lingo, "Obstetrics and Midwifery."
4. Bryan M. Hibbard, *The Obstetrician's Armamentarium: Historical Obstetrical Instruments and Their Inventors*. San Anselmo, California: Norman Publishing, 2000.
5. Dunn, "The Chamberlen Family."
6. Dunn, "The Chamberlen Family."
7. Dunn, "The Chamberlen Family."
8. Sukhera Sheikh *et al.*, "The Birth of Forceps," *Journal of the Royal Society of Medicine Short Reports* 4 (2013): 1–4.
9. Lyle Massey, "Pregnancy and Pathology: Picturing Childbirth in Eighteenth-Century Obstetric Atlases," *The Art Bulletin* 87, 1 (2005): 73–91.
10. Polly F. Radosh, "Midwives in the United States: Past and Present," *Population Research and Policy Review* 5, 2 (1986): 129–146.
11. "Women in Medicine: Agnodice and Childbirth" (University of Virginia: 2007): http://exhibits.hsl.virginia.edu/antiqua/women/.
12. Girl Museum, "STEM Girls: Agnodice" (March 4: 2015): www.girlmuseum.org/stem-girls-agnodice/.
13. Soranus, of Ephesus. *Soranus' Gynecology*. Tr. Owsei Temkin. Baltimore, MD: Johns Hopkins Press, 1956.
14. Tonse N.K. Raju, "The Birth of Caesar and the Cesarean Misnomer," *American Journal of Perinatology* 24, 10 (2007): 567–68.

Chapter 10

1. Brian J. Ford, "The Royal Society and the Microscope," *Notes and Records of the Royal Society of London* 55, 1 (January 2001): 29–49.
2. Lodewijk C. Palm, "The Edition of Leeuwenhoek's Letters: Changing Demands, Changing Policies," *Text* 17 (2005): 265–76.
3. Douglas Anderson, "Still Going Strong: Leeuwenhoek at Eighty," *Antonie van Leeuwenhoek Journal of Microbiology* 105, 4 (2014): lensonleeuwenhoek.net/sites/default/files/avl_at_80.pdf.
4. Ford, "The Royal Society."
5. Palm, "Edition."
6. Howard Gest, "The Discovery of Microorganisms by Robert Hooke and Antoni van Leeuwenhoek," *Notes and Records of the Royal Society of London* 58, 2 (2004): 187–201.
7. Anderson, "Still Going."
8. Palm, "Edition."
9. Gest, "Discovery of Microorganisms."
10. Edward G. Ruestow, "Leeuwenhoek and the Campaign against Spontaneous Generation," *Journal of the History of Biology* 17, 2 (1984): 225–48.
11. Ruestow, "Leeuwenhoek."
12. Henry Baker, "An Account of Mr. Leeuwenhoek's Microscopes," *Philosophical Transactions* 41 (1 January 1739): 503–19.
13. Anderson, "Still Going."
14. Palm, "Edition."
15. Wikipedia, "Gresham College and the Formation of the Royal Society," en.wikipedia.org/wiki/Gresham_College_and_the_formation_of_the_Royal_Society.
16. Royal Society, "History," royalsociety.org/about-us/history/.
17. Royal Society, "History."
18. Anderson, "Still Going."
19. Frank N. Egerton, "A History of the Ecological Sciences, Part 12: Invertebrate Zoology and Parasitology During the 1500s," *Bulletin of the Ecological Society of America* 85, 1 (2004): 27–31.
20. Stephen Porter, *The Great Plague* (Stroud, Gloucestershire: Sutton Publishing, 1999).

Chapter 11

1. Frank Fenner, "Smallpox: Emergence, Global Spread, and Eradication," *History and Philosophy of the Life Sciences* 15, 3 (1993): 397–420.
2. Stephen Coss, *The Fever of 1721: The Epidemic That Revolutionized Medicine and American Politics* (New York: Simon & Schuster, 2016), 171.
3. Cary P. Gross and Kent A. Sepkowitz, "The Myth of the Medical Breakthrough: Smallpox, Vaccination, and Jenner Reconsidered," *International Journal of Infectious Diseases* 3, 1 (1998): 54–60.
4. Gross and Sepkowitz, "Myth of the Medical Breakthrough."
5. Wikipedia, "Smallpox," en.wikipedia.org/wiki/Smallpox.
6. Wikipedia, "Variolation," en.wikipedia.org/wiki/Variolation.
7. Coss, *Fever of 1721*, 83, 84, 87.

8. Coss, *Fever of 1721*, 123.
9. David S. Jones, *Rationalizing Epidemics: Meanings and Uses of American Indian Mortality since 1600* (Cambridge, MA: Harvard University Press, 2004).
10. Coss, *Fever of 1721*, plate.
11. Stefan Riedel, "Edward Jenner and the History of Smallpox and Vaccination," *Proceedings* (Baylor University. Medical Center) 18, 1 (2005): 21–25.
12. Coss, *Fever of 1721*, 268.
13. Coss, *Fever of 1721*, 269.
14. Gross and Sepkowitz, "Myth of the Medical Breakthrough."
15. Cary P. Gross and Kent A. Sepkowitz, "The Myth of the Medical Breakthrough: Smallpox, Vaccination, and Jenner Reconsidered," *International Journal of Infectious Diseases* 3, 1 (1998): 54–60.
16. Parker A. Small and S. Small Natalie, "Mankind's Magnificent Milestone: Smallpox Eradication," *The American Biology Teacher* 58, 5 (1996): 264–71.
17. World Health Organization, "Smallpox."
18. World Health Organization, "Smallpox: Eradicating an Ancient Scourge," Chapter 1 in *Bugs, Drugs, and Smoke: Stories from Public Health*, 3–11 (World Health Organization, 2011).
19. World Health Organization, "Smallpox."
20. Wikipedia, "Smallpox," en.wikipedia.org/wiki/Smallpox.
21. Wikipedia, "Smallpox Demon," en.wikipedia.org/wiki/Smallpox_demon.
22. Angela Ki Che Leung, "'Variolation' and Vaccination in Late Imperial China, Ca 1570–1911," in *History of Vaccine Development*, ed. Stanley A. Plotkin, 5–12 (New York: Springer, 2011).
23. Charles O. Mann, *1491: New Revelations of the Americas Before Columbus* (New York: Vintage, 2011).
24. Adrienne Mayor, "The Nessus Shirt in the New World: Smallpox Blankets in History and Legend," *The Journal of American Folklore* 108, 427 (1995): 54–77.
25. Mayor, "Nessus Shirt."
26. Mayor, "Nessus Shirt."
27. Gross and Sepkowitz, "Myth of the Medical Breakthrough."
28. Small and Small, "Mankind's Magnificent Milestone."

Chapter 12

1. Egon H. Kodicek and Frank G. Young, "Captain Cook and Scurvy," *Notes and Records of the Royal Society of London* 24, 1 (1969): 43–63.
2. Louis Arthur Norton, "Maritime Occupational Disease: 'The Scurvy,'" *The Northern Mariner/le marin du nord* 20, 1 (2010): 57–70.
3. C. C. Lloyd, "The Conquest of Scurvy," *The British Journal for the History of Science* 1, 4 (1963): 357–63.
4. Eleanora C. Gordon, "Scurvy and Anson's Voyage Round the World: 1740–1744—An Analysis of the Royal Navy's Worst Outbreak," *American Neptune* 44 (1984): 155–65.
5. Lloyd, "The Conquest of Scurvy."
6. Jeremy Hugh Baron, "Sailors' Scurvy before and after James Lind—A Reassessment," *Nutrition Reviews* 67, 6 (2009): 315–32.
7. Baron, "Sailors' Scurvy."
8. Arnold Zuckerman, "Scurvy and the Ventilation of Ships in the Royal Navy: Samuel Sutton's Contribution," *Eighteenth-Century Studies* 10, 2 (1976): 222–34.
9. Iain Milne, "Who Was James Lind, and What Exactly Did He Achieve?" *JLL Bulletin: Commentaries on the History of Treatment Evaluation* (2012): www.jameslindlibrary.org/articles/who-was-james-lind-and-what-exactly-did-he-achieve/.
10. Mark Harrison, "Scurvy on Sea and Land: Political Economy and Natural History, 1780–1850," *Journal for Maritime Research* 15, 1 (2013): 7–25.
11. Baron, "Sailors' Scurvy."
12. Lloyd, "The Conquest of Scurvy."
13. Leonard J. Hoenig and Walter H. C. Burgdorf, "Scurvy Aboard Ferdinand Magellan's Voyage of Circumnavigation," *JAMA Dermatology* 150, 7 (2014): 742.
14. MedlinePlus, "Vitamin C," National Library of Medicine, www.nlm.nih.gov/medlineplus/ency/article/002404.htm.
15. Centers for Disease Control and Prevention, "Executive Summary," *Second National Report on Biochemical Indicators of Diet and Nutrition in the U.S. Population* (Atlanta, GA: National Center for Environmental Health, 2012): www.cdc.gov/nutritionreport/index.html.
16. Christiaan Eijkman, "Nobel Lecture," www.nobelprize.org/nobel_prizes/medicine/laureates/1929/eijkman-lecture.html.

Chapter 13

1. William Withering, *An Account of the Foxglove and Some of Its Medical Uses* (Birmingham: Robinson, 1785), 190.
2. Dennis M. Krikler, "The Foxglove, 'The Old Woman from Shropshire,' and William Withering," *Journal of the American College of Cardiology* 5, 5 (1985): 3A–9A.
3. Withering, *Account*, 12–13.
4. Krickler, "Foxglove."
5. "William Withering," *Nature* 3724 (March 15, 1941): 325.
6. Krickler, "Foxglove."
7. Withering, *Account*, 2.
8. Withering, *Account*, xiv-xx.
9. Withering, *Account*.
10. S. H. Rahimtoola, "Digitalis and William Withering, the Clinical Investigator," *Circulation* 52 (1975): 969–71.

11. J. Worth Estes and Paul Dudley White, "William Withering and the Purple Foxglove," *Scientific American* 212 (June 1965): 111–19.
12. Withering, *Account*, 192.
13. Withering, *Account*, 192.
14. Withering, *Account*, vi.
15. Withering, *Account*, 193.
16. Emily K. Teall, "Medicine and Doctoring in Ancient Mesopotamia," *Grand Valley Journal of History* 3, 1 (2014).
17. Teall, "Medicine and Doctoring."
18. R.D. Biggs, "Medicine, Surgery, and Public Health in Ancient Mesopotamia," *Journal of Assyrian Academic Studies* 19, 1 (2005): 1.
19. Rodney H. True, "Folk Materia Medica," *Journal of American Folklore* 14, 53 (1901): 105–14.

Chapter 14
1. Wikipedia, "George Washington," en.wikipedia.org/wiki/George_Washington.
2. David Morens, "Death of a President," *New England Journal of Medicine* 341, 24 (1999): 1845–49.
3. Lois N. Magner, *A History of Medicine*, 2d ed. (New York: Taylor & Francis, 2005), 308.
4. Morens, "Death of a President."
5. Morens, "Death of a President."
6. Ludwig M. Deppisch, "Andrew Jackson and American Medical Practice: Old Hickory and His Physicians," *Tennessee Historical Quarterly* 62, 2 (2003): 130–51.
7. Robert G. W. Kirk and Neil Pemberton, "Re-imagining Bleeders: The Medical Leech in the Nineteenth Century Bloodletting Encounter," *Medical History* 55, 3 (July 2011): 355–60.
8. I.S. Whitaker *et al.*, "Hirudo Medicinalis: Ancient Origins of, and Trends in the Use of Medicinal Leeches throughout History," *British Journal of Oral & Maxillofacial Surgery* 42, 2 (2004): 133–37.
9. Kirk and Pemberton, "Re-imagining Bleeders."
10. Alfredo Morabia, "Pierre-Charles-Alexandre Louis and the Evaluation of Bloodletting," *Journal of the Royal Society of Medicine* 99 (2006): 158–60.
11. Morabia, "Pierre-Charles-Alexandre Louis."
12. Linda Kahn and Alfredo Morabia, "Using the Numerical Method in 1836," *Journal of Clinical Epidemiology* 68, 4 (2014).
13. N. Papavramidou *et al.*, "The Ancient Surgical Bloodletting Method of Arteriotomy," *Journal of Vascular Surgery* 54, 6 (2011): 1842–44; Helen Christopoulou-Aletra and Niki Papavramidou, "Cupping: An Alternative Surgical Procedure Used by Hippocratic Physicians," *Journal of Alternative and Complementary Medicine* 14, 8 (2008): 899–902.
14. Liakat Ali Parapia, "History of Bloodletting by Phlebotomy," *British Journal of Haematology* 143 (2008): 490–95.
15. Howard Tandeter *et al.*, "A Qualitative Study on Cultural Bloodletting among Ethiopian Immigrants," *Israel Medical Association Journal* 3, 12 (2001): 937–39.
16. Mim Dixon and Scott Kirchner, "'Poking,' an Eskimo Medical Practice in Northwest Alaska," *Études/Inuit/Studies* 6, 2 (1982): 109–125.
17. Altaf Hussain, "Kashmir Hospitals Using Leeches," *BBC News* (April 4, 2008): news.bbc.co.uk/2/hi/south_asia/7328369.stm.

Chapter 15
1. Tsung O. Cheng, "How Laënnec Invented the Stethoscope," *International Journal of Cardiology* 118 (2007): 281–285.
2. Lilian R. Furst, "Introduction: From Speculation to Science," 1–21. In *Medical Progress and Social Reality: A Reader in Nineteenth-Century Medicine and Literature*. Albany: State University of New York, 2000.
3. Haragopal Thadepalli, "Women Gave Birth to the Stethoscope: Laennec's Introduction of the Art of Auscultation of the Lung," *Clinical Infectious Diseases* 35, 5 (Sep. 1, 2002): 587–88.
4. John R. Scherer, "Before Cardiac MRI: Rene Laennec (1781–1826) and the Invention of the Stethoscope," *Cardiology Journal* 14, 5 (2007): 518–19.
5. John C. O'Neal, "Auenbrugger, Corvisart, and the Perception of Disease." *Eighteenth-Century Studies* 31, 4 (Summer, 1998): 473–89.
6. Cheng, "How Laënnec Invented the Stethoscope."
7. Jacalyn M. Duffin, "The Medical Philosophy of R.T.H. Laennec (1781–1826)," *History and Philosophy of the Life Sciences* 8, 2 (1986): 195–219.
8. Duffin, "Medical Philosophy."
9. Rachel Hajar, "The Air of History: Early Medicine to Galen (Part I)," *Heart Views* 13, 3 (Jul 2012): 120–28.
10. Nima Ghasemzadeh and A. Maziar Zafari, "A Brief Journey into the History of the Arterial Pulse," *Cardiology Research and Practice* 2011, Article ID 164832 (2011).
11. Hajar, "Air of History (I)."
12. James Finlayson, "Galen [a Biblographical Demonstration in the Library of the Faculty of Physicians and Surgeons of Glasgow,December 9th, 1891] (Concluded)," *The British Medical Journal* 1, 1632 (1892): 771–74.
13. Ghasemzadeh and Zafari, "Brief Journey."
14. Rachel Hajar, "The Air of History (Part V): Ibn Sina (Avicenna)," *Heart Views* 14, 4 (2013): 196–201.
15. Ghasemzadeh N, "A Brief Journey into the History of the Arterial Pulse."

Chapter 16
1. [Thomas Wakley], "The Operation of Lithotomy, by Mr. Bransby Cooper, Which Lasted Nearly One Hour!!" *The Lancet* 1827 – 28, v. 1 (March 29, 1828): 959–60.

2. [Wakley],"The Operation."
3. H. W. Herr, "'I Will Not Cut . . .' : The Oath That Defined Urology," *BJU International* 102, 7 (Sep 2008): 769–71.
4. Lloyd Duhaime, "1828: The First Recorded Medical Malpractice Litigation," duhaime.org/LawMuseum/LawArticle-1324/1828-The-First-Recorded-Medical-Malpractice-Litigation.aspx.
5. J. Shah and H.N. Whitfield, "Urolithiasis through the Ages," *BJU International* 89, 8 (2002): 801–10.
6. Mayo Clinic, "Kidney Stones," mayoclinic.org/diseases-conditions/kidney-stones/basics/definition/con-20024829.
7. Shah and Whitfield, "Urolithiasis."
8. R.C. Chakravorty, "Urinary Stones," *Hist Sci Med* 17, Spec 2 (1982): 328–32.
9. Herr, "I Will Not Cut."
10. Herr, "I Will Not Cut."
11. [Wakley],"The Operation."
12. [Wakley],"The Operation."
13. Roger Jones, "Thomas Wakley, Plagiarism, Libel, and the Founding of *The Lancet*," *The Lancet* 371 (2008): 1410–11.
14. Margaret S. Pearle, "Shock-Wave Lithotripsy for Renal Calculi." *New England Journal of Medicine* 367 (2012): 50–57.
15. Mahmoud M. Osman *et al.*, "5-year-follow-up of Patients with Clinically Insignificant Residual Fragments after Extracorporeal Shockwave Lithotripsy," *European Urology* 47 (2005): 860–864.
16. Wen Zhong *et al.*, "Percutaneous Nephrolithotomy for Renal Stones Following Failed Extracorporeal Shockwave Lithotripsy: Different Performances and Morbidities," *Urolithiasis* 41 (2013): 165–168.

Chapter 17

1. Cristin O'Keefe Aptowicz, *Dr. Mütter's Marvels: A True Tale of Intrigue and Innovation at the Dawn of Modern Medicine* (New York: Avery, 2015), 16.
2. Chauncey D. Leake, "The Historical Development of Surgical Anesthesia," *The Scientific Monthly* 20, 3 (1925): 304–28.
3. E. Ashworth Underwood, "Before and after Morton: A Historical Survey of Anaesthesia," *The British Medical Journal* 2, 4475 (1946): 525–31.
4. Leake, "Historical Development."
5. Aptowicz, *Dr. Mütter's Marvels*, 168.
6. Underwood, "Before and after."
7. Shirley Stallings and Michael Montagne, "A Chronicle of Anesthesia Discovery in New England," *Pharmacy in History* 35, 2 (1993): 77–80.
8. Aptowicz, *Dr. Mütter's Marvels*, 168.
9. A. López-Valverde *et al.*, "The Discovery of Surgical Anesthesia: Discrepancies Regarding Its Authorship," *Journal of Dental Research* 90, 1 (2011): 31–34.
10. Mary Poovey, "'Scenes of an Indelicate Character': The Medical 'Treatment' of Victorian Women," *Representations* 14 (Spring, 1986): 137–168.
11. Aptowicz, *Dr. Mütter's Marvels*, 267.
12. Christopher Hobbs, Medicinal Mushrooms, Overview.
13. Ahmed M. Abdel-Azeem, "The History, Fungal Biodiversity, Conservation, and Future Perspectives for Mycology in Egypt," *IMA Fungus* 1, 2 (Dec. 2010): 123–42.
14. Gaston Guzman, "Hallucinogenic Mushrooms in Mexico: An Overview," *Economic Botany* 62, 3 (2008): 404–12.

Chapter 18

1. Johannes Persson, "Semmelweis's Methodology from the Modern Stand-point: Intervention Studies and Causal Ontology," *Studies in History and Philosophy of Biological and Biomedical Sciences* 40 (2009): 204–09.
2. Donald Gillies, "Hempelian and Kuhnian Approaches in the Philosophy of Medicine: The Semmelweis Case," *Studies in History and Philosophy of Biological and Biomedical Sciences* 36 (2005): 159–81.
3. Patti J. Miller, "Semmelweis," *Infection Control* 3, 5 (1982): 405–09.
4. Cristin O'Keefe Aptowicz, *Dr. Mütter's Marvels: A True Tale of Intrigue and Innovation at the Dawn of Modern Medicine* (New York: Avery, 2015), 255–61.
5. Gillies, "Hempelian and Kuhnian Approaches."
6. Gillies, "Hempelian and Kuhnian Approaches."
7. Gillies, "Hempelian and Kuhnian Approaches."
8. Gillies, "Hempelian and Kuhnian Approaches."
9. Miller, "Semmelweis."
10. Gillies, "Hempelian and Kuhnian Approaches."
11. M. Eileen Magnello, "Victorian Statistical Graphics and the Iconography of Florence Nightingale's Polar Area Graph," *BSHM Bulletin* 27 (2012): 13–37.
12. Christopher J. Gill and Gillian C. Gill, "Nightingale in Scutari: Her Legacy Reexamined," *Clinical Infectious Diseases* 40, 12 (June 15, 2005): 1799–805.
13. Gill and Gill, "Nightingale."

Chapter 19

1. Steven Johnson, *The Ghost Map* (New York: Riverhead Books, 2006), 114.
2. Elizabeth Fee and Theodore M. Brown, "The Public Health Act of 1848," *Bulletin of the World Health Organization* 83, 11 (2005): 866–67.
3. Wikipedia, "Edwin Chadwick," en.wikipedia.org/wiki/Edwin_Chadwick.

4. Johnson, *Ghost Map*, 114.
5. Johnson, *Ghost Map*, 114.
6. C. E. Dolman, "The Sanitarian's Place in Public Health." *Canadian Journal of Public Health / Revue Canadienne de Santé Publique* 39, no. 2 (1948): 41–51.
7. Johnson, *Ghost Map*.
8. M. Jansen, "Water supply and sewage disposal at Mohenjo-Daro," *World Archaeology* 21, 2 (1991): 177–92; Carr, "Harappan Civilization."
9. T.S. Subramanian, "The Rise and Fall of a Harappan City," *Frontline: India's National Magazine* 27, 12 (June 5–18, 2010): www.frontline.in/static/html/fl2712/stories/20100618271206200.htm.
10. Jansen, "Water supply and sewage disposal at Mohenjo-Daro."
11. Harold Farnsworth Gray, "Sewerage in Ancient and Mediaeval Times," *Sewage Works Journal* 12, 5 (1940): 939–46.
12. Jansen, "Water Supply."
13. Gray, "Water Supply and Sewage."

Chapter 20

1. P. Bingham *et al.*, "John Snow, William Farr and the 1849 Outbreak of Cholera That Affected London," *Public Health* 118 (2004): 387–94.
2. Stephen W. Lacey, "Cholera: Calamitous Past, Ominous Future," *Clinical Infectious Diseases* 20, 5 (May, 1995): 1409–19.
3. Steven Johnson, *The Ghost Map* (New York: Riverhead Books, 2006).
4. Ashleigh R. Tuite *et al.*, "Cholera, Canals, and Contagion," *Journal of Public Health Policy* 32, 3 (August 2011): 320–33.
5. Bingham *et al.*, "John Snow, William Farr."
6. Bingham *et al.*, "John Snow, William Farr."
7. Laura Ball, "Cholera and the Pump on Broad Street," *The History Teacher* 43, 1 (2009): 105–19.
8. Johnson, *Ghost Map*.
9. Ball, "Cholera."
10. Johnson, *Ghost Map*.
11. Lacey, "Cholera."
12. Johnson, *Ghost Map*.
13. Ball, "Cholera."
14. Lacey, "Cholera."
15. Johnson, *Ghost Map*.
16. Centers for Disease Control, "Cholera: General Information," cdc.gov/cholera/general/index.html.
17. Sharon Levy, "Cholera's Life Aquatic," *BioScience* 55, no. 9 (2005): 728–32.
18. Rita R. Colwell *et al.*, "Reduction of Cholera in Bangladeshi Villages by Simple Filtration," *Proceedings of the National Academy of Sciences* 100, 3 (2003): 1051–55.
19. Colwell, "Reduction of Cholera."
20. Lacey, "Cholera."

Chapter 21

1. Gavin de Beer, "Mendel, Darwin, and Fisher (1865–1965)," *Notes and Records of the Royal Society of London* 19, 2 (1964): 192–226.
2. P. M. Dunn, "Gregor Mendel, OSA (1822–1884), Founder of Scientific Genetics," *Archives of Disease in Childhood: Fetal and Neonatal Edition* 88, 6 (November 2003): F537–39.
3. de Beer, "Mendel, Darwin, and Fisher."
4. Shannon Hackett *et al.*, "Genes and Genius: The Inheritance of Gregor Mendel," *DNA and Cell Biology* 25, 12 (2006): 655–58.
5. Nelio Bizzo and Charbel N. El-Hani, "Darwin and Mendel: Evolution and Genetics," *Journal of Biological Education* 43, 3 (2009): 108–14.
6. Hackett *et al.*, "Genes and Genius."
7. Mauricio De Castro, "Johann Gregor Mendel: Paragon of Experimental Science," *Molecular Genetics & Genomic Medicine* 4, 1 (2016): 3–8.
8. Hackett *et al.*, "Genes and Genius."
9. Susan Offner, "Mendel's Peas & the Nature of the Gene: Genes Code for Proteins & Proteins Determine Phenotype," *The American Biology Teacher* 73, 7 (2011): 382–87.
10. de Beer, "Mendel, Darwin, and Fisher."
11. de Beer, "Mendel, Darwin, and Fisher."
12. Offner, "Mendel's Peas."
13. World Health Organization, "Sickle-cell Disease and Other Haemoglobin Disorders," Fact Sheet 308 (2011): www.who.int/mediacentre/factsheets/fs308/en/.
14. World Health Organization. "New Report Signals Country Progress in the Path to Malaria Elimination." News Release (December 9, 2015): www.who.int/mediacentre/news/releases/2015/report-malaria-elimination/en/.
15. Lucio Luzzatto, "Sickle Cell Anaemia and Malaria," *Mediterranean Journal of Hematology and Infectious Diseases* 4, 1 (2012).
16. Luzzato, "Sickle Cell."

Chapter 22

1. William T. Clower and Stanley Finger, "Discovering Trepanation: The Contribution of Paul Broca," *Neurosurgery* 49, 6 (December 2001): 1417–25.

2. Stanley Finger and Hiran R. Fernando, "E. George Squier and the Discovery of Cranial Trepanation," *Journal of the History of Medicine* 56 (Oct. 2001): 353–81.
3. Clower and Finger, "Discovering Trepanation."
4. Clower and Finger.
5. Xianli Lv *et al.*, "Prehistoric Skull Trepanation in China," *World Neurosurgery* 80, 6 (2013): 897–99.
6. Lv *et al.*, "Prehistoric Skull Trepanation in China."
7. Manolis J. Papagrigorakas *et al.*, "Neurosurgery During the Bronze Age: A Skull Trepanation in 1900 BC Greece," *World Neurosurgery* 81, 2 (2014): 431–35.
8. G. Tsermoulas *et al.*, "The Skull of Chios," *Journal of Neurosurgery* 121, 2 (2014): 328–32.
9. K. S. Lee, "History of Chronic Subdural Hematoma," *Korean Journal of Neurotrauma* 11, 2 (2015): 27–34.
10. Brian May *et al.*, "The Life and Medical Practice of Hua Tuo," *Pacific Journal of Oriental Medicine* 14 (2000): 40–54.

Chapter 23
1. Wikipedia, "Spontaneous Generation," en.wikipedia.org/wiki/Spontaneous_generation.
2. Harry B. Weiss, "Francesco Redi, the Father of Experimental Entomology," *Scientific Monthly* 23, 3 (1926): 220–24.
3. Edward G. Ruestow, "Leeuwenhoek and the Campaign against Spontaneous Generation," *Journal of the History of Biology* 17, 2 (Summer, 1984): 225–48.
4. Anton E. Lawson, "Human Traits Vs. Crucial Experiments," *The American Biology Teacher* 36, 6 (1974): 334–48.
5. Lawson, "Human Traits."
6. Lilian R. Furst, *Medical Progress and Social Reality: A Reader in Nineteenth-century Medicine and Literature* (Albany: State University of New York Press, 2000): 10.
7. Kendall Smith, "Louis Pasteur, the Father of Immunology?" *Frontiers in Immunology* 3, Article 68 (2012): www.ncbi.nlm.nih.gov/pmc/articles/PMC3342039/.
8. Smith, "Louis Pasteur."
9. Smith, "Louis Pasteur."
10. Prof. [Louis] Pasteur, "On the Germ Theory," *Science* 2, 62 (1881): 420–22.
11. W. W. Keen, "Before and after Lister," *Science* 41, 1067 (1915): 845–53.
12. Hector C. Cameron, "Lord Lister and the Evolution of Modern Surgery," *British Medical Journal* 2, 2189 (1902): 1844–48.
13. Jason R. Francoeur, "Joseph Lister: Surgeon Scientist (1827–1912)," *Journal of Investigative Surgery* 13 (2000): 129–32.
14. Zachary Cope, "Joseph Lister, 1827 – 1912," *British Medical Journal* 2, 5543 (1967): 7–8.
15. Francoeur, "Joseph Lister."
16. S. Robert Lathan, "Caroline Hampton Halsted: The First to Use Rubber Gloves in the Operating Room," *Proceedings* (Baylor University Medical Center) 23, 4 (2010): 389–92.
17. Leslie Hurt, "Dr. Robert Koch: A Founding Father of Biology," *Primary Care Update for OB/Gyns* 10, 2 (2003): 73–74.
18. Steve M. Blevins and Michael S. Bronze, "Robert Koch and the 'Golden Age' of Bacteriology," *International Journal of Infectious Diseases* 14 (2010): e744–e751.

Chapter 24
1. John Frith, "History of Tuberculosis, Part 2: The Sanatoria and the Discoveries of the Tubercle Bacillus," *Journal of Military and Veterans' Health* 22, 2 (2016).
2. Jeanne E. Abrams, "Spitting Is Dangerous, Indecent, and against the Law!" *Journal of the History of Medicine and Allied Sciences* 68, 3 (2013): 416–50.
3. Thomas M. Daniel, "The History of Tuberculosis," *Respiratory Medicine* 100 (2006): 1862–70.
4. Daniel, "The History of Tuberculosis."
5. Steven Johnson, *The Ghost Map* (New York: Riverhead Books, 2006).
6. JoAnne L. Flynn and John Chan, "Tuberculosis: Latency and Reactivation," *Infection and Immunity* 69,7 (2001): 4195–4201.
7. Arthur Stanley Pease, "Some Remarks on the Diagnosis and Treatment of Tuberculosis in Antiquity," *Isis* 31, 2 (1940): 380–93.
8. S. Sabbatani, "[Historical Insights into Tuberculosis]," *Le Infezioni in Medicina* 12, 4 (2004): 284–91.
9. Daniel, "The History of Tuberculosis."
10. Peter Warren, "The Evolution of the Sanatorium," *Canadian Bulletin of Medical History* 23, 2 (2006): 457–70.
11. Daniel, "The History of Tuberculosis."
12. David S. Barnes, "Historical Perspectives on the Etiology of Tuberculosis," *Microbes and Infection* 2 (2000): 431–40.
13. Warren, "Evolution of the Sanatorium."
14. Warren, "Evolution of the Sanatorium."
15. Marc Garetier and Jean Rousset, "Thoracic Balls," *CMAJ/JAMC* 183, 14 (2011): e1091. www.ncbi.nlm.nih.gov/pmc/articles/PMC3185102/.
16. Abrams, "Spitting Is Dangerous."
17. Abrams, "Spitting Is Dangerous."
18. Daniel, "The History of Tuberculosis."
19. World Health Organization, "Tuberculosis: Fact Sheet 104," www.who.int/mediacentre/factsheets/fs104/en/.
20. Barnes, "Historical Perspectives on Etiology."
21. World Health Organization, "Tuberculosis."
22. Stefan Grzybowski and Edward A. Allen, "History and Importance of Scrofula," *The Lancet* 346, 8988 (1995): 1472–74.

23. Wikipedia. "Royal Touch." en.wikipedia.org/wiki/Royal_touch.
24. Michael Bell, "Vampires and Death in New England, 1784 to 1892," *Anthropology and Humanism* 31, 2 (2006): 124–40.

Chapter 25

1. Rosany Bochner, "Paths to the Discovery of Antivenom Serotherapy in France," *Journal of Venomous Animals and Toxins including Tropical Diseases* 22, 1 (2016): 1–7.
2. Wikipedia, "Albert Calmette," en.wikipedia.org/wiki/Albert_Calmette.
3. Annick Guénel, "The Creation of the First Overseas Pasteur Institute, or the Beginning of Albert Calmette's Pastorian Career," *Medical History* 43 (1999): 1–25.
4. Bochner, "Paths."
5. Bochner, "Paths."
6. Guénel, "Creation."
7. Guénel, "Creation."
8. Bochner, "Paths."
9. Raymond L. Ditmars, "Deadly Snakes Now Conquered by Science," *The Science News-Letter* 11, 321 (4 June 1927): 349–50 + 355–56.
10. Centers for Disease Control, "Your Immune System," www.cdc.gov/bam/diseases/immune/immunesys.html.
11. Stefan H.E. Kaufmann, "Elie Metchnikoff's and Paul Ehrlich's Impact on Infection Biology," *Microbes and Infection* 10 (2008): 1417–19.
12. Bochner, "Paths."
13. Guénel, "Creation."
14. Franz Luttenberger, "Arrhenius vs. Ehrlich on Immunochemistry: Decisions about Scientific Progress in the Context of the Nobel Prize," *Theoretical Medicine* 13, 2 (1992): 137–73.
15. Kaufmann, "Elie Metchnikoff's and Paul Ehrlich's Impact."
16. "The Nobel Prize in Physiology or Medicine 1908," *NobelPrize.org*. www.nobelprize.org/nobel_prizes/medicine/laureates/1908/.
17. Paul Ehrlich, "Partial Cell Functions," Nobel Lecture (December 11, 1908): nobelprize.org/nobel_prizes/medicine/laureates/1908/ehrlich-lecture.html
18. "The Immune System: In Defense of Our Lives," Nobel Prize.org (September 6, 2010). www.nobelprize.org/educational/medicine/immuneresponses/overview/.
19. Wikipedia, "Mithridates VI of Pontus," en.wikipedia.org/wiki/Mithridates_VI_of_Pontus.

Chapter 26

1. Peter B. Riesz, "The Life of Wilhelm Conrad Roentgen," *American Journal of Roentgenology* 165 (1995): 1533–37.
2. Otto Glasser, "W. C. Roentgen and the Discovery of the Roentgen Rays," *American Journal of Roentgenology* 165 (1995): 1033–40.
3. Wikipedia, "Crookes Tube," en.wikipedia.org/wiki/Crookes_tube.
4. Riesz, "Life of Wilhelm Conrad Roentgen."
5. Riesz, "Life of Wilhelm Conrad Roentgen."
6. Glasser, "W. C. Roentgen."
7. Richard I. Frankel, "Centennial of Röntgen's Discovery of X-Rays," *Western Journal of Medicine* 164, 6 (1996): 497–501.
8. Frankel, "Centennial."

Chapter 27

1. Edward A. Crawford, Jr., "Paul-Louis Simond and His Work on Plague," *Perspectives in Biology and Medicine* 39, 3 (1996): 446–58.
2. Ludwik Gross, "How the Plague Bacillus and Its Transmission through Fleas Were Discovered: Reminiscences from My Years at the Pasteur Institute in Paris," *Proceedings of the National Academy of Sciences of the United States of America* 92, 17 (August 1995): 7609–11.
3. Crawford, "Paul-Louis Simond."
4. Gross, "How."
5. David J. Bibel and T.H. Chen, "Diagnosis of Plague: An Analysis of the Yersin-Kitasato Controversy," *Bacteriological Reviews* 40, 3 (September 1976): 633–51.
6. Wikipedia, "Waldemar Haffkine," en.wikipedia.org/wiki/Waldemar_Haffkine.
7. Gross, "How."
8. Crawford, "Paul-Louis Simond."
9. Centers for Disease Control, "Plague," www.cdc.gov/plague/index.html.
10. Crawford, "Paul-Louis Simond."
11. Lester K. Little, ed., *Plague and the End of Antiquity: The Pandemic of 541–750* (New York: Cambridge University Press: 2007).
12. National Institute of Allergies and Infectious Diseases, "Plague" (2015): www.niaid.nih.gov/topics/plague/Pages/Default.aspx.
13. Little, *Plague and the End of Antiquity*.
14. Samuel K. Cohn, Jr., "The Black Death: End of a Paradigm," *American Historical Review* 107, 3 (2002): 703–38.
15. Michael McCormick, "Rats, Communications, and Plague: Toward an Ecological History," *Journal of Interdisciplinary History* 34, 1 (2003): 1–25.
16. Graham Twigg, *The Black Death: A Biological Reappraisal* (London: Batsford, 1984).
17. D.M. Wagner *et al.*, "*Yersinia pestis* and the Plague of Justinian 541–543 AD," *The Lancet. Infectious diseases* 14, 4 (2014): 319–26.

18. Stephanie Haensch *et al.*, "Distinct Clones of *Yersinia pestis* Caused the Black Death," *PLoS Pathogens* 6, 10 (2010).
19. T. N. Tran *et al.*, "Brief Communication: Co-detection of *Bartonella quintana* and *Yersinia pestis*," *American Journal of Physical Anthropology* 145, 3 (2011): 489–94.

Chapter 28
1. Thomas M. Rivers, "Viruses and Koch's Postulates," *Journal of Bacteriology* 33, 1 (1937): 1–12.
2. L. Bos, "Beijerinck's Work on Tobacco Mosaic Virus: Historical Context and Legacy," *Philosophical Transactions: Biological Sciences* 354, 1383 (Mar. 29, 1999): 675–85.
3. Bos, "Beijerinck's Work."
4. W. Ian Lipkin, "Microbe Hunting in the 21st Century," *Proceedings of the National Academy of Sciences* 106, 1 (2009): 6–7.
5. Mark Woolhouse et al., "Human Viruses: Discovery and Emergence," *Philosophical Transactions of the Royal Society B: Biological Sciences* 367, 1604 (2012): 2864–71.
6. Rivers, "Viruses."
7. David N. Fredericks and David A. Relman, "Sequence-Based Identification of Microbial Pathogens," *Clinical Microbiology Reviews* 9, 1 (1996): 18–33.
8. World Health Organization, "Yellow Fever," www.who.int/mediacentre/factsheets/fs100/en/.
9. J. H. Bauer, "Yellow Fever," *Public Health Reports (1896–1970)* 55, 9 (1940): 362–71.
10. Porterfield, "Yellow Fever."
11. "Nobel Prize 1951," *The British Medical Journal* 2, 4738 (1951).
12. J. Gordon Frierson, "The Yellow Fever Vaccine: A History," *The Yale Journal of Biology and Medicine* 83, 2 (2010): 77–85.
13. Woolhouse, "Human Viruses."
14. W. M. Stanley, "Progress in the Conquest of Virus Diseases," *Science* 101, 2617 (1945): 185–88.

Chapter 29
1. Sara Rockwell, "The Life and Legacy of Marie Curie," *Yale Journal of Biology and Medicine* 76 (2003): 167–80.
2. Nancy Fröman, "Marie and Pierre Curie and the Discovery of Polonium and Radium," Nobelprize.org (December 1996): www.nobelprize.org/nobel_prizes/themes/physics/curie/.
3. Denise Ham, "Marie Sklodowska Curie: The Woman Who Opened the Nuclear Age," *21st Century* (Winter 2002 – 2003): 30 – 68.
4. Sara Rockwell, "The Life and Legacy of Marie Curie," *Yale Journal of Biology and Medicine* 76 (2003): 167–80.
5. Marie Curie, "The Discovery of Radium," lateralscience.blogspot.com/2012/07/the-discovery-of-radium-by-marie-curie.html.
6. Fröman, "Marie and Pierre Curie."
7. Curie, "The Discovery of Radium."
8. Curie, "The Discovery of Radium."
9. Jean-Jacques Mazeron and Alain Gerbaulet, "The Centenary of Discovery of Radium," *Radiotherapy and Oncology* 49 (1998): 205–16.
10. B. W. Fox, "The History of Radium in Medicine in Manchester," *Clinical Oncology* 10 (1998): 115–24.
11. Jean Dutreix *et al.*, "The Hazy Dawn of Brachytherapy," *Radiotherapy and Oncology* 49 (1998): 223–32.
12. Mazeron and Gerbaulet, "Centenary."
13. Wikipedia, "Marie Curie," en.wikipedia.org/wiki/Marie_Curie.
14. Dutreix, "Hazy Dawn."
15. David I. Harvie, "The Radium Century," *Endeavour* 23, 3 (1999): 100–05.
16. U.S. Department of Commerce, *Measures for Progress: A History of the National Bureau of Standards.*
17. Fox, "History of Radium."
18. Harvie, "Radiation Century."

Chapter 30
1. Kim Pelis, "Blood Clots: The Nineteenth-Century Debate over the Substance and Means of Transfusion in Britain," *Annals of Science* 54 (1997): 331–60.
2. "History of Blood Transfusion," *The British Medical Journal* 1, 4280 (Jan. 16, 1943): 74.
3. Cyrus C. Sturgis, "The History of Blood Transfusion," *Bulletin of the Medical Library Association* 30, 2 (1942): 105–12.
4. Thomas F. Baskett, "The Resuscitation Greats: James Blundell," *Resuscitation* 52 (2002): 229–33.
5. Pelis, "Blood Clots."
6. Baskett, "James Blundell."
7. Pelis, "Blood Clots."
8. Karl Landsteiner, "Individual Differences in Human Blood," *Science , New Series* 73, 1894 (Apr. 17, 1931): 403–09.
9. Landsteiner, "Individual Differences."
10. Wikipedia, "ABO Blood Group System," en.wikipedia.org/wiki/ABO_blood_group_system.
11. Landsteiner, "Individual Differences."
12. Pelis, "Blood Clots."
13. Sturgis, "History of Blood Transfusion."
14. Peter H. Pinkerton, "Norman Bethune, Eccentric, Man of Principle, Man of Action, Surgeon," *Transfusion Medicine Reviews* 21, 3 (2007): 255–64.
15. William DeKleine, "The Blood Plasma Reservoir," *American Journal of Nursing* 41, 5 (1941): 572–73.
16. DeKleine, "Blood Plasma Reservoir."
17. Wikipedia, "Charles R. Drew," en.wikipedia.org/wiki/Charles_R._Drew.

Chapter 31

1. Associated Press, "Tanya Angus," CBS News (January 17, 2013): www.cbsnews.com/news/tanya-angus-woman-who-couldnt-stop-growing-dies-at-34/.
2. MedlinePlus, "Endocrine Diseases," medlineplus.gov/endocrinediseases.html; Wikipedia, "Endocrine System," en.wikipedia.org/wiki/Endocrine_system.
3. Jamshed R. Tata, "100 Years of Hormones," *EMBO Reports* 6, 6 (2005): 490–96.
4. J. H. Henriksen and O. B. Schaffalitzky de Muckadell, "Secretin, Its Discovery, and the Introduction of the Hormone Concept," *Scandinavian Journal of Clinical and Laboratory Investigation* 60 (2000): 463–72.
5. Henriksen and Schaffalitzky de Muckadell, "Secretin."
6. Henriksen and Schaffalitzky de Muckadell, "Secretin."
7. F. López-Muñoz et al., "An Historical View of the Pineal Gland and Mental Disorders," *Journal of Clinical Neuroscience* 18 (2011): 1028–37.
8. Charles L. Ralph, "Evolution of Pineal Control of Endocrine Function in Lower Vertebrates," *American Zoologist* 23, 3 (1983): 597-605.
9. M. Mila Macchi and Jeffrey N. Bruce, "Human Pineal Physiology and Functional Significance of Melatonin," *Frontiers in Neuroendocrinology* 25, 3 (2004): 175–95.
10. W. Michael G. Tunbridge, "La Mujer Barbuda by Ribera, 1631: A Gender Bender." *Quarterly Journal of Medicine* 104, 8 (2011): 733–36.
11. Myron Genel, "The Olympic Games and Athletic Sex Assignment," *JAMA* 316, 13 (October 4, 2016): 1359–60.
12. Simon N. Young, "How to Increase Serotonin in the Human Brain without Drugs," *Journal of Psychiatry & Neuroscience* 32, 6 (2007): 394–99.

Chapter 32

1. George A. Soper, "The Curious Career of Typhoid Mary," *Bulletin of the New York Academy of Medicine* 15, 10 (1939): 698–712.
2. Soper, "Curious Career"; Philip P. Mortimer, "Mr N the Milker, and Dr Koch's Concept of the Healthy Carrier," *The Lancet* 353, 9161 (1999): 1354–56.
3. Soper, "Curious Career."
4. World Health Organization, "Typhoid Fever," www.who.int/topics/typhoid_fever/en/.
5. Robert Moorhead, "William Budd and Typhoid Fever," *Journal of the Royal Society of Medicine* 95, 11 (2002): 561–564.
6. Christopher Brightman, "Typhoid Fever: Yesterday, Today and Unfortunately Still Tomorrow," *Trends in Urology & Men's Health* 6, 6 (2015).
7. Heather Munro Prescott, "Sending Their Sons into Danger: Cornell University and the Ithaca Typhoid Epidemic of 1903," *New York History* 78, 3 (1997): 273–308.
8. Mortimer, "Mr N the Milker."

Chapter 33

1. Florian Winau et al., "Paul Ehrlich—In Search of the Magic Bullet," *Microbes and Infection* 6 (2004): 786–89.
2. Igor Buchwalow et al., "The Contribution of Paul Ehrlich to Histochemistry," *Virchows Archiv* 466 (2015): 111–16.
3. Anthony S. Travis, "Science as Receptor of Technology," *Science in Context* 3 (1989): 383–408.
4. Travis, "Science as Receptor."
5. Travis, "Science as Receptor."
6. Florian Winau et al., "Paul Ehrlich."
7. Fèlix Bosch and Laia Rosich, "The Contributions of Paul Ehrlich to Pharmacology," *Pharmacology* 82 (2008): 171–79.
8. K. J. Williams, "The Introduction of 'Chemotherapy' Using Arsphenamine—the First Magic Bullet," *Journal of the Royal Society of Medicine* 102, 8 (2009): 343–48.
9. Bosch and Rosich, "Contributions of Paul Ehrlich."
10. Bosch and Rosich, "Contributions of Paul Ehrlich."
11. Williams, "Introduction of 'Chemotherapy.'"
12. Williams, "Introduction of 'Chemotherapy.'"
13. Lawrence M. Principe, *The Secrets of Alchemy* (Chicago: University of Chicago Press, 2013).
14. Wikipedia, "William Henry Perkin," en.wikipedia.org/wiki/William_Henry_Perkin.
15. Bruce M. Rothschild, "History of Syphilis," *Clinical Infectious Diseases* 40, 10 (2005): 1454–63.
16. Rothschild, "History of Syphilis."
17. Heinz Hofmann, "Columbus and Epic Recusatio: Fracastoro's Syphilis," in *The Classical Tradition and the Americas*, ed. Wolfgang Haase and Meyer Reinhold (Berlin, New York: Walter De Gruyter, 1994).
18. Charles Webster, "Paracelsus, and 500 Years of Encouraging Scientific Inquiry," *British Medical Journal* 306, 6878 (1993): 597–98.
19. John Parascandola, "From Mercury to Miracle Drugs: Syphilis Therapy over the Centuries," *Pharm Hist* 51, 1 (2009): 14–23.
20. Parascandola, "From Mercury to Miracle Drugs."

Chapter 34

1. Science Museum: Brought to Life, "Leonard Thompson (1908–35)." www.sciencemuseum.org.uk/broughttolife/people/frederickbanting.
2. Wikipedia, "History of Diabetes," en.wikipedia.org/wiki/History_of_diabetes.
3. Lois N. Magner, *A History of Medicine*, 2d ed. (New York: Taylor & Francis, 2005): 18, 60.

4. Nobelprize.org, "The Discovery of Insulin." www.nobelprize.org/educational/medicine/insulin/discovery-insulin.html.
5. Columbia Doctors, "The Pancreas and Its Functions," columbiasurgery.org/pancreas/pancreas-and-its-functions.
6. Michael Bliss, "Dr. Frederick Banting: Getting out of Town," *Canadian Medical Association Journal* (May 1, 1984): 1215–21.
7. Dimitrios T. Karamitsos, "The Story of Insulin Discovery," *Diabetes Research and Clinical Practice* 93S (2011): S2–S8.
8. A. Helmstädter, "Antidiabetic Drugs Used in Europe Prior to the Discovery of Insulin," *Pharmazie* 62, 9 (2007): 717–20.
9. Warren A. Sawyer, "Frederick Banting's Misinterpretations of the Work of Ernest L. Scott as Found in Secondary Sources," *Perspectives in Biology and Medicine* 29, 4 (1986): 611–18.
10. J. Sjöquist, "Physiology or Medicine 1923 – Presentation Speech," Nobelprize.org. www.nobelprize.org/nobel_prizes/medicine/laureates/1923/press.html.
11. M. Bliss, "The Eclipse and Rehabilitation of JRR Macleod, Scotland's Insulin Laureate," *Journal of the Royal College of Physicians of Edinburgh* 43 (2013): 366–73.
12. J. B. Collip, "Frederick Grant Banting, Discoverer of Insulin," *The Scientific Monthly* 52, 5 (1941): 472–74.
13. Bliss, "Dr. Frederick Banting."
14. Collip, "Frederick Grant Banting."
15. Bliss, "Eclipse and Rehabilitation."

Chapter 35
1. Ernst Chain, "Thirty Years of Penicillin Therapy," *Proceedings of the Royal Society of London. Series B, Biological Sciences* 179, 1057 (1971): 293–319.
2. Alexander Fleming, "Penicillin," *British Medical Journal* 2, 4210 (1941): 386.
3. Jos Houbraken *et al.*, "Fleming's Penicillin Producing Strain Is Not *Penicillium Chrysogenum* but *P. Rubens*," *IMA Fungus: The Global Mycological Journal* 2, 1 (2011): 87–95.
4. Edward Abraham, "Penicillin and Its Successors: A Personal View," *Bulletin of the American Academy of Arts and Sciences* 39, 1 (1985): 8–27.
5. Abraham, "Penicillin."
6. H. W. Florey, "Penicillin: A Survey," *British Medical Journal* 2, 4361 (1944): 169–71.
7. B. Lee Ligon, "Penicillin: Its Discovery and Early Development," *Seminars in Pediatric Infectious Diseases* 15, 1 (2004): 52–57.
8. Florey, "Penicillin."
9. Ligon, "Sir Alexander Fleming."
10. Florey, "Penicillin."
11. Ligon, "Penicillin."
12. Abraham, "Penicillin."
13. Milton Wainwright, "Moulds in Ancient and More Recent Medicine," *The Mycologist* (1989): fungi4schools.org/Reprints/Mycologist_articles/Post-16/Medical/V03pp021-023folk_medicine.pdf.
14. Milton Wainwright, "Moulds in Folk Medicine." *Folklore* 100, 2 (1989): 162–66.
15. Sheryl Persson, *Smallpox, Syphilis and Salvation* (Wollombi, NSW: Exisle Publishing, 2009).
16. Persson.

Chapter 36
1. Nobelprize.org. "Egas Moniz—Facts." nobelprize.org/nobel_prizes/medicine/laureates/1949/moniz-facts.html.
2. NPR, "'My Lobotomy': Howard Dully's Journey" (16 November 2005): npr.org/2005/11/16/5014080/my-lobotomy-howard-dullys-journey.
3. Wikipedia, "Rosemary Kennedy," en.wikipedia.org/wiki/Rosemary_Kennedy.
4. A. Miller, "The Lobotomy Patient a Decade Later," *Canadian Medical Association Journal* 96 (April 15, 1967): 1095–1103.
5. Charles Barber, "The Brain: A Mindless Obsession," *The Wilson Quarterly* 32, 1 (2008): 32–44.
6. Siang Yan Tan and Angela Yip, "António Egas Moniz (1874–1955): Lobotomy Pioneer and Nobel Laureate," *Singapore* 55, 4 (2014): 175–76.
7. A. Miller, "The Lobotomy Patient a Decade Later: A Follow-up Study of a Research Project Started in 1948." *Canadian Medical Association Journal* 96 (April 15, 1967): 1095–1103.
8. Cynthia J. Tsay, "Julius Wagner-Jauregg and the Legacy of Malarial Therapy for the Treatment of General Paresis of the Insane." *Yale Journal of Biology and Medicine* 86, 2 (06/13 2013): 245–54.
9. R. Aaron Robinson *et al.*, "Surgery of the Mind, Mood, and Conscious State: An Idea in Evolution," *World Neurosurgery* 80, 3/4 (2013): S2–S26.
10. Barber, "The Brain: A Mindless Obsession."
11. Barber, "The Brain: A Mindless Obsession."
12. Mical Raz, "Psychosurgery, Industry and Personal Responsibility, 1940–1965," *Social History of Medicine* 23, 1 (2010): 116–33.
13. Brianne M. Collins and Henderikus J. Stam, "Freeman's Transorbital Lobotomy as an Anomaly: A Material Culture Examination of Surgical Instruments and Operative Spaces," *History of Psychology* 18, 2 (20154): 119–31.
14. Raz, "Psychosurgery."
15. Brianne M. Collins and Henderikus J. Stam, "A Transnational Perspective on Psychosurgery: Beyond Portugal and the United States," *Journal of the History of the Neurosciences* 23, 4 (2014): 335–54.

Chapter 37
1. Karl Paul Link, "The Discovery of Dicumarol and Its Sequels," *Circulation* 19 (1959): 534–38.

2. Richard L. Mueller and Stephen Scheidt, "History of Drugs for Thrombotic Disease," *Circulation* 89, 1 (Jan 1994): 432–49.
3. Link, "Discovery of Dicumarol."
4. John M. Kingsbury, "Commentary: One Man's Poison," *BioScience* 30, 3 (1980): 171–76.
5. Kingsbury, "One Man's Poison."
6. Kingsbury, "One Man's Poison."
7. Mike Scully, "Warfarin Therapy: Rat Poison and the Prevention of Thrombosis," *Biochemist* (Feb 2002): 15–17.
8. "In Science Fields." *The Science News-Letter* 40, 3 (1941): 40–41.
9. Link, "Discovery of Dicumarol."
10. Scully, "Warfarin Therapy."
11. Link, "Discovery of Dicumarol."
12. A. Lichtenstein, "Award Ceremony Speech," The Nobel Prize in Physiology or Medicine 1943. www.nobel-prize.org/nobel_prizes/medicine/laureates/1943/press.html.

Chapter 38
1. U. S. Army Medical Department, *The Medical Department of the United States Army in the World War*, Chapter XXV, history.amedd.army.mil/booksdocs/wwi/adminamerexp/chapter25.html.
2. National Institutes of Health, "Bacterial Pneumonia Caused Most Deaths in 1918 Influenza Pandemic," www.nih.gov/news-events/news-releases/bacterial-pneumonia-caused-most-deaths-1918-influenza-pandemic.
3. R. J. Dubos, "Oswald Theodore Avery," *Biographical Memoirs of Fellows of the Royal Society* 2 (1956): 35–48.
4. Olga Amsterdamska, "From Pneumonia to DNA," *Historical Studies in the Physical and Biological Sciences* 24, 1 (1993): 1–40.
5. Frank Portugal, "Oswald T. Avery: Nobel Laureate or Noble Luminary?" *Perspectives in Biology and Medicine* 53, 4 (2010): 558–70.
6. Amsterdamska, "From Pneumonia to DNA."
7. Wikipedia, "Griffith's Experiment," en.wikipedia.org/wiki/Griffith%27s_experiment.
8. Dubos, "Avery."
9. Amsterdamska, "From Pneumonia to DNA."
10. Dubos, "Avery."
11. Wikipedia, "Griffith's Experiment."
12. Dubos, "Avery."
13. Florian Maderspacher, "Rags before the Riches: Friedrich Miescher and the Discovery of DNA," *Current Biology* 14, 15 (2004): R608; Ralf Dahm, "Friedrich Miescher and the Discovery of DNA," *Developmental Biology* 278 (2005): 274–88.
14. Maderspacher, "Rags"; Dahm, "Friedrich Miescher."
15. Petter Portin, "The Birth and Development of the DNA Theory of Inheritance: Sixty Years since the Discovery of the Structure of DNA," *Journal of Genetics* 93, 1 (2014): 293–302.
16. Portin, "The Birth and Development of the DNA Theory."
17. Portugal, "Avery."
18. Wikipedia, "DNA," en.wikipedia.org/wiki/DNA.
19. James D. Watson and Francis H.C. Crick. "Molecular Structure of Nucleic Acids: A Structure for Deoxyribose Nucleic Acid." *Nature* 171 (1953): 737–38.
20. Áurea Anguera de Sojo *et al.*, "Serendipity and the Discovery of DNA." *Foundations of Science* 19 (2014): 387–401.
21. Portin, "The Birth and Development of the DNA Theory."
22. Francis S. Collins *et al.*, "The Human Genome Project: Lessons from Large-Scale Biology," *Science* 300, 5617 (2003): 286–90.
23. Bruce Ponder, "Genetic Testing for Cancer Risk," *Science* 278, 5340 (1997): 1050–54.
24. National Cancer Institute, "BRCA1 and BRCA2: Cancer Risk and Genetic Testing," www.cancer.gov/about-cancer/causes-prevention/genetics/brca-fact-sheet.

Chapter 39
1. Milton Wainwright, "Moulds in Folk Medicine," *Folklore* 100, 2 (1989): 162–66.
2. B. Scarpa, "Homage from One Sardinian to Another," *Clinical Microbiology and Infection* 6, S3 (2000): 3–5.
3. G. Bo, "Giuseppe Brotzu and the Discovery of Cephalosporins," *Clinical Microbiology and Infection* 6, S3 (2000): 6–8.
4. Scarpa, "Homage."
5. Beniamino Orrù *et al.*, "Giuseppe Brotzu and the Discovery of Cephalosporins," Cologne: 8th European Conference of Medical and Health Libraries (2002).
6. Scarpa, "Homage."
7. Giuseppe Brotzu, "Research on a New Antibiotic," translated R. Pompei and G. Cornaglia, *Publications of the Cagliari Institute of Hygiene* (1948): 6–19; Orrù *et al.*
8. Brotzu, "Research."
9. Bo, "Giuseppe Brotzu."
10. Edward Abraham, "Penicillin and Its Successors: A Personal View," *Bulletin of the American Academy of Arts and Sciences* 39, 1 (1985): 8–27.
11. Bo, "Giuseppe Brotzu."

Chapter 40

1. Willem J. Kolff, "The Artificial Kidney and Its Effect on the Development of Other Artificial Organs," *Nature Magazine* 8, 10 (October 2002): 1063–65.
2. Theodore H. Stanley, "A Tribute to Dr Willem J. Kolff," *Journal of Cardiothoracic and Vascular Anesthesia* 27, 3 (June 2013): 600–13.
3. Mayo Clinic Staff, "Acute Kidney Failure," www.mayoclinic.org/diseases-conditions/kidney-failure/basics/definition/con-20024029.
4. James H. Shinaberger, "Quantitation of Dialysis," *Seminars in Dialysis* 14, 4 (2001): 238–45.
5. Kolff, "Artificial Kidney."
6. Stanley, "Tribute."
7. Stanley, "Tribute."
8. Stanley, "Tribute."
9. Kolff, "Artificial Kidney."
10. Stephen A. Schwid and Willem J. Kolff, "Closed Sleeve Bandage to Protect Dialysis Shunts," *JAMA* 202, 2 (1967): 156.
11. Kolff, "Artificial Kidney."
12. Lynne M. Dunphy, "Iron Lungs," *American Journal of Nursing* 103, 5 (2003): 64I.
13. Dunphy, "Iron Lungs."
14. Wikipedia, "Iron Lung," en.wikipedia.org/wiki/Iron_lung.
15. Dunphy, "Iron Lungs."
16. Wikipedia, "Iron Lung."

Chapter 41

1. James Whale, director, *Frankenstein: The Man Who Made a Monster*. Clip showing monster animated by electricity: www.youtube.com/watch?v=1qNeGSJaQ9Q.
2. Susan J. Wolfson, "'This Is *My* Lightning' or; Sparks in the Air," *Studies in English Literature 1500 – 1900* 55, 4 (2015): 751–86.
3. Lester D. Friedman, "It's *Still* Alive: Victor Frankenstein," *The Pharos* (Spring 2016): 49–52.
4. Wikipedia, "Artificial Cardiac Pacemaker," en.wikipedia.org/wiki/Artificial_cardiac_pacemaker.
5. Jean B. Rosenbaum and Darwood Hansen, "Simple Cardiac Pacemaker and Defibrillator," *JAMA* 155, 13 (1954): 1151.
6. "Jean Rosenbaum: Health Association Executive, Fitness Physician," Prabook: prabook.org/web/person-view.html?profileId=596729.
7. Oscar Aquilina, "A Brief History of Cardiac Pacing," *Images in Paediatric Cardiology* 8, 2 (2006): 17–81.
8. Aquilina, "Brief History"; Wikipedia, "Artificial Cardiac Pacemaker."
9. Catherine Ward *et al.*, "A Short History on Pacemakers," *International Journal of Cardiology* 169 (2013): 244–48.
10. Ward, "A Short History."
11. Oscar Aquilina, "A Brief History of Cardiac Pacing," *Images in Paediatric Cardiology* 8, 2 (2006): 17–81.
12. Smithsonian. National Museum of American History. "Yorick, the Bionic Skeleton." americanhistory.si.edu/collections/search/object/nmah_1203675.

Chapter 42

1. Mary Patterson McPherson *et al.*, "Baruch S. Blumberg: 28 July 1925–5 April 2011," *Proceedings of the American Philosophical Society* 155, 3 (2011): 301–11.
2. H. Roger Segelken, "Baruch S. Blumberg," *New York Times* (April 6, 2011): nytimes.com/2011/04/07/health/07blumberg.html?_r=0.
3. Baruch S. Blumberg, "The Hepatitis B Virus," *Public Health Reports* 95, 5 (1980): 427–35.
4 Baruch S. Blumberg, "Biographical," Nobelprize.org (1976, 2006): nobelprize.org/nobel_prizes/medicine/laureates/1976/blumberg-bio.html.
5. Baruch S. Blumberg, "The Hepatitis B Virus," *Public Health Reports* 95, 5 (1980): 427-35.
6. Blumberg, "Hepatitis B Virus, the Vaccine, and the Control of Primary Cancer of the Liver," *Proceedings of the National Academy of Science* 94, 14 (1997): 7121–25.
7. Blumberg, "Hepatitis B."
8. B. S. Blumberg *et al.*, "The Relation of Infection with the Hepatitis B Agent to Primary Hepatic Carcinoma," *American Journal of Pathology* 81, 3 (1975): 669–82.
9. Blumberg, "Hepatitis B Virus, the Vaccine."
10. John R. Senior *et al.*, "The Australia Antigen and Role of the Late Philadelphia General Hospital," *Hepatology* 54, 3 (2011): 753–56.
11. Blumberg, "Hepatitis B Virus, the Vaccine."
12. World Health Organization, "World Health Report: Infectious Diseases and Cancer," 1996: who.int/whr/1996/media_centre/press_release/en/index7.html.
13. National Cancer Institute, "Cancer Vaccines," cancer.gov/about-cancer/causes-prevention/vaccines-fact-sheet#q8.

Chapter 43

1. "Ss. Cosmas and Damian, the Patron Saints of Medicine," *The British Medical Journal* 2, 2180 (1902): 1176–77.
2. Christiaan N. Barnard, "Heart Transplants Fell into Disrepute," *New York Times* Arts and Leisure, D1 (November 26, 1972).
3. "First Human Hearts Transplanted." *Science News* 92, 25 (1967): 581.
4. "Balancing the Drug Dosage." *Science News* 93, 1 (1968): 7–8.
5. "First Human Hearts."

6 Thomas E. Starzl, "The Landmark Identical Twin Case," *JAMA* 251, 19 (1984): 2572–73; Thomas E. Starzl and Clyde Barker, "The Origin of Clinical Organ Transplantation Revisited," *JAMA* 301, 19 (May 20, 2009): 2041–43.

7 Lawrence K. Altman, "Christiaan Barnard, Surgeon for First Heart Transplant, Dies," *New York Times* (September 3, 2001).

8. Irving S. Wright, "A New Challenge to Ethical Codes: Heart Transplants," *Journal of Religion and Health* 8, 3 (1969): 226–41.

9. Nobelprize.org. "Peter Medawar - Biographical." www.nobelprize.org/nobel_prizes/medicine/laureates/1960/medawar-bio.html.

10. Thomas E. Starzl, "The Birth of Clinical Organ Transplantation," *Journal of the American College of Surgeons* 192, 4 (2001): 431–46.

11. Thomas E. Starzl, "History of Clinical Transplantation," *World Journal of Surgery* 24, 7 (2000): 759–82.

12. Starzl, "Birth of Clinical Organ Transplantation."

13 Starzl, "History of Clinical Transplantation."

14. Thomas E. Starzl, "Peter Brian Medawar: Father of Transplantation," *Journal of the American College of Surgeons* 180, 3 (1995): 332–36.

15. "Peter Medawar."

16. Starzl, "Birth."

17. C. J. E. Watson and J. H. Dark, "Organ Transplantation," *British Journal of Anaesthesia* 108, suppl 1 (1 January 2012): i29–42.

18. R. N. Ankney, "Miracle in South Africa: A Historical Review of US Magazines' Coverage of the First Heart Transplant." *Ecquid Novi: African Journalism Studies* 19, 2 (1998): 26–38.

19. Wright, "A New Challenge."

20. Wikipedia, "Brain Death," en.wikipedia.org/wiki/Brain_death.

21. U.S. Department of Health and Human Services, "Organ Transplantation: The Process," www.organdonor.gov/about/transplantationprocess.html.

22. Wright, "A New Challenge."

23. Marguerite Holloway, "Graft and Host, Together Forever," *Scientific American*, 2007.

Chapter 44

1. McKenna, Phil. "Malaria's Nemesis." *New Scientist* 212, 2838 (12 November 2011).

2. "From Branch to Bedside: Youyou Tu Is Awarded the 2011 Lasker-DeBakey Clinical Medical Research Award," *Journal of Clinical Investigation* 121, 10 (2011): 3768–73.

3. Louis H. Miller and Xinzhuan Su, "Artemisinin: Discovery from the Chinese Herbal Garden," *Cell* 146, 6 (2011): 855–88.

4. Alan Levinovitz, "Chairman Mao Invented Traditional Chinese Medicine," Slate.com (22 October 2013): www.slate.com/articles/health_and_science/medical_examiner/2013/10/traditional_chinese_medicine_origins_mao_invented_it_but_didn_t_believe.single.html.

5. Tu Youyou, "The Discovery of Artemisinin (Qinghausu) and Gifts from Chinese Medicine," *Nature Medicine* 17, 10 (2011): 1217–20.

6. Tu, "Discovery."

7. Miller and Su, "Artemisinin."

8. Miller and Su, "Artemisinin."

9. Tu, "Discovery."

10. Miller and Su, "Artemisinin."

11. World Health Organization, "WHO/UNICEF Report: Malaria MDG Target Achieved amid Sharp Drop in Cases and Mortality," www.who.int/mediacentre/news/releases/2015/malaria-mdg-target/en/.

12. McKenna, "Malaria's Nemesis."

13. Rhonda Chang, "Making Theoretical Principles for New Chinese Medicine," *Health and History* 16, 1 (2014): 66–86.

14. Brian Dunning, "Mao's Barefoot Doctors: The Secret History of Chinese Medicine," *Skeptoid* Podcast #259 (24 May 2011): skeptoid.com/episodes/4259.

15. Chang, "Making Theoretical Principles."

16. Dunning, "Mao's Barefoot Doctors."

17. Richard Stone, "Lifting the Veil on Traditional Chinese Medicine," *Science* 319, 5864 (February 8, 2008): 709–10.

Chapter 45

1. Robin Marantz Henig, "Lesley Brown, b. 1964," *New York Times* (December 30, 2012): www.nytimes.com/interactive/2012/12/30/magazine/the-lives-they-lived-2012.html?view=Lesley_Brown.

2. Denise Grady, "Lesley Brown, Mother of the World's First 'Test-Tube Baby,' Dies at 64." *New York Times* (June 24, 2012) www.nytimes.com/2012/06/24/health/lesley-brown-mother-of-first-test-tube-baby-dies-at-64.html.

3. Human Fertilisation & Embryo Authority, "About Infertility," (June 1, 2012): www.hfea.gov.uk/infertility.html.

4. Geoff Watts, "IVF Pioneer Robert Edwards Wins Nobel Prize for Medicine," *British Medical Journal* 341, 7776 (2010): 747.

5. John D. Biggers, "IVF and Embryo Transfer: Historical Origin and Development," *Reproductive Biomedicine Online* 25 (2012): 118–27.

6. Martin H. Johnson, "Robert Edwards: Nobel Laureate in Physiology or Medicine," Nobel Lecture, 2010. www.nobelprize.org/nobel_prizes/medicine/laureates/2010/edwards-lecture.html.

7. Johnson, "Robert Edwards."

8. Jessica R. Hoffman, "You Say Adoption, I Say Objection," *Family Law Quarterly* 46, 3 (2012): 397–417.

9. Victoria Ward, "Louise Brown, the First IVF Baby, Reveals Family Was Bombarded with Hate Mail," *The Telegraph* (24 July 2015): www.telegraph.co.uk/news/health/11760004/Louise-Brown-the-first-IVF-baby-reveals-family-was-bombarded-with-hate-mail.html.
10. Robyn Rowland, "Donor Insemination to in Vitro Fertilization," *Politics and the Life Sciences* 12, 2 (1993): 192–93.
11. Bob Simpson, "Managing Potential in Assisted Reproductive Technologies," *Current Anthropology* 54, S7 (2013): S87–S96.
12. Bob Simpson, "Making 'Bad' Deaths 'Good': The Kinship Consequences of Posthumous Conception," *Journal of the Royal Anthropological Institute* 7, 1 (2001): 1–18.
13. Rowland, "Donor Insemination to in Vitro Fertilization."
14. Clare Dyer, "White Couple Can Keep Mixed Race Twins after IVF Blunder," *BMJ* 325, 7372 (2002): 1055.
15. Jacqueline Mroz, "One Sperm Donor, 150 Offspring," New York Times (6 September 2011): www.nytimes.com/2011/09/06/health/06donor.html.
16. Elizabeth B. Connell, "Contraception in the Prepill Era," *Contraception* 59 (1999): 7S–10S.
17. Carol Flora Brooks, "The Early History of the Anti-Contraceptive Laws in Massachusetts and Connecticut," *American Quarterly* 18, 1 (1966): 3–23.
18. Carole Joffe, "Portraits of Three 'Physicians of Conscience,'" *Journal of the History of Sexuality* 2, 1 (1991): 46–67.
19. Kathleen E. Powderly, "Contraceptive Policy and Ethics Illustrations from American History," *The Hastings Center Report* 25, 1 (1995): S9–S11.
20. Powderly, "Contraceptive Policy."
21. Marc Stein, "The Supreme Court's Sexual Counter-Revolution," *OAH Magazine of History* 20, 2 (2006): 21–25.
22. Linda Greenhouse and Reva B. Siegel, "Before (and after) Roe V. Wade: New Questions About Backlash," *Yale Law Journal* 120, 8 (2011): 2028–87.

Chapter 46

1. Monica J. Casper and Adele E. Clarke, "Making the Pap Smear into the 'Right Tool' for the Job," *Social Studies of Science* 28, 2 (1998): 255–90.
2. Siddhartha Mukherjee, *The Emperor of All Maladies: A Biography of Cancer* (New York: Scribner, 2010): 287.
3. Casper and Clarke, "Making the Pap Smear."
4. Lynette Denny *et al.*, "Cervical Cancer," in *Cancer: Disease Control Priorities*, Third Edition (Volume 3). Washington (DC): The World Bank, 2015. ncbi.nlm.nih.gov/books/NBK343648/.
5. Harald zur Hausen, "Papillomaviruses in the Causation of Human Cancers—A Brief Historical Account," *Virology* 384 (2009): 260–65.
6. Ernest L. Wynder, "Environmental Factors in Cervical Cancer: An Approach to Its Prevention," *British Medical Journal* 1, 4916 (1955): 743–47.
7. Zur Hausen, "Papillomaviruses."
8. Harald zur Hausen, "Biographical," Nobelprize.org, nobelprize.org/nobel_prizes/medicine/laureates/2008/hausen-bio.html.
9. Zur Hausen, "Nobel Lecture."
10. Zur Hausen, "Biographical."
11. Meenakshi Dawar *et al.*, "Human Papillomavirus Vaccines Launch a New Era," *Canadian Medical Association Journal* 177, 5 (2007): 456–61.
12. National Cancer Institute, "Causes and Prevention: Infectious Agents," cancer.gov/about-cancer/causes-prevention/risk/infectious-agents.
13. Chester M. Southam *et al.*, "Homotransplantation of Human Cell Lines," *Science, New Series* 125, 3239 (1957): 158–60.
14. L.J. Sandlow, "Oaths, Codes, and Charters in Medicine over the Ages," *Hektoen International* (Fall 2011): hektoeninternational.org/index.php?option=com_content&view=article&id=399:oaths-codes-and-charters-in-medicine-over-the-ages&catid=71&Itemid=716.
15. Susan Lederer, "Experimentation on Human Beings," *OAH Magazine of History* 19, 5 (2005): 20–22.
16. Jochen Vollmann and Rolf Winau, "Informed Consent in Human Experimentation before the Nuremberg Code," *BMJ: British Medical Journal* 313, 7070 (1996): 1445–47.
17. George J. Annas and Edward R. Utley, *The Nazi Doctors and the Nuremberg Code: Human Rights in Human Experimentation* (New York: Oxford University Press, 1992).
18. Wikipedia, "Nuremberg Code," en.wikipedia.org/wiki/Nuremberg_Code.
19. Gregory J. Higby, "Tuskegee Syphilis Study Revisited," *Pharmacy in History* 41, 4 (1999): 169–70.
20. Lederer, "Experimentation."

Chapter 47

1. Cynthia Stark, "MMR Vaccine and Autism—A Mother's Journey to Heal Her Child," Vaccine Choice Canada (February 2013): vaccinechoicecanada.com/personal-stories/mmr-vaccine-and-autism-a-mothers-journey-to-heal-her-child/.
2. Centers for Disease Control, "Autism Spectrum Disorder (ASD) Facts." www.cdc.gov/ncbddd/autism/facts.html.
3. Centers for Disease Control, "Autism Spectrum Disorder (ASD) Data & Statistics." www.cdc.gov/ncbddd/autism/data.html.
4. Dennis K. Flaherty, "The Vaccine-Autism Connection: A Public Health Crisis Caused by Fraudulent Science," *Annals of Pharmacotherapy* 45 (October 2011): 1302–04.
5. William Meacham, "Postinfection Immunity to Measles Was Known to Common Folk Well Before Its Discovery by Science," *American Journal of the Medical Sciences* 347, 6 (June 2014): 502–03.
6. World Health Organization, Media Centre, "Measles Fact Sheet" (2016): www.who.int/mediacentre/factsheets/fs286/en/.

7. St. Louis Children's Hospital, "Case Study: July 'First Disease,'" www.stlouischildrens.org/
health-care-professionals/publications/doctors-digest/september-october-2013/case-study-july-first-d.
8. World Health Organization, Media Centre, "Rubella Fact Sheet," (2016): www.who.int/mediacentre/
factsheets/fs367/en/.
9. Meacham, "Postinfection Immunity."
10. Jan Hendriks and Stuart Blume, "Measles Vaccination before the Measles-Mumps-Rubella Vaccine," *American Journal of Public Health* 103, 8 (August 2013): 1393–1401.
11. Flaherty, "The Vaccine-Autism Connection."
12. Anjali Jain *et al.*, "Autism Occurrence by MMR Vaccine Status Among US Children With Older Siblings With and Without Autism," *Journal of the American Medical Association* 313, 15 (2015): 1534–40.
13. Flaherty, "The Vaccine-Autism Connection."
14. Gregory A. Poland, "MMR Vaccine and Autism: Vaccine Nihilism and Postmodern Science," *Mayo Clinic Proceedings* 86, 9 (September 2011): 869–71.
15. Wikipedia, "Leo Kanner," en.wikipedia.org/wiki/Leo_Kanner.
16. Flaherty, "The Vaccine-Autism Connection."

Chapter 48
1. Stacy Theobald, "Custom Surgery Creates Normal Hips for 30-Year-Old," Mayo Clinic (October 27, 2011): sharing.mayoclinic.org/discussion/custom-surgery-creates-normal-hips-for-30-year-old/.
2. Thomas Kohnen *et al.*, "Cataract Surgery with Implantation of an Artificial Lens," *Deutsches Ärzteblatt International* 106, 43 (10/23/2009): 695–702.
3. Mark Spangehl, "Hip Resurfacing: An Alternative to Conventional Hip Replacement?" Mayo Clinic (2014): www.mayoclinic.org/hip-resurfacing/expert-answers/faq-20057913.
4. Kohnen *et al.*, "Cataract Surgery."
5. Spangehl, "Hip Resurfacing."
6. Hans Van Brabandt *et al.*, "Transcatheter Aortic Valve Implantation (TAVI): Risky and Costly," *BMJ: British Medical Journal* 345, 7868 (2012): 24–27.
7. Theobald, "Custom Surgery."
8. C. Lee Ventola, "Medical Applications for 3D Printing: Current and Projected Uses," *Pharmacy and Therapeutics* 39, 10 (2014): 704–711.
9. Stephen Chen, "'This Is Just the Beginning': China Approves World's First 3D-Printed Hip Joint for General Use," *South China Morning Post* (1 September 2015): www.scmp.com/tech/science-research/article/1854369/just-beginning-china-approves-worlds-first-3d-printed-hip.
10. Ventola, "Medical Applications."
11. Thomas K. Grose, "Human Spare Parts," ASEE Prism 24, 6 (2015): 24–29.
12. Grose, "Human Spare Parts."
13. Ventola, "Medical Applications."
14. "Advanced Delivery Devices: Implantable Drug-Eluting Devices," *Drug Development and Delivery* (2015): www.drug-dev.com/Main/Back-Issues/ADVANCED-DELIVERY-DEVICES-Implantable-DrugEluting-1006.aspx.
15. "Sbu Systematic Review Summaries," In *Drug-Eluting Stents in Coronary Arteries* (Stockholm: Swedish Council on Health Technology Assessment, 2014).
16. Advanced Delivery Devices.
17. Advanced Delivery Devices.
18. Bob Roehr, "Vaginal Ring Offers Hope in HIV Prevention," *Scientific American* (February 24, 2016): www.scientificamerican.com/article/vaginal-ring-offers-hope-in-hiv-prevention/.
19. Wolfgang Hohenforst-Schmidt *et al.*, "Drug Eluting Stents for Malignant Airway Obstruction: A Critical Review of the Literature." *J Cancer* 7, 4 (2016): 377–90.
20. E. Dabizzi and P. G. Arcidiaco, "Update on Enteral Stents," *Current Treatment Options in Gastroenterology* 14, 2 (2016): 178–84.
21. Moy, Brian T. and John W. Birk. "An Update to Hepatobiliary Stents." *Journal of Clinical and Translational Hepatology* 3, 1 (2015): 67–77.
22. Advanced Delivery Devices.
23. Advanced Delivery Devices.

Chapter 49
1. William Hsiao and Claire Fraser-Liggett, "Human Microbiome Project," *Drug Discovery Today* 14, 7 (2009): 331–33.
2. Robert Orenstein *et al.*, "Moving Fecal Microbiota Transplantation into the Mainstream," *Nutrition in Clinical Practice* 28, 5 (2013): 589–98.
3. CDC Press Room, "Nearly Half a Million Americans Suffered from *Clostridium difficile* Infections in a Single Year." (Feb. 25, 2015): www.cdc.gov/media/releases/2015/p0225-clostridium-difficile.html.
4. Giovanni Cammarota *et al.*, "Gut Microbiota Modulation," *Internal and Emergency Medicine* 9 (2014): 365–73.
5. Cammarota *et al.*, "Gut Microbiota Modulation."
6. Els van Nood *et al.*, "Duodenal Infusion of Donor Feces for Recurrent *Clostridium difficile*," *New England Journal of Medicine* 368, 5 (2013): 407–15.
7. Carl Zimmer, "Fecal Transplants Can Be Life-Saving, but How?" *New York Times* (July 15, 2016): nytimes.com/2016/07/15/science/fecal-transplants-bacteria-viruses.html?_r=0.
8. Trevor C. Van Schooneveld *et al.*, "Duodenal Infusion of Donor Feces: To the Editor," *New England Journal of Medicine* 368, 22 (May 30, 2013): 2143.
9. van Nood *et al.*, "Duodenal Infusion."
10. Dinesh Vyas *et al.*, "Fecal Transplant Policy and Legislation," *World Journal of Gastroenterology* 21, 1 (Jan 7, 2015): 6–11.

Chapter 50

1. Donald G. McNeil, Jr., *Zika: The Emerging Epidemic* (New York: W. W. Norton, 2016), 42–45.
2. Enny S. Paixão *et al.*, "History, Epidemiology, and Clinical Manifestations of Zika," *American Journal of Public Health* 106, 4 (April 2016): 606–12.
3. McNeil, *Zika*, 53.
4. McNeil, *Zika*, 66.
5. Brazil, "Ministry of Health Confirmed 1,709 Cases of Microcephaly." (16 July 2016): translate.google.com/translate?hl=en&sl=pt&u=portalsaude.saude.gov.br/&prev=search.
6. Paixão *et al.*, "History, Epidemiology, and Clinical Manifestations of Zika."
7. CDC, "Zika Virus," cdc.gov/zika/index.html.
8. World Health Organization, "Zika Virus and Complications," who.int/emergencies/zika-virus/en/.
9. Weaver, "Zika Virus."
10. McNeil, *Zika*.
11. Scott C. Weaver *et al.*, "Zika Virus: History, Emergence, Biology, and Prospects for Control," *Antiviral Research* 130 (2016): 69–80.
12. Brazil, "Ministry of Health."

Conclusion

1. Simon Brooker, "Estimating the Global Distribution and Disease Burden of Intestinal Nematode Infections: Adding up the Numbers – a Review," *International Journal for Parasitology* 40, 10 (04/27/2010): 1137-44.
2. Jan Andersson *et al.*, "Avermectin and Artemisinin: Revolutionary Therapies against Parasitic Diseases," www.nobelprize.org/nobel_prizes/medicine/laureates/2015/advanced-medicineprize2015.pdf.
3. "Ancient Chinese Anti-fever Cure Becomes Panacea for Malaria: An Interview with Zhou Yiqing." *Bulletin of the World Health Organization* 87 (2009): 743–744. www.who.int/bulletin/volumes/87/10/09-051009.pdf.
4. World Health Organization, "Malaria Fact Sheet," April, 2016: www.who.int/mediacentre/factsheets/fs094/en/.
5. Elisabeth Hsu, "Reflections on the 'Discovery' of the Antimalarial Qinghao," *British Journal of Clinical Pharmacology* 61, 6 (2006): 666–70.
6. "Ancient Chinese Anti-fever Cure."
7. World Health Organization, "WHO Position Statement" (2012): www.who.int/malaria/publications/atoz/position_statement_herbal_remedy_artemisia_annua_l/en/.
8. A. Falodun, "Herbal Medicine in Africa: Distribution, Standardization and Prospects," *Research Journal of Phytochemistry*, 4 (2010): 154–161.
9. Ambrose O. Talisuna *et al.*, "The Affordable Medicines Facility-malaria," *Malaria Journal* 11 (2012): 370.
10. Novartis Malaria Initiative, "First-in-Class Treatment," www.malaria.novartis.com/malaria-initiative/treatment/first-in-class-treatment/index.shtml.
11. Caroline Meier zu Biesen, "The Rise to Prominence of *Artemisia Annua* L.—The Transformation of a Chinese Plant to a Global Pharmaceutical," *African Sociological Review* 14, 2 (2010): 24–46.

Index

abortion, 218
Abraham, Edward, 187–188
Accomplish't Midwife, The, 37
Account of the Foxglove and Some of Its Medicinal Uses, An (Withering), 60
acquired immunological tolerance, 204
ACT (Artemisinin-based combination therapy), 245–246
Affordable Medicines for Malaria (AMFM) program, 246
Agnodice, 39
alleles, 100*ph*, 103
Allison, Anthony, 199
Alpert, Richard, 81
Al-Rashid, Harun, 27–28
Al-Razi (Rhazes), 27–30, 28*ph*
Amherst. Lord Jeffrey, 50, 50*ph*
André the Giant, 149*ph*
anesthetics, 77–80, 79*ph*, 107, 107*ph*
Angus, Tanya, 147
animalcules, 108–110
Anrep, Gleb V., 149–150
anthrax, 110–111
antibiotics, 116, 185–188, 235–237
antibodies, 121, 122, 136, 203
anticoagulants, 174–176
antigens, 121, 122, 136, 198, 203
anti-rejection drugs, 203–204
antisepsis, 85
antitoxins, 119–121
antivenom seratherapy, 119–121, 122
Aristotle, 23, 24, 108
artemisia, 208–210, 210*ph*, 244–245
artemisinin, 209–210, 211*ph*
arteries, hardening of, 31
artificial joints, 230
Asclepiades, 9
Ashurbanipal, King, 9
Asklepios, 17–20, 18*ph*, 19*ph*, 20, 21
assisted reproductive technology (ART), 217
atoxyl, 158–159
Auenbrugger, Leopold, 68
auscultation, 68
Australia antigen (Au), 198, 199–201
autism spectrum disorder (ASD), 224–228, 225*ph*, 229
Avery, Oswald, 178–181, 180*ph*, 181*ph*
Ayurvedic texts, 26

bacteria, discovery of, 42
Bakken, Earl, 193, 194–195, 195*ph*
Bakken Museum, 194*ph*
Banting, Frederick, 163–165, 163*ph*, 164*ph*

Barnard, Christiaan, 202, 204*ph*, 205, 206
Baylis, William M., 148–150
Beck, Lewis, 93
Becquerel, Henri, 137, 139
Beijerinck, Martinus Willem, 133
beriberi, 55, 56, 56*ph*
Best, Charles, 163*ph*, 165
Bichat, Xavier, 67–68
Billingham, Rupert, 204
birth control, 218, 234
birth stools, 39
Black Death, 34, 127–132
bladder stones, 72–76, 73*ph*
Blane, Sir Gilbert, 54
Blavatsky, Helena P., 151*ph*
Blood, Diane, 217
blood donation and storage, 146
blood pressure cuff, 71
blood transfusions, 142–146, 143*ph*, 144*ph*, 146*ph*
blood types, 144–145, 145*ph*
bloodletting, 62–66, 63*ph*, 65*ph*
Blum, Theodore, 141
Blumberg, Baruch S., 198–-201, 199*ph*
Blundell, James, 142–143, 143*ph*
Boivin, Melanie, 217
Bosch, Hieronymus, 171*ph*
Boylston, Zabdiel, 46–49
brain death, 205
breast cancer, 184
breathing tubes, 79*ph*
Brent, Leslie, 204
Brinkan, Robert, 190
Broca, Paul, 104–106
Brooke, Blythe, 187
Brotzu, Giuseppe, 185–188, 186*ph*, 188*ph*, 212
Broussais, François-Joseph-Victor, 64, 64*ph*
Brown, George, 117
Brown, Lesley, 213, 216
Brown, Louise, 213, 215*ph*
Brueghel, Pieter, the Elder, 132*ph*
bubonic plague, 127–132, 129*ph*
Budd, William, 154–155
Burnet, Macfarlane, 204

Caesarean section, 35, 38, 38*ph*
Calmette, Albert, 116, 118–121, 122
Campbell, Harold, 175
cancer prevention, 219–222
canopic jars, 15*ph*
cardiac pacemakers, 193–196, 195*ph*, 196*ph*
care effect, 21

Carlson, Ed, 174, 176, 176*ph*
Carter, Howard, 14*ph*
Cartier, Jacques, 51
case reporting, 15
cathode rays, 123–124
Celsus, Aulus Cornelius, 9, 11, 121
cervical cancer, 220–221
Chadwick, Edwin, 85, 87–91, 88*ph*
Chain, Ernst Boris, 167–169
Chamberland, Charles, 136*ph*
Chamberlen, Hugh the Elder, 36–37
Chamberlen, Hugh the Younger, 37
Chamberlen family, 35–38, 38*ph*
chemotherapy, 157–160
Cheselden, William, 75
childbed (puerperal) fever, 82–85, 83*ph*, 84*ph*
childbirth, 35–38, 78–79, 82–85
Chinese medicine, 207–212
chloroform, 78–79
cholera, 91, 93–97, 94*ph*, 95*ph*
chromosomes, 180–181, 183, 214
circulatory system, 31–34
Clostridium difficile infections (CDI), 235–237, 236*ph*
coal tar dyes, 157
Collip, John, 165
complementary medicine, 20
Comprehensive Book of Medicine (Al-Razi), 29
computed tomography (CT) scan, 232, 232*ph*
Comstock, Anthony, 218
confirmation bias, 66
congestive heart failure, 57–60, 59*ph*
consumption (tuberculosis), 114–116
context effect, 21
contraception, 218, 234
Cooper, Bransby, 73–74, 75, 75*ph*
correlation vs. causation, 91
cortisol, 11
Cosmas, Saint, 203*ph*
coumarin, 174–176
cowpox, 48*ph*
Crick, Francis H. C., 182–183, 182*ph*
Crile, George Washington, 145
Crookes tubes, 123–124, 125*ph*
cupping, 64, 66, 66*ph*
Curie, Marie Sklodowska, 137–141, 139*ph*, 140*ph*
Curie, Pierre, 137, 138*ph*, 139, 139*ph*, 140*ph*
Curie Electrometer, 138*ph*

da Gama, Vasco, 51
da Vinci, Leonardo, 31–34, 32*ph*, 33*ph*
Daily, Cynthia, 217
Dam, Henrik, 177
Damascenus, Alexander, 23
Damian, Saint, 203*ph*

Darwin, Charles, 98, 198
Darwin, Erasmus, 57–58
Davy, Sir Humphry, 78
demons, 7, 9
Descartes, René, 151*ph*
diabetes, 162–165
dialysis, 189–191, 190*ph*, 191*ph*
dicoumarol, 174–176
digitalis (foxglove), 57–59, 59*ph*
diphtheria vaccination, 229*ph*
dissection, 15, 16, 23, 31, 34, 34*ph*
DNA, 178–184, 182*ph*, 183*ph*
Doisy, E. A., 177
double blind trials, 21
Doubts about Galen (Al-Razi), 29
Douglass, William, 47
Drew, Charles, 146
dropsy, 58, 58*ph*
drug-eluting implants, 234, 234*ph*
Duchesne, Ernest, 169
Dully, Howard, 170
Dully, Lou, 170
dyes, 157

Eberth, Karl, 155
Edgbaston Hall, 60*ph*
Edkins, John Sydney, 149
Edwards, Robert, 213–215, 214*ph*, 215*ph*, 216, 217–218
Edwin Smith Papyrus, 14–15
Egyptians, ancient, 13–15
Ehrlich, Paul, 122, 122*ph*, 157–160, 158*ph*
Eijkman, Christiaan, 56
Einthoven, Willem, 197
Eiseman, Ben, 237
Eisenhower, Dwight D., 176*ph*, 177
electrocardiogram (EKG), 197
Enders, John, 225
endocrinology, 147–151
Enlightenment, 43
entheogens, 81
Epidauros, 20*ph*
epidemiology, 96
evidence-based medicine, 27–30, 54
extracorporeal shock-wave lithotripsy (ESWL), 76

Fabric of the Human Body, The (Vesalius), 34
Farr, William, 93–95
fecal microbiota therapy (FMT), 237
Finlay, Carlos, 134
Finsen, Niels Ryberg, 141*ph*
Finsen lamp, 141*ph*
Fleming, Alexander, 166–169, 167*ph*, 168*ph*, 185, 212
Florey, Howard Walter, 167–169, 187
fluid replacement, 96
folk healing/remedies, 5–8, 245–246
forceps, 36–38, 36*ph*, 37*ph*, 38*ph*

forensic analysis of iceman, 1–4
foxglove, 57–59, 59*ph*
Fracastoro, Girolamo, 44, 44*ph*, 116, 161
Frankenstein (Shelley), 193, 194*ph*, 197
Franklin, Rosalind E., 182–183
Frederick II, 34
Freeman, Walter, 170, 172–173, 173*ph*
fumigators, 91*ph*
fungi, 3–4, 81, 81*ph*, 243

Gaffky, Georg, 155
Galen, 22–25, 23*ph*, 24*ph*, 29, 30, 33, 34,
    62, 71, 114, 116
Galvani, Luigi, 197, 197*ph*
gametes, 100–101
Gardasil, 221
Ge Hong, 209, 237
genetic counseling, 184
genetics, 98–101, 103, 178–184
genital warts, 220
germ theory, 44, 85, 91, 108–113, 110*ph*
germ warfare, 50, 50*ph*
Greatbatch, Wilson, 195
Griffith, Frederick, 179–180, 181*ph*
Guérin, Camille, 116
Guillain-Barré Syndrome (GBS), 238–240

Haffkine, Waldemar, 128
Haldane, J. B. S., 102
Halley, Edmond, 44
hand washing, 82–86
Hansen, Darwood, 194
Harappan civilization, 92, 92*ph*
Harington, Sir John, 92
Harvey, William, 25, 31, 33, 142
Hata, Sahachiro, 158*ph*, 159
Hausen, Harald zur, 220–222, 222*ph*
Hayes, Brooke, 230–231, 232, 232*ph*
healthy carriers, 153–154, 156
heart, 31–34, 57–60. *see also* pacemakers
heart transplants, 202–206, 204*ph*, 205*ph*
heart valves, artificial, 233*ph*
hepatitis B, 198–201, 200*ph*, 201*ph*
Herbalome Project, 212
herd immunity, 228, 228*ph*
Herodotus, 13
Herophilus, 31, 39
Hérrison, Jules, 71, 71*ph*
Hilleman, Maurice, 226, 227*ph*
Hinsey, Joseph C., 219–220
hip replacements, 230–231, 231*ph*
Hippocrates, 9, 20, 24, 30, 114
Hippocratic Oath, 73
Hoffmann, Erich, 159
Holmes, Oliver Wendell, Sr., 82
Hooke, Robert, 41, 43*ph*, 44
hormones, 147–151, 148*ph*, 149*ph*
hospitals
    childbed (puerperal) fever and, 82–85

Islamic, 27–28
    Nightingale and, 85–86
    see also Asklepios
Human Fertilization and Embryology
    Authority, 218
Human Genome Project, 183
human growth hormone (HGH), 147
human leukocyte antigen (HLA) system, 204
human papillomavirus (HPV), 220–221,
    222*ph*
humors, 24–25, 25*ph*, 26, 26*ph*, 29, 53, 62
Humphrey, Roy, 146*ph*
Hunter, William, 143–144
hydrodynamics, 32–33
Hyginus, 39
Hyman, Albert, 194
hyperandrogenism, 150

Ibn Al-Nafis, 33
Ibn Sīnā, 71
iceman, 1–4
iceman, forensic analysis of, 1–4
immune system, 120*ph*
immunology, 120–121
impetigo, 169*ph*
in vitro fertilization (IVF), 213–218, 214*ph*,
    216*ph*
India, 16, 26
influenza, 135, 180*ph*
informed consent, 223
inherited traits, 98–101
inoculation, 45–49
*Inquiry into the Sanitary Conditions of the
    Labouring Population of Great Britain*
    (Chadwick), 85
Institutional Review Boards, 223
insulin, 163
intestinal worms, 243
iron lung, 192, 192*ph*
Ivanovsky, Dimitrii, 133
Ivermectin, 243

Jackson, Andrew, 64
Jackson, Charles, 78
Jackson, James, 65–66
Jenner, Edward, 50
Johnson, Anna, 217
Jundi-Shapur, 30
Justinian's Plague, 132

Kelvin, Lord (William Thomson), 137,
    138*ph*
Kenner, Leo, 229
kidney, artificial, 189–191, 190*ph*
kidney stones, 72–76, 73*ph*, 74*ph*
kidney transplants, 202, 203–204
King, Charles Glen, 55
Kitasato, Shibasaburo, 127
Klein, Johann, 82, 84

Koch, Robert, 96, 110–111, 113, 116, 122, 133, 153, 156, 157, 158
Kolff, Willem, 189–191, 190*ph*

Laennec, René, 67–71, 68*ph*, 69*ph*, 70*ph*, 115
Lancet, The, 75
Landsteiner, Karl, 144–145
Langerhans, Paul, 162
Larsson, Arne, 195
Latta, Thomas, 96
laughing gas, 77–80
Law of Independent Assortment, 101
Law of Segregation, 100*ph*
Leary, Timothy, 81
leeches, 64, 64*ph*, 66
Lenard, Philipp, 123–124
leukemia, 199–200
Li Shizhen, 237
Lidwell, Mark, 193–194
Lillehei, C. Walton, 194, 195*ph*
Lind, James, 52–53, 53*ph*, 54
Link, Karl Paul, 174, 176–177, 177*ph*
Lister, Joseph, 85, 112, 112*ph*, 126, 143, 169
Liston, Robert, 77
lithotomy, 72–73
lithotripsy, 76*ph*
lobotomy, 170–173
Louis, Pierre-Charles-Alexandre, 63*ph*, 65–66
Lower, Richard, 142
Lunar Society, 57–58, 60*ph*
Ly, Larry, 238
lysozyme, 167

Ma Fei San, 107
Macleod, J. R. R., 163–165, 164*ph*
Magdalena Ventura with Her Husband and Son (Ribera), 150*ph*
malaria, 102, 102*ph*, 186*ph*, 199, 207–211, 208*ph*, 244–246, 244*ph*
Mallon, Mary, 153–156, 154*ph*, 155*ph*
malnutrition, 51–55
Mao Zedong, 207–208, 212
Marey, Etienne, 71
Martland, Harrison, 141
massage, 9–12, 10*ph*, 12*ph*
Mather, Cotton, 45–46, 47*ph*, 48
measles, 224–225, 226*ph*, 227*ph*
Mechnikov, Ilya, 122
Medawar, Peter, 202–204
medicinal fungi, 3–4
melatonin, 151
Mendel, Gregor Johann, 98–101, 99*ph*, 100*ph*, 101*ph*, 180
MERS virus, 135*ph*
miasma theory, 44, 53, 88–90, 91*ph*, 93–94
microbial antagonism, 167
microcephaly (MC), 238–242, 241*ph*, 242*ph*

microchimerism, 206, 206*ph*
Micrographia (Hooke), 41, 43*ph*, 44
microscopes, 40–44, 42*ph*
Middle East Respiratory Syndrome, 135*ph*
midwifery, 36–37, 39
Miescher, Friedrich, 180
Miller, Louis, 211
Millman, Irving, 201
Minkowski, Oskar, 162
Mithridates VI, 121, 121*ph*
MMR vaccine, 224–228, 229
molds, 169, 175, 212. *see also* penicillin
Moniz, António Egas, 170–172
Montagu, Lady Mary Wortley, 48–49
Morgagni, Giovanni, 67
Morton, William T. G., 78
mosquitoes, 134*ph*, 208*ph*, 240–241. *see also* malaria; yellow fever; Zika virus
moxibustion, 244
Mueller, Ed, 196
mummies and mummifiers, 13–15, 14*ph*, 15*ph*, 46*ph*, 116*ph*
mumps, 227*ph*
mushrooms, 81, 81*ph*
Müter, Thomas, 79

National Institutes of Health, 11–12
National Research Act, 223
Needham, John, 109–110
nerves, 22–25, 24*ph*
Nestorians, 30
neurotransmitters, 152
Newton, Isaac, 44
Nightingale, Florence, 85–86, 85*ph*
nitrous oxide, 77–80, 79*ph*, 80*ph*
Nobel Prizes, 122
nocebo effect, 21
Noguchi, Hideyo, 134
Nuremberg Code of Medical Ethics, 223
nutritional deficiencies, 55

occupational medicine, 15
Oldenburg, Henry, 42
On the Motion of the Heart and Blood (Harvey), 142
On the Origin of Species (Darwin), 98
Onesimus, 46
osteoarthritis, 230
Ötzi the Iceman, 1–4, 2*ph*, 3*ph*, 243

pacemakers, 193–196, 195*ph*, 196*ph*
Pacini, Filippo, 96
paleopathology, 106
pancreas, 165*ph*
Pap smears, 219–220, 220*ph*, 221*ph*
Papanicolaou, George, 219–220
Paracelsus, 61, 77, 161
parental rights, 217
Pasteur, Louis, 85, 96, 110–111, 110*ph*,

111*ph*, 112, 122, 166–167
Pauling, Linus, 182
Pavlov, Ivan, 148, 148*ph*, 149
Pavlov Museum, 148*ph*
penicillin, 166–169, 168*ph*, 185
Pepys, Samuel, 74*ph*
percussion, 68
percutaneous nephrolithotomy (PCNL), 76
Perkin, William Henry, 160
Perutz, Max, 182
phagocytes, 122
pharmaceuticals, ancient, 61
Philosophical Transactions, 44
Phisalix, Césaire, 122
physicians
    in ancient Egypt, 14–15
    in ancient India, 16
Pidoux, Hermann, 115
piezoelectricity, 137
piezoelectroscope, 140*ph*
pill, the, 218
Pincus, Gregory Goodwin, 218
pineal gland, 151, 151*ph*
pitchblende, 137, 138, 139*ph*
pituitary gland, 147
placebo effect, 21
Pliny the Elder, 121
plombage, 116
pneumonia, 178–180, 179*ph*, 180*ph*, 181*ph*
polio, 192
Pollard, Steven, 72, 73–74, 75
polonium, 138
poop transplants, 237
Popielski, Leon, 148
Pott's disease, 116*ph*
prefrontal lobotomy, 170–173
Priestley, Joseph, 58, 78
Principia Mathematica (Newton), 44
prothrombin, 175
Prunières, P. Barthélemy, 105
psilocybin, 81, 81*ph*
psychosurgery, 170–173, 173*ph*
Public Health Act, 87, 88*ph*, 91
pulse, taking, 71, 71*ph*

qinghao, 208–210, 210*ph*

radiation therapy, 139–141
radioactivity, 137–141
radium, 138–140, 139*ph*, 140*ph*, 141, 141*ph*
Raistrick, Harold, 167
Ramses V, 46*ph*
rat fleas, 127–131, 128*ph*, 131*ph*
red cure, 49
Redi, Francecso, 108, 109*ph*
Reed, Walter, 134, 223
"Removing the Stone of Folly" (Bosch), 171*ph*
Renaissance, 34

Ribera, José de, 150*ph*
Rigoni-Sterm, 220
Roderick, L. M., 175
Roe v. Wade, 218
rondelles, 105
Röntgen, Wilhelm, 123–124, 124*ph*, 125*ph*, 126*ph*
Rosenbaum, Jean, 193, 194
Roux, Emile, 119
Royal Society for Improving Natural Knowledge, 40, 41–42, 42*ph*, 43–44, 60
rubella, 224–225
Rush, Benjamin, 62–63

Salvarsan, 158*ph*, 159, 161, 223
sanatoria, 115–116
Sanger, Margaret, 218
sanitation, 82–86, 87–91, 92
Sassanid Empire, 30
Schaudinn, Fritz, 159
Scientific Revolution, 43, 44
Scott, Ernest Lyman, 162–163, 164
scrofula, 117, 117*ph*
scurvy, 51–54, 52*ph*, 53*ph*, 54*ph*
Semmelweis, Ignatz, 82–85, 84*ph*, 112
serotonin, 11, 152
serum, 119
sewerage and drainage systems, 87–91, 88*ph*, 89*ph*, 90*ph*, 92, 92*ph*
shamans, 5–8, 6*ph*, 7*ph*, 8*ph*
Shelley, Mary, 197
Shitala, 46*ph*
sickle-cell disease, 102, 102*ph*, 199
side-chain theory, 122*ph*
Simond, Paul-Louis, 127–131, 131*ph*
Simpson, James Young, 78, 85
skin grafts, 202–203
sleep therapy, 17–20
smallpox, 45–50, 46*ph*, 50*ph*
Smellie, William, 37, 37*ph*
snake venom, 118–121, 119*ph*, 122
Snow, John, 94–96, 94*ph*
Society for the Suppression of Vice, 218
Soper, George, 153
Soranus of Ephesus, 39
Southam, Chester, 222
Spallanzani, Lazzaro, 109–110
Spanedda, Antonio, 187
sperm donors, 217
sphygmograph, 71, 71*ph*
sphygmomanometer, 71
sphygmometer, 71, 71*ph*
spondyloepiphyseal dysplasia congenita (SEDC), 230
spontaneous generation, 108–110, 109*ph*, 111*ph*
Squibb, Edward Robinson, 80
Squier, Ephraim George, 104–105, 106*ph*
staining, 157–160, 159*ph*

Starling, Ernest H., 147–150
Starzl, Thomas, 206
stents, 234, 234*ph*
Steptoe, Patrick, 213–215, 214*ph*, 216
steroids, 204
stethoscope, 67–71, 68*ph*, 70*ph*
stones, 72–76
"substance P," 11
sulfa drugs, 167
suppuration, 112, 112*ph*
surgery
    in ancient India, 16
    germ theory and, 112
    lobotomy, 170–173
    skull, 104–106
    for stones, 72–75, 73*ph*
Sushruta, 16, 72–73
Sushruta Samhita, 16*ph*
swan-necked flask experiment, 110, 111*ph*
sweet clover, 174–176, 175*ph*
syphilis, 158*ph*, 159–160, 160*ph*, 161,
    161*ph*, 223*ph*
Szent-Györgi, Albert, 55

test-tube babies, 213–218
Theiler, Max, 134
theosophy, 151*ph*
thiamine (vitamin B1), 55, 56
Thompson, Leonard, 162–163
3D printing, 232–233, 232*ph*
thrombosis, 176
Thyphoid Mary, 153–156, 154*ph*, 155*ph*
tobacco mosaic disease, 133
Torre, Marcantonio della, 32
tracheotomy, 63
Traditional Chinese Medicine (TCM), 212
transcatheter aortic valve implantation
    (TAVI), 232
transfusions, 142–146, 143*ph*, 144*ph*, 146*ph*
transorbital icepick lobotomy, 173, 173*ph*
transplantable artificial heart (TAH), 191
transplants, 202–206, 203*ph*, 204*ph*, 205*ph*
trench fever, 132
trepanation, 104–106, 105*ph*, 172*ph*
Triumph of Death, The (Brueghel), 132*ph*
Trotter, Thomas, 54
tryptophan, 152
Tu Youyou, 207–211, 244–245
tuberculosis, 114–116, 115*ph*
tuberculous spondylitis, 116*ph*
Tuo, Hua, 107, 107*ph*, 209*ph*, 210*ph*
Tuskegee Study of Untreated Syphilis, 223,
    223*ph*
Tutankhamun's tomb, 14*ph*
typhoid fever, 153–156, 186–187

uranium, 137–138
urea, 189

vaccines, 48*ph*, 118–120, 134–135, 224–
    228, 227*ph*, 229*ph*
vampires, 117
van Leeuwenhoek, Antonie, 40–44, 41*ph*,
    42*ph*, 108
Van Roonhuysen family, 37
ventilators, 192*ph*
Ventura, Magdalena, 150
Vermeer, Johannes, 41*ph*
Vesalius, Andreas, 25, 34
Villemin, Jean-Antoine, 115
viruses, 133–136. *see also individual viruses*
vitamin C, 51, 54, 55, 55*ph*
vitamin K, 176–177, 177*ph*
"Vitruvian Man" (da Vinci), 32*ph*
von Mering, Joseph, 162

Wakefield, Andrew, 227–228, 229, 229*ph*
Wakley, Thomas, 75, 75*ph*
Waller, August Desiré, 197
warfarin, 176–177
Warren, General, 153
Washington, George, 62–63, 63*ph*, 135*ph*
wastewater, 92
Watschinger, Bruno, 191
Watson, James D., 182–183, 182*ph*
Watson, Lyall, 5
Watt, James, 58, 173*ph*
Wells, Horace, 78
Whitehead, Henry, 95
Wilkins, Maurice, 182–183
Withering, William, 57–60, 61
Witsen, Nicolaes, 6*ph*
Wren, Christopher, 43
Wright, Almorth, 166–167

X-rays, 123–126, 124*ph*, 140*ph*

Yellow Emperor's Classic of Internal Medicine,
    26
yellow fever, 134–135, 134*ph*, 135*ph*
Yersin, Alexandre, 127, 128
yi, 212
Yorick, 196, 196*ph*

Zika virus, 238–242, 240*ph*

About the Authors

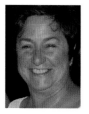

MARGUERITE VIGLIANI, MD is Clinical Professor of Obstetrics and Gynecology at the Warren Alpert Medical School at Brown University. She has been a private solo OB/GYN practitioner for the last 36 years in Rhode Island, where she lives with her family. She has authored a number of medical case reports and clinical opinions for peer-reviewed journals, and she has taught medical students, residents, and fellows in OB/GYN.

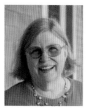

GALE EATON has spent a lifetime with books for children and young adults, first as a children's librarian at the Boston Public Library and the Berkshire Athenaeum, and later as a professor of children's literature at the University of Rhode Island Graduate School of Library and Information Studies. She is the author of *A History of Civilization in 50 Disasters* and *A History of Ambition in 50 Hoaxes,* as well as academic books and journal articles. Raised in Maine, Gale lives in Wakefield, Rhode Island. *(Photo by Tony Balko, the Harrington School of Communication and Media, University of Rhode Island)*

About the History in 50 Series Editor

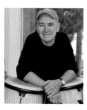

PHILLIP HOOSE is the widely acclaimed author of books, essays, stories, songs, and articles, including the National Book Award and Newbery Honor winning book *Claudette Colvin: Twice toward Justice* and the Boston Globe–Horn Book Honor winner *The Boys Who Challenged Hitler: Knud Pedersen and the Churchill Club.* A graduate of Indiana University and the Yale School of Forestry and Environmental Sciences, Hoose was for 37 years a staff member of The Nature Conservancy, dedicated to preserving the plants, animals, and natural communities of the Earth. Find out more at www.philliphoose.com. *(Photo by Gordon Chibrowski, Maine Newspapers)*